HEALTH TAXES

Policy and Practice

Imperial College Business School | Centre for Health Economics & Policy Innovation

World Health Organization

HEALTH TAXES

Policy and Practice

Editors

Jeremy A Lauer
University of Strathclyde, UK
formerly World Health Organization, Switzerland

Franco Sassi
Imperial College London, UK

Agnès Soucat
Agence Française de Développement, France
formerly World Health Organization, Switzerland

Angeli Vigo
World Health Organization, Switzerland

World Scientific

NEW JERSEY • LONDON • SINGAPORE • BEIJING • SHANGHAI • HONG KONG • TAIPEI • CHENNAI • TOKYO

Published by

World Scientific Publishing Europe Ltd.

57 Shelton Street, Covent Garden, London WC2H 9HE

Head office: 5 Toh Tuck Link, Singapore 596224

USA office: 27 Warren Street, Suite 401-402, Hackensack, NJ 07601

Library of Congress Cataloging-in-Publication Data

Names: Lauer, Jeremy A., editor. | Sassi, F., editor. | Soucat, Agnes L. B., editor. | Vigo, Angeli, editor. | World Health Organization, issuing body.

Title: Health taxes : policy and practice / editors, Jeremy A Lauer, Franco Sassi, Agnès Soucat, Angeli Vigo.

Description: Hackensack, New Jersey : World Scientific, [2022] | Includes bibliographical references.

Identifiers: LCCN 2022025017 | ISBN 9781800612389 (hardcover) | ISBN 9781800612396 (ebook for institutions) | ISBN 9781800612402 (ebook for individuals)

Subjects: MESH: Health Policy--economics | Taxes--economics | Economics, Medical | Health Promotion--economics

Classification: LCC RA410.53 | NLM WA 525 | DDC 338.4/73621--dc23/eng/20220708

LC record available at https://lccn.loc.gov/2022025017

British Library Cataloguing-in-Publication Data

A catalogue record for this book is available from the British Library.

For any available supplementary material, please visit
https://www.worldscientific.com/worldscibooks/10.1142/Q0365#t=suppl

Typeset by Diacritech Technologies Pvt. Ltd.
Chennai - 600106, India

https://doi.org/10.1142/9781800612396_fmatter

Forewords

Each year, 41 million people die from preventable non-communicable diseases (NCDs) such as cardiovascular diseases, cancers, chronic respiratory diseases and diabetes. Most of these deaths occur in low- and middle-income countries, and could have been avoided by eliminating tobacco use and alcohol misuse and by improving unhealthy diets.

One of the most cost-effective ways of addressing NCDs is through the intelligent use of health taxes. One of the aims of health taxes is to reduce the consumption of unhealthy products; another is to disincentivise unhealthy behaviours that are typically associated with such products. Health taxes achieve both these aims by changing the price faced by consumers so that healthier choices are promoted.

Health taxes can also serve as a revenue booster for governments, a fact which is particularly relevant now, as governments are facing the challenges of financing the Sustainable Development Goals. Now more than ever health taxes can play a vital role in achieving the twin goals of improving health outcomes and in raising public-sector revenues.

Despite their demonstrated benefits, health taxes remain underutilised globally. To address this problem, WHO (through its health system teams and with the support of its health promotion teams), spearheaded a multi-year programme of knowledge exchange with leading experts in the field of health, tax policy, public financial management, trade law and public governance. The discussions are now chronicled in this book, *Health Taxes: Policy and Practice.*

This book represents the first coherent discussion of health taxes as an independent domain, and authoritatively addresses the expressed concerns of policymakers, and fiscal-sector practitioners, in particular. It also provides a long-needed bridge between global health and fiscal policy concerns.

Zsuzsanna Jakab
Deputy Director-General
World Health Organization

Health taxes (excise taxes on tobacco, alcohol and sugar-sweetened beverages) are an important tool to simultaneously improve health and fiscal outcomes. Introducing or reforming health taxes can improve health by reducing the consumption and associated negative externalities of health-harming commodities. They can also improve fiscal balances by increasing tax revenue and reducing health care costs associated with illnesses and injuries in the long run. These taxes are a pro-poor and progressive policy once one accounts for health and productivity benefits of reduced consumption on households.

In this current environment where health and fiscal systems are under serious strain, health taxes are more important than ever before. However, to achieve maximum benefit, health taxes need to be designed and administered well. We emphasise here the importance of looking at health taxes in a holistic manner, including the structure of the tax system and the incidence of these taxes, all while aiming at rate levels that maximise health and fiscal benefits. Equally important, reforms must be underpinned by the understanding that tax policies are only as effective as the tax administration systems that implement them.

I welcome the publication of *Health Taxes: Policy and Practice*. This timely publication presents a broad perspective and rich set of contributions from a wide-ranging group of experts on health taxes. It is a useful resource for researchers, policymakers and practitioners, and will be an important reference to all of them as we continue to support policies that bring about sustainable economic development and greater welfare – including in terms of health outcomes – for all.

Marcello Estevão
Global Director
Macroeconomics, Trade & Investment, World Bank

https://doi.org/10.1142/9781800612396_fmatter

Contents

https://doi.org/10.1142/9781800612396_fmatter

Acknowledgements

This publication was developed in close coordination with the WHO's Fiscal Policies for Health Team, led by Jeremias Paul Jr.

The editors are especially grateful to **Jack Olney**, Executive Director of Imperial College's Centre for Health Economics & Policy Innovation (CHEPI), for his tireless efforts in driving the development and production of the book, and to **Lorraine Sheehy** (CHEPI), **Vida Gyamerah** and **Gael Kernen** (WHO) for their administrative support.

The editors also acknowledge the contributions of the following reviewers, who have provided invaluable comments on chapters of this book and participated in review meetings (listed in alphabetical order):

WHO reviewers: **Hélène Barroy**, **Delia Itziar Belausteguigoitia**, **Evan Blecher**, **Katrin Engelhardt**, **Kaia Engesveen**, **Mark Goodchild**, **Joseph Douglas Kutzin**, **Juliette McHardy**, **Anne-Marie Perucic**, **Michal Stoklosa** and **Temo Waqanivalu**.

Reviewers from other organisations: **Eduardo Banzon** (Asian Development Bank, Philippines), **Mark Blecher** (National Treasury, South Africa), **Alan Carter** (Her Majesty's Revenue and Customs, United Kingdom), **Michele Cecchini** (Organisation for Economic Co-operation and Development, France), **Amandine Garde** (University of Liverpool, United Kingdom), **Juan Nicolas Guerrero-Peniche,** (WHO Framework Convention on Tobacco Control), **Knut-Inge Klepp** (Norwegian Institute of Public Health), **Mpho Legote** (National Treasury, South Africa), **Aik Hoe Lim** (World Trade Organization, Switzerland), **Lauro Locks** (World Trade Organization,

Switzerland), **Mick Moore** (International Centre for Tax and Development, United Kingdom), **Rachel Nugent** (RTI International, United States), **Nicholas Stacey** (University of the Witwatersrand, South Africa) and **Anne-Marie Thow** (University of Sydney, Australia).

The production of this book has been supported by the Making Country Health Systems Stronger programme of the Department for International Development (now Foreign, Commonwealth & Development Office) of the United Kingdom and the Government of Norway.

https://doi.org/10.1142/9781800612396_0001

Chapter 1

Introduction

Franco Sassi*, Jeremy A Lauer†, Agnes Soucat‡, Angeli Vigo§, and Jeremias Paul§

1.1. Background

Virtually all fiscal measures can (or have the potential to) influence people's health, through shaping behaviour, consumption, income and wealth. A subset of fiscal measures, however, can be identified as more directly linked to improving health by targeting behaviours and risks that are known to be strongly associated with health outcomes. Some of these measures, which we define as 'health taxes' in this book, have existed for a long time, although only in recent years have they been consistently framed as means of improving the health of individuals and populations. Taxes on alcoholic beverages have existed for over two millennia, for example, starting in ancient China. But these taxes have mostly been used to raise public revenues and control some of the detrimental social consequences, or negative externalities, of alcohol use. As evidence of the adverse health impacts of alcohol use has been consolidating, the rationale for alcohol taxation has

* Imperial College London, UK.

† University of Strathclyde, UK (formerly World Health Organization, Switzerland).

‡ Agence Française de Développement, France (formerly World Health Organization, Switzerland).

§ World Health Organization, Switzerland.

increasingly focused on health promotion and improvement, and today alcohol taxes are widely used worldwide as health taxes.

The narrative of health taxes began with the concept of 'sin taxes' on sugar, tobacco and alcohol. A focus on the taxation of 'unnecessary' consumption goods has been reflected in the work of economists since Adam Smith's widely quoted statement 'sugar, rum, and tobacco are commodities which are nowhere necessaries of life, which are become objects of almost universal consumption, and which are therefore extremely proper subjects of taxation'.[1] The classical rationale for taxing such commodities was to raise the revenues necessary for collective use without interfering with essential forms of consumption. The work of Frank Ramsey,[2] a century ago, added the concept that efficient commodity taxation requires a focus on goods whose demand is not sensitive to price changes, holding firm the principle in Adam Smith's quote. Arthur Pigou further strengthened the rationale for commodity taxation by linking it to negative externalities, or socially undesirable consequences not reflected in the market price, that are associated with the production or consumption of the goods to be taxed.[3] Products that today we know are associated with poor health outcomes happen to have all these characteristics: they are not necessities, their demand is relatively insensitive to price and they generate negative externalities. The fact that such commodities have been taxed long before evidence of their health impacts emerged makes it possible to pursue health goals in fiscal policies simply by repurposing existing taxes, that is, adapting their design to ensure they generate meaningful health impacts; it is not necessary to identify new objects of taxation.

In recent years, we have seen a considerable change in government attitudes towards the taxation of products with adverse health impacts, and the health rationale has increasingly taken centre stage. Thus, taxes often discussed in the past as 'sin taxes', based on a narrative focused on individual responsibility for unhealthy and socially stigmatised consumption, have been embraced and rebranded as *health* taxes that have broad societal benefits and externalities and can thus be considered as Common Goods for health.[a,b] Other taxes, such as environmental taxes, can also fit into a health taxes framework, as we shall see in the following.

Consumption taxes typically involve uniform tax rates across a wide range of products, to ensure an efficient tax administration and to not cause 'distortions' in consumption patterns; however, rate differentiation is used in many taxation systems, either through differentiation of general consumption tax rates or by imposing excise taxes on specific goods. An international review[4] chaired by Nobel Prize winner James Mirrlees provided a vision for tax system reforms in the 21st century, dwelling at length on the issue of consumption tax rate differentiation. The review concluded that 'There are convincing arguments for [...] differentiated tax rates where the consumption of a particular good or service creates spill-over costs or benefits', including costs or benefits faced by one's future self. Such future spill-over effects, realised within an individual, can be identified as 'internalities'. In practice, therefore, in addition to addressing traditional market externalities, 'taxes can encourage people to avoid acting against their own self-interest' [op. cit.] as well. Internalities, however, vary between individuals and addressing consumer heterogeneity in the design of consumption taxes is challenging.

1.2. Scope of the book

This book is the result of knowledge exchange between the staff of the World Health Organization (WHO) and a multidisciplinary team of researchers and policymakers. Its purpose is to bring sharper focus to the subject of health taxes and to expose its various facets in turn. We aim to enumerate the key health taxes of interest, explore their effects, both

[a] Yazbeck AS, Soucat A. When both markets and governments fail health. *Health Systems & Reform*. 2019; 5(4): 268–279.

[b] Soucat A. Financing common goods for health: fundamental for health, the foundation for UHC. *Health Systems & Reform*. 2019; 5(4): 263–267.

positive and negative, and how these effects are influenced by the design of these taxes and by the context in which they are applied. We ask how and where they can be implemented. Critically, we build throughout the book an argument for why policymakers across government should care about health taxes.

As such, this book is intended for those who have primary responsibility for the design and implementation of health taxes, namely fiscal policymakers, and for those who have primary responsibility for the health of individuals and populations, namely health policymakers. The former will benefit from this book through an improved understanding of the conditions required for health taxes to have meaningful health impacts, and of the factors that may affect the success of health taxes as fiscal policy instruments. The latter, on the other hand, will benefit from an improved understanding of the wider fiscal policy context in which health taxes are used, and of the constraints within which health taxes operate, and the book should accordingly put health policymakers in a stronger position to be effective advocates for health taxes within government. Beyond these core constituencies, we also hope to engage the interest of officials in health and finance ministries, stakeholders and activists in civil society, staff in international organisations, young professionals and students in global health and fiscal policy, and academic researchers.

Health taxes exist within a universe of policy tools (Figure 1.1). We will not consider all fiscal policies, notably excluding 'negative' taxation such as subsidies, some of which are widely discussed in the public health policy debate, and we will not consider all revenue-raising fiscal policies, although most of them have at least some effect on health. As explained further in Chapter 2, the focus of this book will be on indirect taxes that target consumption (primarily excise taxes), and affect the market prices of the products concerned, thus shaping consumer behaviour. However, the book will not address all government policies designed to influence the prices of products that may have detrimental health effects. In particular, regulatory

Fig. 1.1. The specific emphasis of this book within related policy spheres.

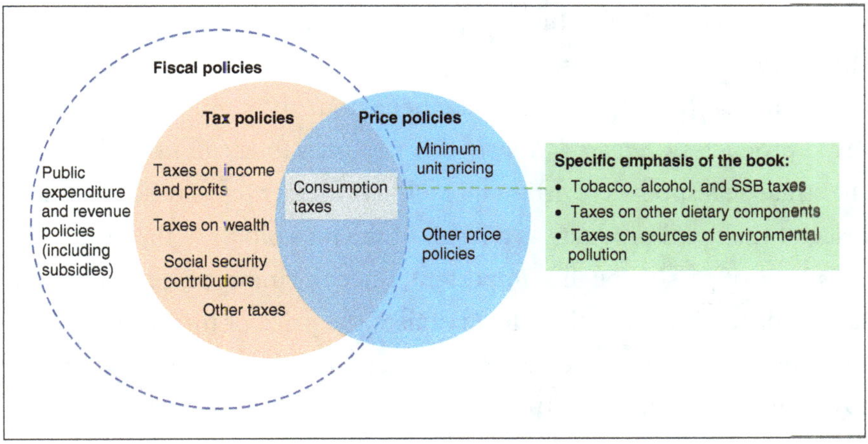

policies such as minimum pricing, which are applied to alcoholic beverages and tobacco products in a number of jurisdictions, are beyond the scope of this book. While we recognise the importance of price regulation for health policy, and while some of the contents of this book will be applicable both to price regulation and to health taxes, we feel that the fiscal policy context of health taxes warrants a detailed examination of its own.

1.3. Questions addressed by this book

The book reflects discussions among public health experts, economists and other experts, and it represents, perhaps, the first attempt to discuss health taxes comprehensively. The book aims to address the following questions.

1.3.1. Can taxes be used as health interventions?

Taxes, which have been historically used as revenue-raising measures, can also be designed to help achieve health-related objectives. *Chapter 3: Protecting and promoting health through taxation: Evidence and gaps* explains the pathways through which taxes on tobacco, alcohol and sugar-sweetened beverages (SSBs) impact consumption and health outcomes and how substitution and tax avoidance behaviours may affect the net impact of the taxes.

Can health taxes influence the behaviour of manufacturers of the taxed products? *Chapter 4: Supply-side responses to health taxes* describes the strategic responses of firms and looks at whether firms raise the selling price of the taxed products as a result of the imposition of the health tax. This issue of pass-through is important, since the impact on consumption largely depends on whether the tax raises the price of the taxed product relative to others. The same chapter also examines whether taxes can be used to encourage manufacturers to reformulate their products, or to increase the promotion of products with a lower concentration of the taxed ingredient.

What about taxes on other activities which negatively affect health (e.g. the increased use of cars)? *Chapter 7: Expanding health taxation to other unhealthy behaviours and harmful activities* explores the application of taxes to discourage other unhealthy behaviours, looking at examples on air pollution, gambling, farming practices and others.

1.3.2. What are the economic impacts of health taxes?

Governments have long relied on tobacco and alcohol taxes as steady streams of revenue. If taxes on these products are designed with a health goal in mind, can taxes on these products still generate stable revenue for countries? *Chapter 2: The place for health taxes in the wider fiscal system* explores this question and examines the revenue-raising potential of health taxes and how general principles of tax policy may be applied in this context.

Opponents of health taxes often claim that these measures will have negative labour impacts and result in economic downturn, particularly in lower income contexts. *Chapter 5: The labour market impact of health taxes* assesses whether these claims are supported by evidence. The chapters delve into the impact of health taxes on employment and productivity using empirical and modelled evidence.

1.3.3. Can health taxes advance the achievement of the sustainable development goals?

The SDGs represent a shared blueprint for peace and prosperity for people and the planet, now and into the future. Can health taxes help countries achieve their SDG-related targets? *Chapter 6: Impacts of health taxes on the attainment of the SDGs* examines health taxes using a wider lens and explores the links between health taxes and broader development goals.

1.3.4. What are the considerations for designing and implementing health taxes?

These considerations are explained extensively in three chapters. *Chapter 8: The design of effective health taxes* explains how tax type, tax structure, tax rate affect the impact of the tax on consumption and its implications on revenue. *Chapter 9: Public governance and financing, and earmarking health taxes* places health taxes within the broader context of public financing systems and also explains the considerations around earmarking of health tax revenue. *Chapter 10: Monitoring and measuring health taxes* explains the importance of tracking health taxes implementation and proposes an approach for monitoring taxes on alcoholic beverages and SSBs, based on the methodology used in the field of tobacco taxation.

1.3.5. Do health taxes affect countries' commitments under international trade law?

To effectively design and structure health taxes in compliance with international obligations, policymakers must understand the rules of international trade law. *Chapter 11: Health taxes and trade law* examines how the rules of international trade law and agreements governing customs and monetary unions and how these may affect the implementation of health taxes.

1.3.6. What is the political economy of health tax policy?

Chapter 12: A political economy analysis of health taxes examines the key players in the health taxes arena and how these actors influence the policy environment. The chapter also lists recommendations for interacting with industries affected by health taxes.

1.4. A brief history of health taxes

The idea of health taxes was born before the term. At the end of the last century, it began to be commonplace to talk about a limited set of excise taxes as health interventions.[5,6] This innovation can be seen as presaging an idea subsequently popularised by the WHO early in the era of the Millennium Development Goals (MDGs), namely that the health system is the sum of 'all the activities whose primary purpose is to promote, restore or maintain health.'[7] This concept, although clearly in line with the thinking of the drafters of the WHO Constitution, nevertheless represented a broadening of the predominantly medical-and-public-health focus of previous thinking. Shortly afterwards, staff at the WHO and others[8,9] began to analyse the cost-effectiveness of the taxation of alcohol and tobacco, and to make explicit comparisons with that of other usual health-system activities, giving further impetus to the concept.

Later, comparative studies of hundreds of interventions[10,11] helped establish the idea that alcohol taxes and tobacco taxes were not only cost-effective ways of improving population health but were in fact more cost-effective than many widely recognised health interventions. Prior to these publications, alcohol tax, cigarette tax, but also road-safety measures and a host of other actions outside of the healthcare sector as narrowly understood — were not routinely thought of as 'health policies'. Yet it soon became impossible to ignore them. This represented a fundamental change in thinking about the health system and about health interventions.

That thinking is now being extended, and part of that story involves the birth of health taxes as a term. However, it is helpful to recognise that, at least prior to the increased regulation of tobacco products and smoking following the adoption of the WHO Framework Convention on Tobacco Control (FCTC), there were few interventions in the medical or public-health repertoires capable of addressing the harms caused by alcohol and tobacco, as well as by a host of other causes outside of the range of proximal risk factors, such as pathogens or poor sanitation, that had been the traditional focus of public health. It is said that out of necessity comes invention and so two of the humble fiscal instruments originally designed to constitute the revenue backbone for the early modern state (i.e. alcohol and tobacco taxes) acquired new lustre as leading health interventions.

The imperative of a globalising epidemiological transition, along with an increasing prevalence of non-communicable diseases (NCDs), reinforced this trend. Tobacco use (in any of its many forms), the harmful use of alcohol, unhealthy diet and physical inactivity are among the main causes of ill-health. Rapidly rising obesity and overnutrition in particular became increasingly understood as causes of ill-health intermediate between the distal behavioural-and-social factors and the proximal biomedical ones.

A series of studies conducted by the OECD and by the WHO[12,13] were early in linking these trends (i.e. taxation, on the one hand, and diet and obesity, on the other). The resulting publications demonstrate that by the end of the first decade of this century it was possible to talk meaningfully about a previously unheard-of concept, namely 'fiscal measures for health'. The use of the term 'fiscal measures' was intended to include health-promoting *subsidies*, such as for fruits and vegetables, alongside health-promoting *taxes*, for example on foods high in fat. 'Fiscal measures', traditionally the domain of specialists in tax and public finance, became thenceforth words frequently in the mouths of public health professionals, most of whom would have barely noticed the term in its traditional domain of application.

Following a High-level Meeting on NCDs held in Moscow in 2010, taxes on sweetened products (sometimes referred to as 'sugar taxes') — as well as fat taxes and other taxes directed at reducing the consumption of various dietary components — began to be implemented by numerous governments, supported by a public health rationale. Everywhere in the world it is safe to say that alcohol and tobacco taxes had as their original purpose not the improvement of health but rather the raising of public revenues. Conversely, however, it is safe to affirm that in most countries where taxes on SSBs have been implemented (i.e. in very many jurisdictions[14]), the foremost aim of such taxes has been to improve health by incentivising a more balanced diet, and not to raise public revenues (although the 2008 international financial crisis that left governments scrambling for revenues to cover budget deficits was among the factors that created the conditions for this trend). Though under-recognised at the time, taxes on SSBs proved in the years following 2010 to be a thought innovation, much as the work of others on tobacco and alcohol had been decades earlier. It was a game-changing innovation for one overwhelming reason: in the wake of the introduction of SSB taxes it became possible — at least in principle — to reimagine taxes, or even fiscal policies altogether, primarily as health interventions.

1.5. The rationale for health taxes

1.5.1. The neoclassical rationale for taxation: Public goods and externalities

The original notion of taxation has everywhere been that of an obligation ('duty') owed to an authority, with little notion of reciprocity. For most of human history, taxation has been conceived as the right of the strong to extract resources from the weak. Some of the first forms of (direct) taxation were 'corvee' (forced labour) and 'tithe' (a share of income, or 'rent'). Later, taxation buttressed the power of mercantilist states in the form of tariffs and excises on trade. With the Enlightenment, however, the concept of taxation changed. For the first time, a duty of the state towards the individual was needed to justify the levy of taxes. This revolution in thought arose in part in response to revolutions in deed, against the French and British crowns, motivated in part by burdensome taxation.

Reducing the harms of financing the state remains a central concern of tax policy.[15] A related view is that those who benefit the most from the state should contribute more to its finances [op. cit.]. The thinking of Smith, Ramsey and Pigou falls squarely into this classical policy frame. The main additions to it are the twin ideas of neoclassical economics that (i) unfettered markets in perfect competition result in a kind of social optimum and (ii) the goal of taxation should therefore be to distort market prices and the behaviour of economic agents as little as possible. Neoclassical tax policy thus seeks to finance the state for a narrow set of purposes ancillary to the action of the free market: fixing externalities (Pigouvian taxes), correcting market failures, supplying public goods and eliminating tariffs and barriers to trade.

Most work on tax policy has adopted the reference point of economic efficiency: taxation, a necessary evil perhaps, should be designed so as to determine the least distortionary yet still viable tax regime enabling the state to perform its role. The most efficient form of taxation is a lump-sum tax. As the latter has a number of undesirable properties, the next-best forms of taxation in the neoclassical concept are direct taxes on income or generalised consumption taxes (e.g. value-added tax, VAT) that do not change the relative prices of consumption goods. In OECD countries, income taxes, both individual and corporate, make up on average about a third of government revenue, generalised consumption taxes on goods and services make up another third, social security contributions contribute about a quarter, and property taxes provide the balance.[16] The picture differs in developing countries, but, in general, excise taxes on tobacco and alcohol account for a small share of government revenue since, in the lens of neoclassical economic theory, such taxes are relatively undesirable as interfering with (relative) market prices.

1.5.2. An independent rationale for health taxes

The idea of health taxes represents a development from the concept that efficient markets, redistribution and addressing externalities are the primary aims of fiscal policy in the area of consumption taxation. Health taxes require that future harms to consumers themselves, particularly to their health, must also be considered, provided that those harms are not otherwise factored into consumer choices. Health taxes thus enhance the concept of market efficiency as a policy goal because at least one of their objectives is to promote and protect a non-market-traded good, namely health. Health taxes can also be means of progressive redistribution when health benefits are considered as well as income effects.[17] As argued by Grossman,[18] health is one of a limited set of goods (as education) that we both experience directly (i.e. as a constituent of our 'well-being') but which is also an enabler (or, a 'factor of production') for many other goods that people value, such as visits with friends, decent work or performance in family role.

In consultations surrounding the WHO Commission on Ending Childhood Obesity,[19] Partha Dasgupta noted that health *per se* cannot be bought or sold and lamented that there is no readily understandable metric ('vulgar metric') of intrinsic health, but rather merely *post hoc* measures of its realisation such as life expectancy.[20] Amartya Sen[21,22] and others, notably Martha Nussbaum,[23,24] develop rich health-related concepts in the theory of capabilities[c,25] but the absence of a precise, and prospective, measure of health is not thereby addressed.

Health is widely recognised, at a minimum, as a fundamental component of welfare, or well-being. In the WHO definition, however, health is intrinsically linked with well-being ('Health is a state of complete physical, mental and social well-being and not merely the absence of disease or infirmity'). This makes health a special kind of good, one

[c] 'Capability theory involves two normative claims, first the claim that the freedom to achieve well-being is of primary moral importance, and second, that freedom to achieve well-being is to be understood in terms of people's capabilities, that is, their real opportunities to do and be what they have reason to value'.[26]

deserving of special consideration, and fiscal policy should offer no exception to this rule.

A health tax might be considered as any tax designed to promote health as one of its primary objectives. Taking health into account, however, does not mean abandoning other social goals, such as raising government revenues, effecting socially desirable redistribution, internalising market externalities or repairing market failures. So, while health taxes may represent an incremental change in policy, they can also be seen as a quantum leap in vision.

1.5.3. Correcting demand-side failures in health

The sustainable development goals (SDGs) are now, perhaps, out of reach in light of the economic impact of the COVID-19 pandemic. In April 2020, the Chief Economist of the IMF, Gita Gopinath, wrote,

> It is very likely that the global economy will experience its worst recession since the Great Depression.... A partial recovery is projected for 2021... with considerable uncertainty about the strength of the rebound. Much worse growth outcomes are possible and maybe even likely... if the pandemic and containment measures last longer, emerging and developing economies are even more severely hit, tight financial conditions persist, or if widespread scarring effects emerge due to firm closures and extended unemployment.[26]

The report continues, 'Many countries face a multi-layered crisis comprising a health shock, domestic economic disruptions, plummeting external demand, capital flow reversals, and a collapse in commodity prices. Risks of a worse outcome predominate'. This picture has become somewhat more nuanced in the intervening years, as external demand, for example, has proved to be more durable than anticipated in early 2020; nevertheless, negative consequences, including inflationary cycles, still predominate global economic prospects in the post-pandemic era.

In a post-pandemic world, the relationship between the individual and the state seems sure to change. In particular, if the SDGs are not to be retired as obsolete aspirations, the state's tax system will have to negotiate new models to enable these goals in the face of possibly stagnant growth in real incomes, rising international uncertainty and durable disruptions to travel, commerce and trade. While these changes pose numerous threats, they also open opportunities for the development of health taxes.[27]

Seen in this light, health taxes are not merely instruments to diminish the demand for unhealthy products. Rather, health taxes can be conceived as increasing and enabling demand for longer, healthier lives. There are fundamental reasons why individuals are not themselves necessarily effective demanders of longer, healthy lives for themselves; these reasons can be summarised in the concept, previously mentioned, of internalities: since uncertainty, asymmetric information, hyperbolic discounting and incomplete markets cloud the foresight of the rational agent, negative behavioural spill-over effects can be realised by one's own future self. One of the main results of such internalities is to cause suboptimal demand for longer, healthier lives.

A social contract fostering capabilities

The prevailing view of the social contract holds that broadly based income or consumption taxes are preferable to tariffs on trade or narrow-based consumption taxes such as excises. According to the tax handle theory,[28] as countries develop they tend to implement first numerous narrow-based consumption and trade taxes primarily based on reasons of administrative convenience; whereas in countries with more developed systems of governance and tax administration, broad-based consumption taxes (e.g. VAT) and income taxes (both individual and corporate) predominate.[29–33] That said, in all countries with developed systems of tax administration the bulk of state revenues were originally raised from excises and tariffs.

Thus, the link to public governance and administration, both in cross-section and longitudinally, is made for two reasons: (i) broad-based consumption taxes such as the VAT require a comprehensive ledger of transactions along the production-and-consumption value chains, while (ii) income taxes require high levels of voluntary compliance, an effective withholding system or both. Direct taxes on income and generalised taxes on consumption are held to be the least distortionary but are the hardest to implement. On the other hand, taxes on commodities are potentially more distortionary but easier to implement.

The main Enlightenment philosophical tradition regarding the social contract[34] is based on the idea of the consent of the governed to a set of principles to which all can agree. Kant gave this principle expression in his categorical imperative, 'Act only according to that maxim whereby you can, at the same time, will that it should become a universal law'.[35] Thus, a set of symmetric rights and duties is often held to be one of the fundamental bases of the post-Enlightenment social contract. Sometimes these goals are made explicit in constitutions, for example, in affirming certain 'inalienable' rights, such as to life, liberty and the pursuit of happiness.

There might seem to be relatively few social goals regarding which there is nearly universal consensus. We might however expand on the foregoing list by adding the following: The avoidance of lives needlessly impoverished and foreshortened through illness and disease of all kinds.

This principle is in fact enunciated in the 1946 Constitution of the World Health Organization, where it is held to be 'basic to the happiness, harmonious relations and security of all peoples': 'The enjoyment of the highest attainable standard of health is one of the fundamental rights of every human being without distinction of race, religion, political belief, economic or social condition'.

While the WHO has achieved some notable successes, one possible reason why it has not been more successful in the pursuit of this paramount constitutional goal may be that it has failed so far to enunciate a set of duties, such as health taxes, that are symmetric to the presumed right to 'the highest standard of health'. Expediency and opportunity have recently become more aligned in favour of the principle of health taxes, however, which not only are being adopted by governments but often benefit from strong public support.

Individual-level enabling factors

Health taxes are a population-wide public health policy based on the delivery of enabling incentives to individuals. Health taxes directly improve health by reducing the consumption of unhealthy products and the health impacts that others may suffer as a result of that consumption. Not only are health taxes a cost-effective means of improving health, but they are also feasible, acceptable and affordable.[36]

Health taxes convey important information to consumers. That information helps individuals to understand how to demand longer, healthier lives (to correct internalities). As with cigarette-package warnings, individuals understand the reasons for the imposition of a health tax, and they take this into account in making their consumption decisions, independently of the impact of health taxes on their pocketbook. Health taxes also convey useful information to producers. In the case of SSB taxes, the information conveyed helps producers to understand how to reformulate their products, which, at least for SSB taxes, is one of the main effects intended.

Finally, health taxes correct externalities by internalising the cost of health impacts in the market price paid by the consumer. When a smoker gets ill and insurance needs to pays for treatment, the other insured individuals all contribute to pay for increased healthcare costs. Representing this cost directly in the price of cigarettes is one of the main functions of health taxes, although estimating the value of externalities is often very challenging.

Health taxes are enablers of sustainable development

Broad-based tax reform will be required to reach the SDGs and health taxes will be an important part of it. Health taxes allow the pursuit of social welfare goals beyond redistribution and the provision of public goods, so they broaden the range of social welfare objectives that can be pursued through fiscal policies. Significantly, health taxes are to date the only fiscal instrument to have been approved in international normative law such as resolutions of the World Health Assembly or the high-level political declarations of the United Nations.[37–39] Health taxes are easier to administer than other kinds of taxes and they are *a fortiori* suitable for states with lower tax capacity and lower capacity for public financial management.

Indeed, the World Bank has found that achieving a minimum size of the tax to GDP ratio of around 15% is associated with major development gains, although health taxes will be only a part of a broader fiscal programme capable of achieving this level of tax revenue.[40] However, health taxes boost revenues both by broadening the tax base and by strengthening the credibility of the public sector. Health taxes effectively link — both conceptually and politically — revenue to expenditure and thereby reinforce the implicit social contract.

Health taxes can thus be seen as "third-generation tax reforms" with health, environmental (e.g. when aimed at pollutants) and economic dividends. As stated by Dr Rakesh Mohan, former Deputy Governor of the Reserve Bank of India, the 'third generation of economic reforms must focus on a similar empowerment of the government to deliver growth-enhancing public goods and services for the benefit of all segments of the public, private sector and corporate entities alike'.[d]

1.6. Tax reform for health: Reconciling expenditure and income adjustments

Health taxes, as they are defined in this chapter and book, belong to the domain of consumption taxes, and all consumption taxes are generally more regressive, or at least less progressive, than income or wealth taxes. In

[d] Mohan R. A third-generation strategy for accelerated growth and development in India: Need for government strengthening and institutional development (CSEP Working Paper-3), Centre for Social and Economic Progress, New Delhi, January 2021.

addition, the types of consumption targeted by health taxes are typically more common among people of low socio-economic status. However strongly justified health taxes may be on internality and externality grounds, their income distribution impacts make them vulnerable to claims of inequity and exacerbating poverty.

In fact, there should be no expectation for health taxes to be progressive. They are small addition to a much larger pool of consumption taxes, which may be either progressive or regressive as a whole, but which represent a fundamental component of any fiscal system, raising substantial shares of all tax revenues. The fairness of a fiscal system must be assessed globally, based on the extent to which the distributional effects of different types of taxes can be balanced. However, in many instances, fiscal systems have become less progressive in recent years, partly because of an increased reliance on consumption taxes (e.g. the weight of VAT has increased considerably after the 2008 financial crisis in many countries), partly because of the flattening of income tax schedules or the reduced use of wealth taxes, not to mention the corporate tax base erosion and loopholes, especially for major multinational businesses. This has created an especially hostile environment for measures like health (and environmental) taxes, which are designed to be salient and highly visible to consumers in order to accomplish their goal of deterring the consumption of products that have potentially detrimental health and environmental impacts.

Amidst increasing social inequalities within and across countries, fiscal systems ought to provide the means to mitigate inequalities and their impacts. When, in 2018, the French government slashed wealth taxes and increased fuel taxes, the latter measure gave rise to the so-called yellow vest protest.[41] Despite a strong environmental and health rationale, fuel taxes were highly visible and strongly perceived as hitting low-income rural workers whose livelihoods depend on fuel.

As argued extensively in this book, any assessment of the distributional impacts of health taxes must consider the welfare effects of those taxes globally, that is, their effects on health and well-being and their distribution, as well as their effects on income and its distribution. Beyond the complexity of assessing the wide-ranging impacts of health taxes and their distribution, the evidence available today from health taxes that have been implemented across the world points consistently to an overall welfare effect in the direction of a mitigation, rather than exacerbation, of inequalities. Yet, health taxes will continue to attract criticism on the grounds of their potentially regressive financial impacts, boosted by their high visibility and polarising effects, and policymakers will have to design a coherent set of policy measures and a consistent narrative to support them in order to forestall such criticism.

References

1. Smith A. *The Wealth of Nations: An Inquiry into the Nature and Causes of the Wealth of Nations.* Petersfield: Harriman House Limited; 2010, p. 731.
2. Ramsey FP. "A contribution to the theory of taxation." *The Economic Journal.* 1927; 37(145): 47–61.
3. Pigou AC, Aslanbeigui N. *The Economics of Welfare.* New York: Routledge, 2017, p. 68.
4. Mirrlees J, Adam S, Besley T, Blundell R, Bond S, Chote R, Gammie M, Johnson P, Myles G, Poterba JM. *Tax by Design.* London: Institute for Fiscal Studies; 2011.
5. Chaloupka FJ, Warner KE. The economics of smoking. *Handbook of Health Economics,* Vol. 1, Part B; 2000, pp. 1539–1627.
6. Chaloupka FJ and Jha P. *Curbing the Epidemic: Governments and the Economics of Tobacco Control.* Washington: World Bank; 1999.
7. World Health Organization. *The World Health Report 2000: Health Systems: Improving Performance.* Geneva: World Health Organization; 2000.
8. Chisholm D, Doran D, Shibuya K, Rehm J. Comparative cost-effectiveness of policy instruments for reducing the global burden of alcohol, tobacco and illicit drug use. *Drug and Alcohol Review.* 2006; 25: 553–565.
9. Lai T, Habicht J, Reinap M, Chisholm D, Baltussen R. Costs, health effects and cost-effectiveness of alcohol and tobacco control strategies in Estonia. *Health Policy.* 2007; 84(1): 75–88.
10. Evans DB, Adam T, Tan-Torres Edejer T, Lim SS, Cassels A, Evans TG. Achieving the millennium development goals for health: time to reassess strategies for improving health in developing countries. *BMJ.* 2005; 331: 1133–1136.
11. Chisholm D, Baltussen R, Evans DB, Ginsberg G, Lauer JA, Lim S, Ortegón M, Salomon J, Stanciole A, Tan-Torres Edejer T. What are the priorities for prevention and control of non-communicable diseases and injuries in sub-Saharan Africa and South East Asia? *BMJ.* 2012; 344: e586.
12. Sassi F, Cecchini M, Lauer JA, Yong YL, Guajardo-Barron V, Chisholm D. Tackling of unhealthy diets, physical inactivity and obesity: health effects and cost-effectiveness. *Lancet.* 2010; 376: 1775–1784.

13. Sassi F, Cecchini M, Lauer J, Chisholm D. *Improving Lifestyles, Tackling Obesity: The Health and Economic Impact of Prevention Strategies.* Paris: OECD; 2009 (OECD Health Working Papers, No. 48).
14. World Cancer Research Fund International. Building momentum: lessons on implementing evidence-informed nutrition policy; 2018, www.wcrf.org/buildingmomentum (accessed 9 October 2018).
15. Weinzierl M. Revisiting the classical view of benefit-based taxation. *The Economic Journal.* 2018; 128(612): F37–F64.
16. OECD. Tax revenue statistics, https://stats.oecd.org/ (accessed 1st September 2021).
17. Sassi F, Belloni A, Mirelman AJ, et al. Equity impacts of price policies to promote healthy behaviours. *Lancet.* 2018 (published online April 4).
18. Grossman M. On the concept of health capital and the demand for health. *The Journal of Political Economy.* 1972; 80(2): 223–255.
19. Report of the Commission on Ending Childhood Obesity. World Health Organization; 2016.
20. Sir Alleyne G. Keynote speech: health, NCDs, and human capital. World Bank Non-Communicable Diseases and Human Capital Workshop, Toronto, 9–10 July 2019.
21. Sen A. Informational bases of alternative welfare approaches: aggregation and income distribution. *Journal of Public Economics.* 1974; 3(4): 387–403.
22. Sen A. Equality of what? In McMurrin S (ed) *Tanner Lectures on Human Values.* Cambridge: Cambridge University Press; 1979, pp. 197–220; Sen A. Issues in the measurement of poverty. *The Scandinavian Journal of Economics.* 1979; 81(2): 285–307.
23. Nussbaum M. *Women and Human Development: The Capabilities Approach.* Cambridge: Cambridge University Press; 2000; Nussbaum M. *Frontiers of Justice: Disability, Nationality, Species Membership.* Cambridge, MA: Harvard University Press; 2006.
24. Nussbaum M. *Creating Capabilities.* Cambridge, MA: Harvard University Press; 2011.
25. Sen A. "Development as freedom." *Development in Practice-Oxford.* 2000; 10(2): 258–258.
26. World Economic Outlook: The Great Lockdown, Washington, DC: International Monetary Fund; 14 April 2020.
27. Summers LH. Taxes for health: evidence clears the air. *Lancet.* 2018; 391(10134): 1974–1976.
28. Mansfield CY. Tax administration in developing countries: an economic perspective. *IMF Staff papers* 1988; 35(1): 181–197.
29. Hinrichs HH. A General Theory of Tax Structure Change During Economic Development, Cambridge, MA: Law School of Harvard University; 1966.
30. Lotz JR, Morss ER. *Measuring "Tax Effort" in Developing Countries. Staff Papers.* Washington: International Monetary Fund, Vol. 14; 1967, pp. 478–497.
31. Chelliah RJ. *Trends in Taxation in Developing Countries. Staff Papers.* Washington: International Monetary Fund, Vol. 18; 1971, pp. 254–327.

32. Chellah RJ, Baas HJ, Kelly MR. *Tax Ratios and Tax Effort in Developing Countries, 1969-71.*" Staff Papers. Washington: International Monetary Fund, Vol. 22; 1975, pp. 187–205.
33. Tait AA, Gratz WLM, Eichengreen BJ. *International Comparisons of Taxation for Selected Developing Countries. Staff Papers.* Washington: International Monetary Fund, Vol. 26; 1979, pp. 123–156.
34. Rousseau JJ. Social Contract. Oxford; 1999.
35. Kant I. *Groundwork for the Metaphysics of Morals.* Yale University Press; 2008.
36. World Health Organization. "Constitution of the World Health Organization"; 1995.
37. World Health Organization. *Global Action Plan for the Prevention and Control of Noncommunicable Diseases 2013–2020 (Appendix 3).* Geneva: World Health Organization; 2013.
38. Political declaration of the third high-level meeting of the General Assembly on the prevention and control of non-communicable diseases, Resolution adopted by the General Assembly on 10 October 2018, A/RES/73/2.
39. Political Declaration for the UN High-Level Meeting Meeting on UHC, Resolution adopted by the General Assembly on 10 October 2019, A/RES/74/2.
40. Junquera-Varela RF, Verhoeven M, Shukla GP, Haven B, Moreno-Dodson B. *Strengthening Domestic Resource Mobilization: Moving from Theory to Practice in Low-and Middle-Income Countries.* World Bank Publications; 2017.
41. Sassi F. Global public health challenges, fiscal policies, and yellow vest. *The Lancet.* 2019; 393(10173): 745–746.

https://doi.org/10.1142/9781800612396_0002

Chapter 2

The Place for Health Taxes in the Wider Fiscal System[a]

Céline Colin*, Gioia de Melo*, and Bert Brys*

Health taxes on tobacco and alcohol have a long history and on average raise significant amounts of revenues across countries. Moreover, interest in – and adoption of – taxes on sugar-sweetened beverages has increased in recent years as evidence of the negative health effects of unhealthy diets has become more prevalent. Overall, there is a trend towards a wider use of health taxes as part of countries' health protection and promotion policies. On average, Health tax revenues account for 0.8% of GDP in high and middle-income countries and 0.4% of GDP in low-income countries. Scope exists to enhance the role of health taxes, but health tax reform needs to be embedded within the design and functioning of the broader tax system. Together with environmental taxes that aim at reducing practices which cause damage to the environment and people's health, health taxes could play a role helping restore public finances once economies are on a more solid path to recovery from the COVID-19 crisis. In addition to increasing health tax rates, there might be substantial revenue potential from extending health taxes to other products that generate negative externalities linked to health. We begin by

* Organisation for Economic Co-operation and Development (OECD), France.

[a] The authors wish to thank David Bradbury, Stéphane Buydens and Alastair Thomas from the OECD Centre for Tax Policy and Administration and Alan Carter from the UK HMRC for their input, comments and suggestions.

describing how health taxes are generally levied and we then consider their revenue-raising capacity. We consider general tax policy design principles and discuss how health taxes may interact with these principles.

From an economic perspective, health taxes can be justified where they internalise the external costs and correct for internalities associated with the consumption of products for which all consumption has a negative impact on health, such as tobacco, and products for which excessive consumption is harmful, such as sugar.

Health taxes raise revenues that generally flow to general budgets and can support the financing of the health sector. Health taxes on tobacco and alcohol have a long history and raise, on average, significant amounts of revenues across countries. Moreover, interest in – and adoption of – taxes on sugar-sweetened beverages (SSBs) has increased significantly in recent years as evidence of the negative health effects of unhealthy diets has become more prevalent. Overall, there is a trend towards a wider use of health taxes as part of countries' health protection and promotion policies. This then raises the question on how to design health taxes aligned with best tax practice.

This chapter starts by describing how health taxes are generally levied and considers their revenue-raising capacity. The chapter argues that there is scope to enhance the role of health taxes but that this needs to be embedded within the design and functioning of the broader tax system. The chapter then considers general tax policy design principles and applies these principles to health taxes.

2.1. Health taxes in the broader tax system

Taxes are compulsory, unrequited payments made to the general government. Taxes are unrequited in the sense that benefits provided by the government to taxpayers are not normally in proportion to their payment. They can be classified according to the economic function of their base: income and profits; payroll and workforce; property; goods and services; and compulsory social security contributions.[1]

Taxes on goods and services (GST) include, amongst others, sales taxes, value-added taxes (VAT), excise taxes and taxes levied on the import and export of goods and services. They are levied on the production, extraction, sale, transfer, leasing or delivery of goods and the rendering of services; or in respect of the use of goods, permission to use goods or to perform activities. They are often categorised as indirect taxes as they are generally not levied directly on the person who is supposed to bear the burden of the tax, but are rather imposed on certain transactions, products or events. Governments generally collect the tax from producers and distributors at various points in the value chain, while the burden of the tax falls in principle on consumers assuming that it will be passed on to them in the prices charged by suppliers.[2]

Health taxes are generally levied in the form of excise duties. Excise duties, unlike other general goods and services taxes, are levied only on specific goods and are usually assessed by reference to the weight, volume, strength or quantity of the product and may be combined in some cases with the value or sometimes calculated on a value basis only.[2] Health taxes are levied on goods that adversely affect health such as alcohol, tobacco, SSBs and certain foods (e.g. confectionaries, chocolate, ice creams, salt, fats, etc.). They can be levied directly on the component that creates negative health effects (e.g. alcohol volume, gram of sugar, salt or saturated fat) or on the product that contains the component that is harmful to consumer health (e.g. per litre of soft drink or alcoholic beverage or per pack of cigarettes). They can also be levied when these components or products are used as inputs in the production process.

Environmentally related taxes typically overlap with health taxes in that they correct externalities linked to the environment and often to health as well. Environmentally related taxes are taxes whose tax base is a physical unit that has a proven, specific, negative impact on the environment.[3] They include taxes on energy (CO_2 taxes, taxes on energy products such as fossil fuels and electricity), transport, pollution (taxes on air pollution, ozone-depleting substances, water pollution or waste management) and resources (mining, freshwater, sand, etc.). Some of those taxes have an indirect positive impact on health and, in this respect, they could be considered as health taxes.

The VAT interacts with excise duties. Excise duties are part of the VAT base, meaning that VAT is usually levied on the total value of the products, inclusive of excise duties. Therefore, an increase in excise duties will also increase the VAT that has to be paid.[2]

2.2. The revenue-raising capacity of health taxes

Tax-to-GDP ratios and tax structures vary significantly across countries and by country income groups. Across the countries covered by the OECD Global Revenue Statistics database, on average, the tax-to-GDP ratio is 14.8% in 2017 for low-income countries, 18.6% for lower-middle-income countries, 21.5% for upper-middle-income countries and 32.6% for high income.[b] Tax structures also vary widely across countries and country groups. Even if all countries rely extensively on taxes on goods and services (between 9% and 11% of GDP) (Figure 2.1), countries use a more diversified range of taxes to raise revenues when their per capita income increases (Figure 2.2). Taxes on goods and services represented 63% of tax revenues in low-income countries in 2017, but only 34% in high-income countries. High-income countries rely significantly on personal income taxes and social security contributions, while these tax categories are utilised less in less developed countries.

[b] The OECD Global Revenue Statistics database covers 98 countries. Based on World Bank income groups: 8 low-income countries, 22 lower-middle-income countries, 26 upper-middle-income countries and 42 high-income countries.

Fig. 2.1. Level and structure of taxes, as a % of GDP, 2017.

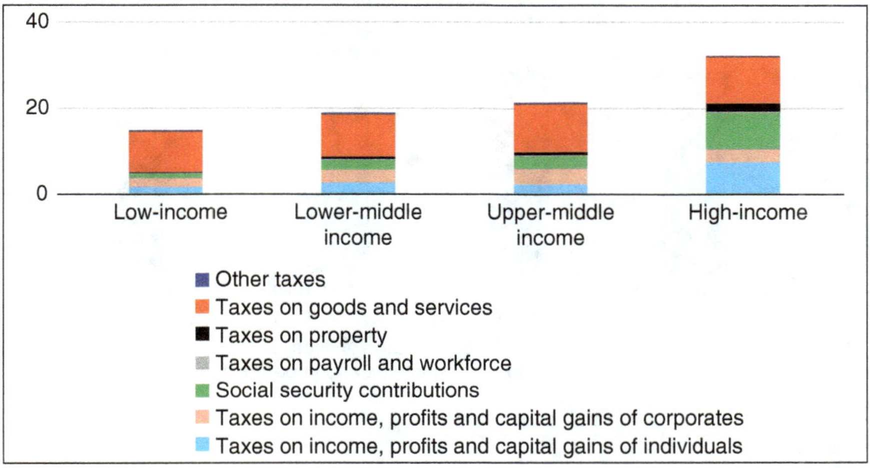

Source: OECD Global Revenue Statistics database.

Note: This figure includes only countries for which there is information available in the OECD Global Revenue Statistics database.

Fig. 2.2. Tax structure, as a % of total tax revenues, 2017.

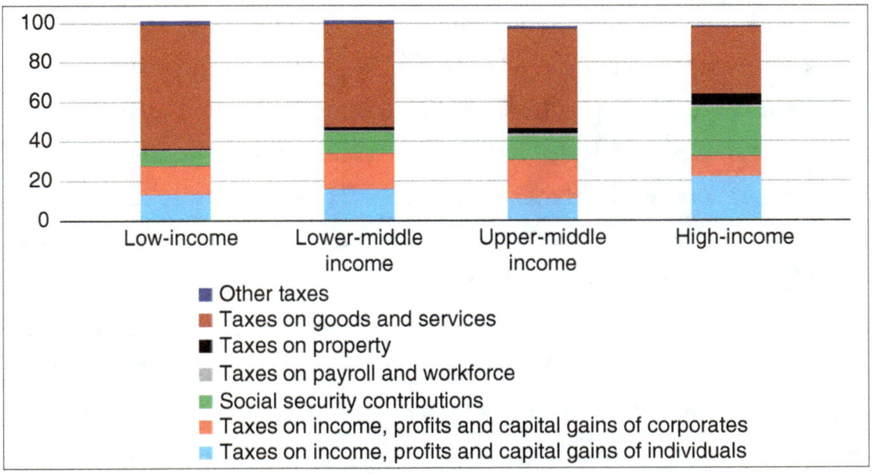

Source: OECD Global Revenue Statistics database.

Note: This figure includes only countries for which there is information available in the OECD Global Revenue Statistics database. For some categories, the total does not exactly round up to 100% as averages are considered.

Fig. 2.3. Decomposition of taxes on goods and services, as a % of GDP, 2017.

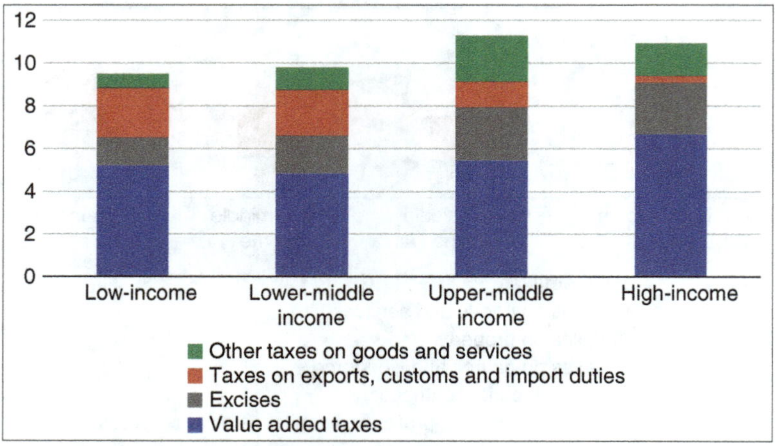

Source: OECD Global Revenue Statistics database.

Note: This figure includes only countries for which there is information available in the OECD Global Revenue Statistics database. Other taxes on goods and services include sales taxes, taxes on profit of fiscal monopolies, on investment goods, on specific services and taxes on the use of goods and perform activities.

In all income groups, on average, revenues from taxes on goods and services (i.e. consumption taxes) primarily come from the VAT. The VAT represents 5–7% of GDP across all country income groups (Figure 2.3). Excise taxes are the second largest consumption tax in high-income and upper-middle-income countries (2.5% of GDP), while in low and lower-middle-income countries taxes levied on the import and export of goods (at 2.2% of GDP) raise more revenues than excise taxes. Excise taxes raise 1.3% of GDP and 1.8% of GDP in low and lower-middle-income countries, respectively.

Health taxes raise limited revenues. Health tax revenues account for less than 1% of GDP in all income groups (Figure 2.4).[c] As a share of tax revenues, they represent 2.5% of total tax revenues in high-income countries to about 4% in middle-income countries, which remains relatively low. While health tax revenues as a share of total tax revenues have not varied significantly over time (Figure 2.5), they have increased for middle-income countries when measured as a share of GDP (Figure 2.6).

[c] The annex provides detailed information on which types of taxes are considered health taxes in this section. While taxes levied on goods that adversely affect health such as alcohol, tobacco, SSBs, certain foods (e.g. confectionaries, chocolate, ice creams, salt, fats, etc.) are considered health taxes, environmental taxes are not included due to a lack of disaggregated data. Health social contributions are not included, as they are not considered as health taxes.

Fig. 2.4. Health tax revenues, as a % of GDP and total tax revenues, 2017.

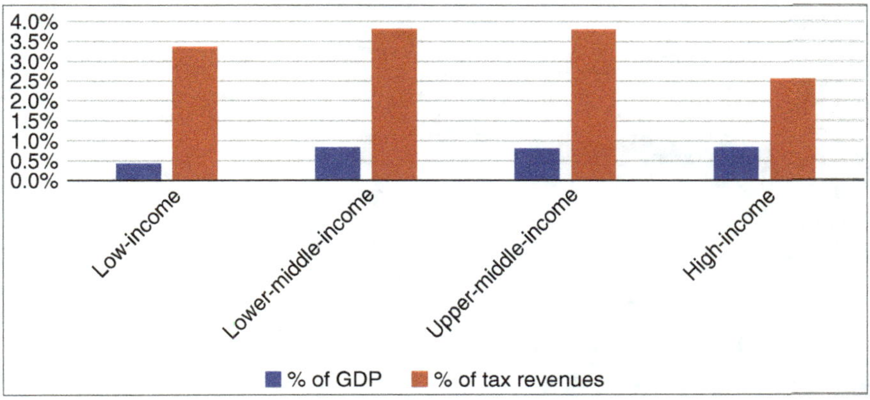

Source: OECD Global Revenue Statistics database.

Note: This figure covers 5 low-income countries, 10 lower-middle-income countries, 11 upper-middle-income countries and 37 high-income countries for which disaggregated data on health taxes are available – see Annex for more information on health taxes considered in this figure.

Fig. 2.5. Evolution of health tax revenues, as a % of total tax revenues, 2003–2016.

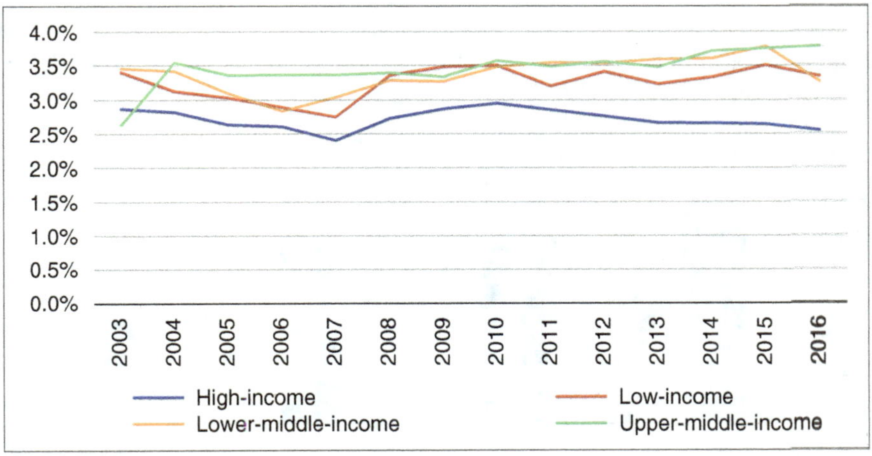

Source: OECD Global Revenue Statistics database.

Note: This figure covers 5 low-income countries, 10 lower-middle-income countries, 11 upper-middle-income countries and 37 high-income countries for which disaggregated data on health taxes are available – see Annex for more information on health taxes considered in this figure.

Health tax revenues account for a significant share of public health expenditure. On average, health tax revenues represent 25% of domestic government health expenditure in low-income countries, 31% in lower-middle-income countries, 23% in upper-middle-income countries and 16% in high-income countries (Figure 2.7). However, these aggregated figures hide significant differences across countries (Figures 2.8 and 2.9).

Fig. 2.6. Evolution of health tax revenues, as a % of GDP.

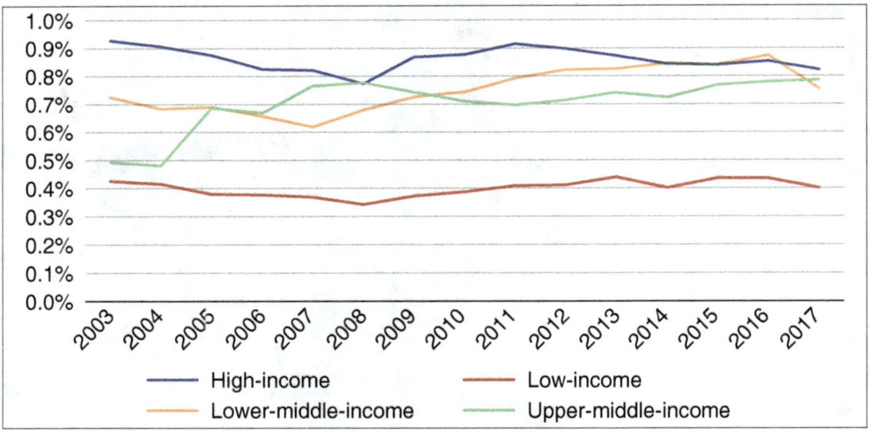

Source: OECD Global Revenue Statistics database.

Note: This figure covers 5 low-income countries, 10 lower-middle-income countries, 11 upper-middle-income countries and 37 high-income countries for which disaggregated data on health taxes are available – see Annex for more information on health taxes considered in this figure.

Fig. 2.7. Share of public health expenditure financed by health taxes, as a %, 2017.

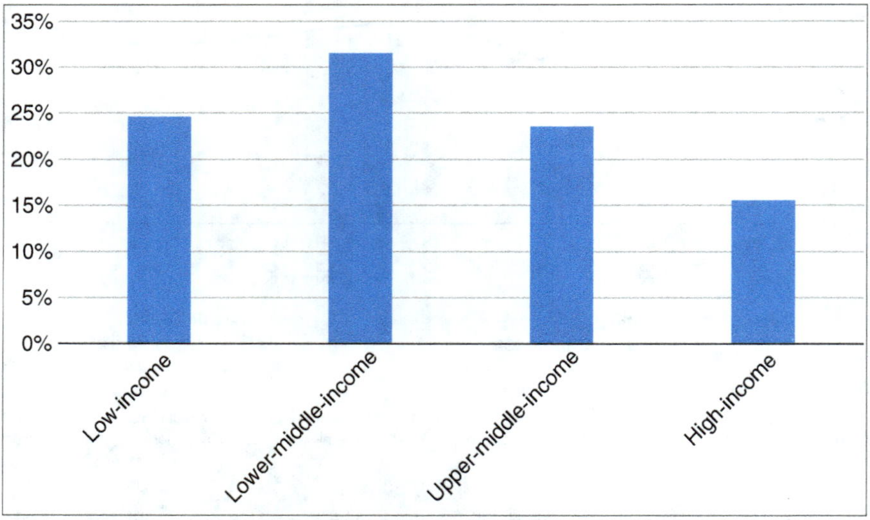

Source: OECD calculation based on OECD Global Revenue Statistics database and WHO Global Health Expenditure database.

Note: This figure covers 4 low-income countries, 10 lower–middle-income countries, 11 upper-middle-income countries and 37 high-income countries for which disaggregated data on health taxes are available – see Annex for more information on health taxes considered in this figure.

Fig. 2.8. Share of health taxes, as a % of public health expenditure, 2017.

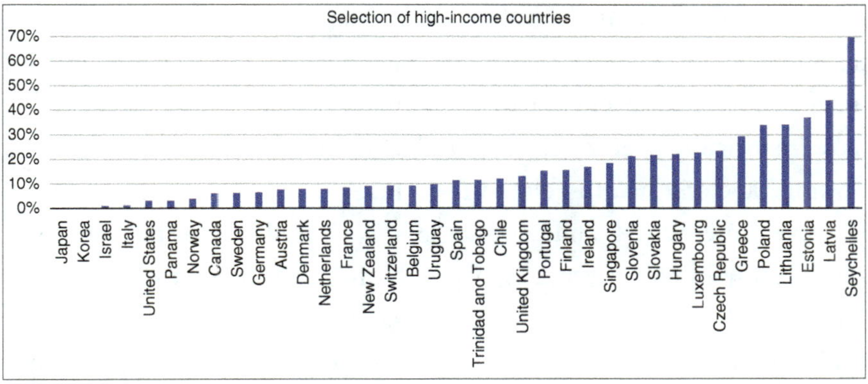

Source: OECD calculation based on OECD Global Revenue Statistics database and WHO Global Health Expenditure database.

Note: This figure covers 37 high-income countries for which disaggregated data on health taxes are available – see Annex for more information on health taxes considered in this figure.

Fig. 2.9. Share of health taxes, as a % of public health expenditure, 2017.

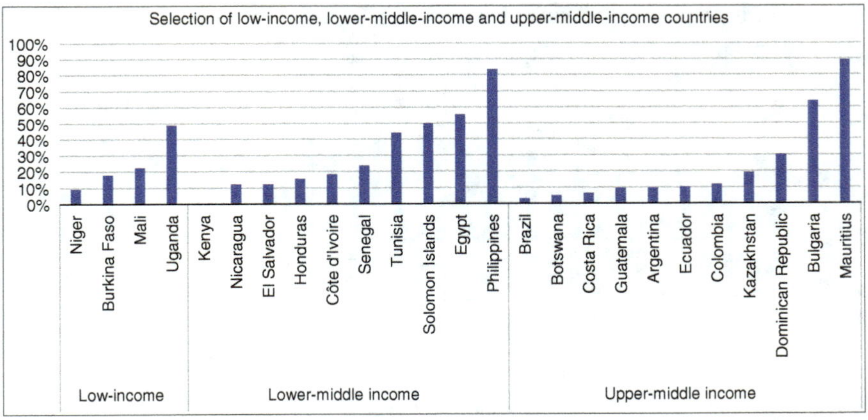

Source: OECD calculation based on OECD Global Revenue Statistics database and WHO Global Health Expenditure database.

Note: This figure covers 4 low-income countries, 10 lower–middle-income countries, 11 upper-middle-income countries for which disaggregated data on health taxes are available – see Annex for more information on health taxes considered in this figure.

For all country income groups, health tax revenues are predominantly raised on tobacco and alcohol products (Figures 2.10 and 2.11). While taxes on alcohol and tobacco products have been widely used by countries for many years as revenue-generating measures, taxes on food and SSBs have historically been rarely imposed, and a large majority of countries do not have any health-related food taxes or taxes on SSBs in place. However, interest in – and adoption of – such health taxes has increased significantly in recent years as evidence of the negative health effects of unhealthy diets has become more prevalent. Indeed, there is now strong evidence that the excess consumption of products high in sugar, salt and saturated fats have negative impacts on long-run health outcomes.[4] At least 14 OECD countries as well as India, Peru, Saudi Arabia, South Africa and some developing countries have imposed some form of taxation on SSBs or other types of food.[5]

Fig. 2.10. Decomposition of health tax revenues, as a % of health tax revenues, 2017.

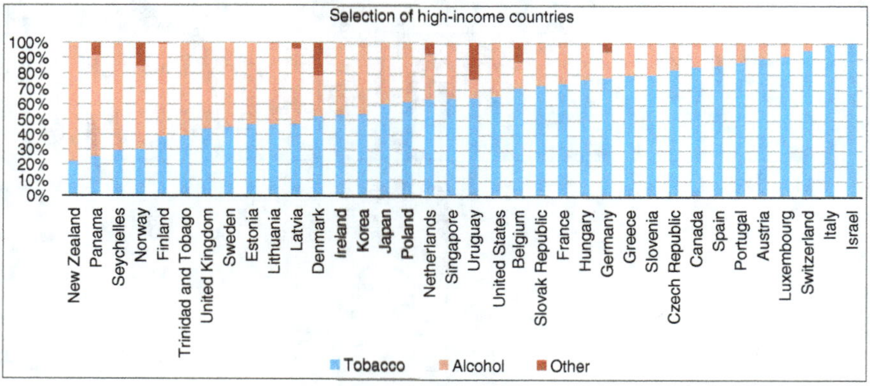

Source: OECD calculation based on OECD Global Revenue Statistics database.

Note: This figure does not include health social security contributions. Chile is not represented in this figure because of the difficulty to disentangle tobacco taxes from alcohol taxes in the OECD Global Revenue Statistics database. Turkey is not represented either due to insufficient data. The category "other" includes taxes on SSBs, sugar, chocolate, ice creams etc. – see Annex for more information.

Fig. 2.11. Decomposition of health tax revenues, as a % of health tax revenues, 2017.

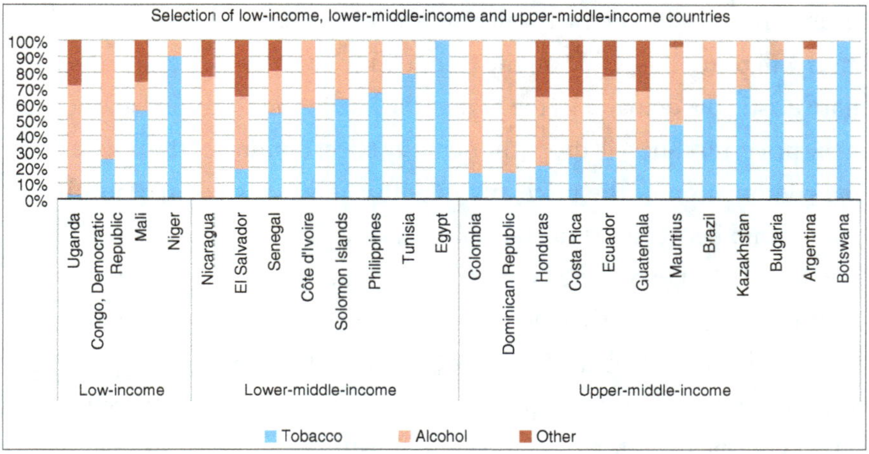

Source: OECD calculation based on OECD Global Revenue Statistics database.

Note: This figure does not include health social security contributions. Kenya is not represented due to insufficient data. The category "other" includes taxes on SSBs, sugar, chocolate, ice creams etc. – see Annex for more information.

2.3. The use of health taxes can be enhanced

Scope exists to strengthen the role of health taxes. While many countries could increase the rates and broaden the base of the health taxes they currently levy on invariably unhealthy consumption, there is also scope to enlarge the tax base by taxing other goods that are unhealthy when consumed excessively and/or the inputs that are used in the production of these unhealthy consumption goods. While the revenue potential of increasing tax rates and broadening tax bases seems higher in low- and middle-income countries given the current low revenues these taxes raise as a percentage of GDP, high-tax rate countries do have scope to enlarge their health tax base.

The relation between health tax rates and health tax revenues is non-linear. The revenue impact from increases in health taxes will depend crucially on the elasticity of the demand for the taxed goods, as health taxes are typically consumption taxes. A higher tax rate results in higher revenue for each unit sold (price effect) as excise taxes are generally almost fully passed through to prices.[d] The higher price also leads to a drop in the

[d] See Ref.[13] for a review of pass through of tax increases applied to SBBs.

quantity sold (quantity effect). A drop in demand will not only reduce the revenue from health taxes, it will also result in lower VAT revenues. Which effect will prevail depends on the price elasticity of the demand curve. The more elastic the demand is, the higher the likelihood that upon an increase in the price, revenue will drop (the quantity effect dominates the price effect). The combination of the price and quantity effects results in a non-linear relationship between the tax rate and tax revenues.[6]

A wide range of other factors determines the relationship between health tax rates and tax revenues. An increase in tax rates may induce households to avoid the tax increase by shifting to other more lightly taxed consumption goods. The revenue impact of a tax increase will therefore also depend on the tax rates levied on close substitutes and the extent to which tax bases are broad or narrow. The impact of a health tax increase will also depend on the extent to which the tax increase is passed onto consumers in the form of higher after-tax prices. If producers reduce the consumption good's before-tax price in response to a health tax increase, the consumer might not have to pay a higher after-tax price; instead, producers would absorb (partially or fully) the tax increase through a reduction in their profit margin or by lowering the wages they pay to their workers. The increase in health tax revenues may then be offset by lower income tax revenues. In fact, the revenue impact in response to a change in the before-tax price will depend on whether health taxes are levied on an "ad quantum" or "ad valorem" basis, and this effect is further enhanced through the VAT, which is levied on top of health excise taxes. Finally, illicit trade and opportunities for cross-border shopping are other factors that might have an impact on the revenue potential of health taxes.

In theory, one could try to find the level of a health tax rate that would maximise health tax revenues. However, the discussion in the previous paragraphs indicates that a wide range of factors has to be taken into account and that in practice, this is less straightforward than it looks at first sight. In addition, tax economists would argue that governments should not set tax rates to maximise tax revenues but that they should set rates to maximise social welfare. A revenue maximising tax rate is indeed not necessarily an "optimal" tax rate as it, for instance, does not take into account the main health tax goal (i.e. correcting for negative externalities and internalities).

Nevertheless, increasing health tax rates is expected to increase tax revenues as empirical evidence shows that, in many countries, the tax rates are very likely not set at their tax revenue maximising point. For alcoholic beverages, the empirical literature suggests that the price elasticity of demand is relatively inelastic.[7] Evidence for France, Poland and Spain suggests that tax rates for beer and wine are well below the revenue maximising point while the evidence for spirits is inconclusive.[6] Regarding cigarettes, the price elasticity of demand also seems to be relatively inelastic.[8,9] The relatively inelastic demand of tobacco has induced many OECD countries to increase tax rates on cigarettes gradually over time to relatively high levels. This gives rise to the question: does the tax rate remain below the negative spill-over effects induced by smoking? However, tax rates in developing and emerging countries are typically far below the rates set in OECD countries. Studies for both Indonesia and Latin America and the Caribbean have found that health tax revenues could increase by about 30% from raising tobacco excise taxes by 50% per pack.[8,10] On the other hand, for taxes on SSBs the capacity of raising revenue by increasing tax rates could be more limited as the demand for SSBs seems considerably more elastic.[11,12] However, as the tax base for SSBs is larger than for other products, there is potential to raise a moderate amount of tax revenue from increasing the taxation of these products as well.

In addition to increasing tax rates, there might be substantial revenue potential from extending health taxes to other products that generate negative externalities linked to health. Health taxes could aim at reducing negative externalities on health outcomes generated from the consumption of food or inputs used in the production of certain types of food that are harmful to health such as plastic and pesticides.

The relation between environmentally related taxes and health taxes remains an area that has received little attention in the tax policy debate. Environmentally related excise taxes penalise the production and consumption of environmental "bads" to improve environmental outcomes. Certain environmentally related taxes could be considered as health taxes to the extent that some pollutants have a direct negative impact on health. Furthermore, there is increasing evidence that excessive consumption of certain food items, such as meat, can be harmful for health while at the same time its production plays a significant role in the emission of CO_2 and therefore generates negative externalities both linked to health and the environment. Higher taxes on fossil fuels may induce people to leave their car at home and cycle or walk, which will create positive health externalities. How to design green and health-friendly tax reforms remains an area that deserves further work.

The COVID-19 crisis creates an opportunity for a "health-friendly and green" tax reform. The crisis should induce countries to reconsider the use and design of health taxes, including in developing countries. Public revenues as a share of GDP are expected to decrease worldwide, including in low- and middle-income countries. As countries move to restore their public finances beyond the COVID-19 crisis, many of them will have to implement tax measures at some stage in the future. While it is now widely acknowledged that the recovery from the COVID-19 crisis should be green, the public debate has put less emphasis on the fact that the recovery should also be health-friendly. Health taxes are particularly attractive tax instruments to increase revenue in the short run in countries with low administrative capacity and with narrow income tax bases because of a large informal economy. In fact, the arguments in favour of health taxes are particularly strong in the context of the COVID-19 pandemic as smoking and obesity, as well as local air pollution, are linked to increased risk factors of COVID-19.

2.4. Health taxes interact with other taxes

A discussion on the optimal level of health tax rates should include in its scope and evaluation of the optimal mix between health (and other) excise taxes and the VAT. While the level of indirect tax revenues in the OECD has been relatively constant over time, this trend hides a change in the mix of consumption taxes. Countries have gradually moved away from specific consumption taxes, including trade-related import and export duties, towards an increased use of the VAT. The strengthened role of the VAT has been overall a story of great success.

The optimal design of health taxes and the VAT needs to be integrated. Optimal tax policy calls for a broad VAT base where all goods and services are levied at a standard VAT rate without the use of reduced rates. Health excise taxes that are levied in addition to the VAT play then a central role in the taxation of unhealthy goods. In reality, however, many countries implement reduced VAT rates and these generally cover food and, in some countries, beverages. In these circumstances, there are arguments to exclude alcoholic beverages and SSBs from the list of products that benefit from the reduced VAT rates, despite the fact that this may increase tax complexity. Similarly, countries that decide to levy a reduced rate on raw food may still consider taxing processed food at the standard VAT rate. In practice, almost all OECD countries apply a standard VAT rate to alcoholic beverages while many apply a reduced VAT rate to other beverages.[2] If, in turn, unhealthy consumption items benefit from a reduced VAT rate (as is the case for SSBs in many countries) and a VAT reform is not (e.g. politically) feasible, this tax reduction could be compensated by using higher excise taxes. Tax differentiation for unhealthy products can also be implemented through higher VAT rates, which is for instance the case in India where tobacco products and sugary drinks are taxed at higher VAT/GST rates, although the use of excise taxes remains the preferred tax policy choice.

Countries may consider rebalancing the tax mix towards more health excise taxes rather than increasing VAT rates further. After the 2008–2009 crisis, many OECD countries raised their standard VAT rates in order to restore their budgets, and rates are now relatively high in many countries. This raises the question of whether and to what extent there is scope to continue increasing standard VAT rates. On the other hand, there remains scope to broaden VAT bases in many countries. In relation to health, there is an additional argument that needs to be considered. Many health-friendly consumption goods such as bio-products are typically more expensive to produce and are therefore relatively more expensive for the consumer to buy. This effect is exacerbated by the VAT, which is levied on the price irrespective of the quality of the product. This suggests that excise (including health taxes) may have an important role to play in the tax mix.

High import tariffs levied on unhealthy imported products will not lead to better health outcomes if consumers can shift to locally produced goods that are a close substitute to the imported goods. Import duties result in price differentiation between domestically and foreign-produced goods and thereby merely encourage consumers to substitute consumption towards items produced locally (see also Chapter 8). Instead, it may prove more effective from a health perspective to lower import tariffs on the unhealthy products and introduce excise taxes on foreign and domestically produced unhealthy items. However, higher import tariffs may prove effective in small countries that do not produce close substitutes in the domestic economy. Indeed, small islands such as Bermuda, Palau, Fiji and Seychelles levy import tariffs on SSBs.[13]

2.5. General tax considerations providing guidance when designing taxes

This section describes the general principles that are applied to design individual taxes and the overall tax system. The following section will then apply these principles to health taxes.

2.5.1. Efficiency

Tax policies should aim at being efficient. An efficient tax system is designed in such a way that the after-tax market equilibrium stays as close as possible to the market equilibrium that would have occurred in the absence of taxation. Put differently, the tax system should induce agents to change their behaviour as little as possible in response to the taxes levied. The efficiency criterion induces tax systems to be as neutral as possible to minimise discrimination in favour of, or against, any particular economic choice. In certain cases, however, there are good reasons to distort behaviour. This is the case in the presence of positive or negative spill-over effects where an efficient tax system would induce agents, for instance, to internalise externalities, as well as in the presence of other market failures. In this case, there are efficiency arguments for taxes to create a distortion. Finally, for taxes to be effective in internalising external effects, the tax would ideally be levied as close as possible to the source of the externality.

2.5.2. Equity

A parallel but potentially conflicting objective of tax policy is equity. There are different forms of equity: horizontal equity, which requires that taxpayers in an equal situation pay an equal amount of tax; and vertical equity, which requires that taxpayers with a greater ability to contribute, pay relatively more tax. Greater efficiency in tax systems is usually consistent with stronger horizontal equity, while governments are often faced with trade-offs between efficiency and vertical equity.

While looking at efficiency-equity trade-offs on a tax-by-tax basis is critical, it is not sufficient. To ensure a coherent tax system, it is essential to view the tax system as a whole rather than consider its different elements in isolation. Individual parts of the tax system may be well-designed, but looking in isolation at one tax provision or one type of tax can lead to poor tax policy choices and sub-optimal economic and social outcomes.[14] For instance, an individual tax can be progressive (regressive), while the whole tax system is regressive (progressive).

The distributional consequences of tax mix shifts should be examined in concert with the public spending mix. Greater reliance on taxes that may be regressive may actually increase the amount of overall redistribution due to the tax and transfer system if the spending associated with the reform has progressive effects. Indeed, a tax that raises significant amounts of revenue but is slightly regressive can help to increase the overall progressivity of the tax and benefit system if the tax revenue is spent in a manner that benefits the poor.

The distributional impact of the tax system should also be considered from a lifetime perspective. Some taxes such as income taxes may be highly progressive when considered in a given period, but may be less progressive from a lifetime perspective, as individuals who may have low incomes at one time might have higher incomes later in life.[15]

Finally, the ability to shift the final tax burden onto other taxpayers will affect the distributional impact and the efficiency-equity trade-offs of a tax reform. The taxpayers directly paying the tax may not be the ones ultimately bearing the burden of the tax. The incidence of the tax not only depends on behavioural responses but also on the degree of competition and the linkages across markets.[16]

2.5.3. Administrative simplicity, transparency and tax certainty

Administrative capacity needs to be taken into account when designing the tax system. Tax rules should be clear and designed with as much simplicity as possible in order to minimise the tax compliance costs for households and businesses and the enforcement costs for tax administrations. Tax rules need to be transparent and give individuals and businesses tax certainty. Tax rules that have nice efficiency and equity characteristics when designed on the tax policy drawing board might achieve just the opposite if the tax administration does not have the data, income tax tools and overall human and technical capacity to make the tax work in practice. Tax compliance costs can also be impacted by the tax collection process and, in return, impact the incidence of a tax.[16]

2.5.4. Tax revenue-raising potential

The amount of revenues that can be collected does matter. Taxes allow governments to raise revenues, but the marginal cost of raising these funds can be larger than the amount of the tax revenue itself. As pointed out, taxes might distort behaviour and result in compliance and enforcement costs. This explains why optimal tax policy does not aim at maximising tax revenues, but takes broader welfare considerations and compliance costs into account.

2.5.5. Non-tax system factors that affect the efficiency and equity implications of taxes

A number of non-tax system factors also have an impact on the efficiency and equity implications of taxes, which need to be taken into consideration when designing efficient and inclusive tax systems.[16] These include, among others:

- The economic structure, which includes the functioning of the industry that is affected by the tax, the economy's labour and capital intensity and returns, the distribution of income and wealth, the purchasing power of households across the income distribution, informality levels, productivity levels, etc.
- The informal economy. The informal sector has an impact on how countries have designed and can reform their tax systems. The tax system should be designed such that it provides incentives to the informal sector to formalise and prevents formal businesses from becoming informal.
- Time horizons. Equity-efficiency trade-offs tend to be more significant in the short term than in the long run. For instance, individuals who are considered as poor today might not be poor in the future and the negative distributional implications of a pro-growth tax reform may be overestimated when looking only at short-term impacts. On the other hand, behavioural effects of high tax rates may be higher in the longer run as it typically takes time before agents change their behaviour.
- The political economy. Tax decisions, such as the level of the tax rate imposed, may be influenced by political economy considerations (e.g. supra-national setting; industry lobbying; public opposition; popularity of the measures; the political parties in power and the time to the next election).

2.6. Designing health taxes to address externalities

2.6.1. Ensuring that the design of health taxes is efficient and effective

The costs of the negative health outcomes generated by harmful products for health are often not borne only by the consumer, but also by society as a whole. This market failure is the main justification for the imposition of a corrective health tax that aims at inducing consumers to internalise these external costs. Other tax policy reasons for implementing health taxes include time inconsistency of preferences (a preference for short-term gratification over long-term health) and information constraints (a lack of knowledge of the underlying health implications of consumption of certain products). Standard economic theory suggests setting the tax rate at a level that internalises, at the margin, the negative external effects of the consumption, or to higher levels if the aim is to also correct for time inconsistency of preferences or other market failures.[17,18]

Determining the size of the negative external effects is important but extremely challenging. Significant work to estimate negative external effects has been undertaken regarding consumption of tobacco and alcohol. However, even in the case of tobacco – where there is a direct link between consumption of a unit of product and the external cost due to passive smoking, for example – empirical estimates vary widely. For alcohol and SSBs, it is even more difficult as external costs depend on excess consumption. With SSBs, negative external effects are mainly associated to financial healthcare costs, which are shared through public insurance. Empirical evidence that guides the setting of tax levels to internalise the negative external effects of consumption of SSBs has increased in recent years (see e.g. Refs.[19,20]).

The aim of the tax is to offset externalities and internalities without preventing the consumption of the unhealthy good altogether. Regulation can be a more effective way of preventing unhealthy behaviour, and in this case the challenge lies in determining which goods should or should not be banned.[12]

The effectiveness of a health tax will depend on a number of factors, including the extent to which it is passed on by businesses to consumers in terms of higher prices; the responsiveness of consumers to those higher prices, which also will depend on the salience of the tax and the impact of those behavioural responses on long-run health. While a detailed analysis is needed in each case, empirical evidence does suggest that, in general, health taxes are to a large degree passed on to consumers via higher prices, if introduced at a rate that is sufficiently high, they do alter consumption behaviour, and they can positively impact health outcomes.[4,17,18,21]

A key decision countries face in designing a health tax is whether to apply the tax to a product or to a nutrient or product content (e.g. alcohol volume, quantity of sugar, salt or saturated fat). Applying a content-based tax can be expected to better target the negative health effects of consumption than a product-based tax. In addition, it will also encourage product improvement and innovation by producers to reduce the content of the taxed nutrient (see e.g. Ref.[22]).

If a product-based tax is chosen, a key choice is whether to apply it on an ad quantum or ad valorem basis. Overall, ad quantum excises – also referred to as "specific" excises – are preferred to ad valorem excise taxes for a number of reasons. An ad quantum product-based tax can target the negative health externality more closely than an ad valorem tax. This is because the quantity of the product, rather than its value, is more closely linked to the amount of the unhealthy product of concern (e.g. sugar, tobacco, alcohol). Ad valorem taxes may encourage consumers to switch to lower cost brands rather than reducing the quantity consumed of the unhealthy product ("trading down"). Ad quantum excise taxes also provide producers less opportunities to attract consumers and stimulate consumption of unhealthy products through price adjustments.[23] Ad valorem taxes would also discourage expensive product innovation by producers. Another argument that favours ad quantum taxes is that healthier products might be more expensive and that an ad valorem tax would therefore discourage consumption of the healthier product. In addition, empirical evidence has found that ad quantum taxes tend to be more than fully passed through to the consumer (price rises by more than the tax increase), whereas ad valorem taxes tend to be less than fully passed through.[17]

2.6.2. Introducing health taxes in an equitable and fair manner

An often-cited concern in implementing health taxes is their potential distributional impact. In particular, poorer households may have more unhealthy lifestyles and spend a greater proportion of their current income on products subject to health taxes than richer households do (see, e.g. Ref.[24] for the United Kingdom). However, this may not necessarily be the case as a percentage of their current expenditure.[25] That being said, there will still be many households that are both current and lifetime poor, and health taxes can be expected to be regressive for these households whether measured as a proportion of income or expenditure.

Even when the poor do bear a greater tax burden than the rich, they can still be expected to benefit significantly, and possibly even more, from improvements in health outcomes. To evaluate who benefits or is disadvantaged by health taxes it is necessary to evaluate not only which income groups will bear the higher tax burden but also which households will benefit the most from a reduction in negative health outcomes.[12,26] If low-income consumers are more responsive to after-tax price changes of unhealthy consumption items, then the corrective benefits are large relative to the financial burden, making the regressivity of the tax less of a concern.[12,27] Progressive health gains can be expected because smoking and consumption of SSBs cause diseases that disproportionately affect low-income households.[21,28]

Moreover, as mentioned previously, the progressivity of the tax and benefit system has to be analysed as a whole and the distributional consequences of tax mix shifts should be examined in concert with the public spending mix. Even a regressive health tax can still lead to an overall progressive outcome if its revenues are spent particularly on the poor (also referred to as progressive revenue recycling).

While ad quantum taxes are preferred to ad valorem health taxes from an efficiency perspective, the outcomes might be different from an equity and tax revenue perspective (Chapter 8 discusses in detail the pros and cons of these two types of excises). Although ad quantum taxes might discourage unhealthy consumption by lower income, they might be too low to induce high-income earners to change behaviour. Ad valorem taxes, in contrast, would lead to a higher tax burden for high-income earners under the assumption that high-income taxpayers purchase more expensive products. The exact distributional impact will depend on consumption patterns, and even with an ad valorem tax, high-income taxpayers may still end up paying less tax relative to their income than poor households.

In summary, there might be a strong case for a combination of ad quantum and ad valorem taxes when looking at health taxes from an efficiency, equity and tax revenue perspective. Where there are large differences in prices of a product, an ad quantum tax will comprise a significantly lower proportion of the price of a high-value product, and therefore be less likely to reduce demand for the high-value product, and will raise less revenue from it than an ad valorem tax. Additionally, higher income consumers who are more likely to consume high-value products may be less responsive than low-income groups to the health tax. Imposing a higher aggregate tax on these expensive products will therefore be necessary to affect behaviour. To achieve this, an ad valorem tax may be adopted, but in order to reduce the likelihood of trading down, an ad quantum tax may still be imposed as well. Such an approach is common with tobacco taxation. See Chapter 8 for an in-depth discussion on equity and distributional effects of health taxes.

2.6.3. Minimising administrative, enforcement and collection costs of health taxes

A well-designed health tax keeps administrative and compliance costs as low as possible. Tax administration considerations need to be taken into account with respect to a wide range of health tax design choices, including a product- or nutrient-based tax, the type of product to tax, an ad quantum or an ad valorem tax, the tax rate, whether or not to use a minimum threshold and the point of collection of the tax (see Chapter 8).

- An ad quantum tax may be administratively easier to implement than an ad valorem tax, as it is based on the quantity of a product and not its price, thereby reducing abuse and administrative costs. That said, an ad quantum tax needs to be monitored and updated to adjust for inflation whereas an ad valorem tax automatically increases with inflation.
- Gradual phasing-in of health taxes is more administratively costly (to both government and businesses) than immediately introducing the tax at the desired level, but may increase the visibility of the tax as consumers must adjust a number of times over a longer time period to the tax and may be politically unpopular.
- Adopting a minimum threshold[e] to better target unhealthy products may result in an increase in administrative costs due to the need to police this boundary between taxable and non-taxable products.
- Imposing health taxes at the producer/importer level minimises administrative costs, as the tax can be levied on a relatively small number of agents compared to when it would be levied at the retailer level.
- In the case of SSBs, concerns exist regarding the administrative costs of a nutrient-based tax. Applying a tax to the nutrient content within a product will result in significantly greater compliance and administrative costs than a product-based tax that can simply be applied on the total (and easily observable) quantity of the product. This can explain the relative popularity of product-based taxes on soft drinks.

[e] Where a minimum content of the relevant unhealthy content is specified, and only products with content above this threshold are subject to the tax.

2.6.4. The health tax revenue potential might be significant

Health taxes have a significant tax revenue potential that governments could use. Optimal tax policy indicates that goods that are inelastic in demand can be taxed at relatively high tax rates (following the so-called Ramsey rule). Because empirical evidence shows that the demand for unhealthy goods such as tobacco and alcohol is relatively inelastic, at least in the short run, this creates opportunities to use these taxes also for revenue-raising objectives. Governments have a wide range of taxes at their disposal in order to collect a set amount of tax revenue needed to finance public spending. In that sense, health taxes are not different from any other tax, and governments should determine an optimal tax structure of which health taxes are an integral part.

2.6.5. A wide range of non-tax factors will impact the design of a health tax

Political economy factors have to be incorporated into the design of a health tax, including the relations with industry and lobbying efforts. Large firms in a given industry can dilute the impact of fiscal policies with aggressive marketing campaigns and lobbying efforts,[29] as discussed in Chapters 4 and 12. When dialogue with the industry concerned is possible, a health tax should ideally be designed collaboratively, as this may be an effective way of inducing businesses to change their production processes towards more health-friendly products.

Addressing potential public opposition should also be considered when designing health taxes. While consumers are now well aware of the negative external effects of smoking and alcohol consumption, they might be less aware of the negative external effects of unhealthy food consumption. This might reduce their willingness to pay such a tax, which might be perceived as paternalistic. Tax design and information campaigns should therefore go hand in hand such that government can explain the reasons why the health tax is introduced. In fact, the narrative used upon the introduction of the tax may have significant behavioural effects in itself.

Another way of increasing support for a health tax may be to earmark the revenue from the tax for a specific health-related purpose, either formally (via legislation) or informally (by public political commitment) (see also Chapters 9, SF3 and 10 for a discussion on earmarking). For example, in Mexico, the revenue from the tax on soft drinks is earmarked for health expenditure. In Hungary, the revenue from the health tax goes to a health fund. The United Kingdom also earmarks the revenue raised from the tax on SSBs to fund sports activities in schools and healthy living programmes for children. A significant concern with earmarking – particularly formal earmarking – is that it reduces flexibility in government budgeting. For example, if more revenue is raised in a particular year from an earmarked tax than is necessary for the related expenditure, the excess revenue cannot be used to address budget shortfalls elsewhere. This concern may be less of an issue if revenue from the tax is earmarked broadly for healthcare expenditure where it will only ever comprise a small component of total government healthcare expenditure.[30]As the recent COVID-19 crisis has led to increased pressure on tax revenues and health financing in most countries, soft earmarking of (additional) health tax revenues for health spending could be considered, despite of the overall disadvantages of earmarking, to ensure a sufficient level of funding for the health sector. The soft earmarking might be introduced with a sunset clause in order to ensure that the provisions are re-evaluated regularly. Moreover, some degree of revenue earmarking may contribute to increased political acceptability of the tax.

Increases in prices of harmful products for health may have an impact on illicit markets and smuggling (see Chapter SF2). In developing countries where tax administration capacities are weaker, increases in health taxes rates might lead to increased smuggling and illicit trade. However, even in the presence of illicit trade, a rise in excise taxes may decrease the consumption of unhealthy goods and even raise revenues as was the case of the 2011 Brazil tobacco reform.[31] In addition, increases in health tax rates can lead to cross-border shopping (see Chapter 3).

A final issue in designing health taxes is the alignment of the tax design with international tax commitments and obligations, such as World Trade Organisation (WTO) and European Union rules. For example, the General Agreement on Tariffs and Trade prevents WTO members from introducing taxes to protect domestic production. If, for example, a health tax was imposed on food products that are predominantly imported, whereas similar domestic products do not face a similar tax then this could potentially constitute a breach to the WTO rules (see Chapter 11 for an in-depth discussion).

Key messages

- Health taxes are generally justified as a way to correct for the externalities from negative health outcomes generated by harmful products. Other tax policy reasons for implementing health taxes include time-inconsistency of preferences (a preference for short-term gratification over long-term health) and information constraints (a lack of knowledge of the underlying health implications of consumption of certain products).
- Health taxes are generally levied in the form of excise duties. Applying a content-based tax can be expected to better target the negative health effects of consumption than a product-based tax.
- Increasing health tax rates is expected to increase tax revenues as empirical evidence shows that, in many countries, the tax rates are very likely not set at their tax revenue maximising point.
- There might be substantial revenue potential from extending health taxes to other products that generate negative externalities linked to health.

Annex

Table A2.1 presents disaggregated information on health taxes at the country level that is considered in the descriptive analysis of health tax revenues. Some countries might levy other health taxes other than those listed in Table A2.1 but, as disaggregated information was not available in the database, they were not considered in the revenue analysis.

Table A2.1. Health taxes considered in the revenue analysis.

Country	Tobacco	Alcohol	Other
High-income countries			
Austria	Tobacco	Beer; wine; sparkling wine; special duty alcoholic drinks	Beverage tax
Belgium	Tobacco	Spirits; consumption tax on alcohol and spirits; beer; Intermediate alcoholic products	Fermented sparkling beverages; fermented fruit beverages; non-alcoholic beverages; coffee, sugar and syrup
Canada	Tobacco (federal and provincial taxes)	Liquor (federal taxes)	
Chile	Cigarettes and tobacco		
Czech Republic	Tobacco products	Alcohol and liquor; beer; wine	
Denmark	Cigarettes and tobacco duties; duties on cigars, cheroots and cigarillos	Duty on beer; duty on wine; duty on spirits; duty on restaurant sales of alcoholic beverages	Sales duties on chocolate and sugar; raw material duty on chocolate and sugar; special tax on chocolate and sugar; duty on ice cream; duty on coffee
Estonia	Tobacco	Alcohol	
Finland	Excise on tobacco products	Excise on medium, strong beer; tax on alcoholic beverages	Excise on sweetmeats; excise on non-alcoholic beverages; excise on certain foodstuffs; excise on margarines; excise on sugar products
France	Taxes on tobaccos and matches; fees on tobacco stores	Taxes on wines, ciders and meads; taxes on alcohol; taxes on beer and mineral water	Tax on cereals; fees on potash salt; tax on flour; surtax on appetisers; tax on beet, sugar and alcohol; tax on food fats; tax on meat; sugar market fund tax

Table A2.1. *(Continued)*

Country	Tobacco	Alcohol	Other
Germany	Duty on tobacco	Duty on alcohol; duty on beer; duty on champagne	Duty on coffee; duty on sugar; duty on tea; duty on salt; duty on beverages; duty on ice cream
Greece	Duty on tobacco products	Duty on alcohol and spirits	Duty on sugar
Hungary	Tobacco (central budget excise)	Alcohol production duty; alcohol (central budget excise)	Coffee (central budget excise)
Ireland	Tobacco	Beer; spirits; wine, cider, perry	
Israel	On domestically processed tobacco products		
Italy		Duty on spirits; duty on beer; alcohol, spirits, liquor	Duty on sugars; duty on bananas; duty on coffee; duty on cocoa; duty on olive oil; meat
Japan	Prefectural tobacco tax; municipal tobacco tax; tobacco tax; special tobacco tax	Liquor tax	Sugar excises
Korea	Tobacco sales tax (local); tobacco consumption tax (local)	Liquor tax	
Latvia	Excise duty on tobacco	Excise duty on alcoholic beverages; excise duty on beer	Excise duty on coffee and non-alcoholic beverages
Lithuania	Manufactured tobacco	Alcoholic beverages; wine and sparkling wine; beer; other alcoholic beverages	Sugar
Luxembourg	Excise duties on tobacco (part on national production); excise duties on tobacco	Tax on the consumption of national alcoholic beverages and spirits; excise duties on imported alcoholic beverages; excise duties on beers (part on national production); excise duties on nationally produced alcoholic beverages	Excise duties on fermented sparkling beverages; excise duty on sugar

(Continued)

Table A2.1. *(Continued)*

Country	Tobacco	Alcohol	Other
The Netherlands	Excise on tobacco	Excise on spirits; excise on beer; excise on wine	Excise on sugar; excise on soft drinks
New Zealand	Tobacco	On alcoholic beverages; beer; wine; spirits	Refined sugar
Norway	Stamp duty on tobacco	Taxes on spirits and wines; excise on beer	Chocolate and sweets; sugar; non-alcoholic beverages
Panama	Cigarettes	Beer; wine and liquor	Soft drinks
Poland	On domestic and imported excise products of tobacco	On domestic and imported excise products of spirits, beer, wine	
Portugal	Excise duties on tobacco	Excise duties on beer; excise duties on alcoholic beverages; excise duties on alcohol	
Seychelles	Tobacco	Alcohol (beverages spirits and vinegar)	
Singapore	Tobacco	Liquors	
Slovak Republic	On tobacco products	On alcohol and liquors; on beer; on wine	
Slovenia	Tobacco; duty-free shops – tobacco	Alcohol and alcoholic drinks; duty-free shops – alcohol and alcoholic drinks	
Spain	Tobacco	Beer; wine; alcohol	
Sweden	Tobacco tax	Tax on spirits; tax on wine; tax on beer and soft drinks	
Switzerland	Excises on tobacco	Beer tax	
Trinidad and Tobago	Cigarette products	Beer; alcohol products; malt beverages	
Turkey			Sugar consumption taxes
United Kingdom	Tobacco	Beer; wines, spirits, cider and perry	
United States	Tobacco taxes federal government; Tobacco taxes state and local government	Alcohol taxes federal government; alcohol taxes state and local government	Sugar tax federal government
Uruguay	Tobacco products	Beer	Non-alcoholic beverages
Upper-middle-income countries			
Argentina	Tobacco products	Alcoholic beverages; beers	Non-alcoholic beverages
Botswana		Alcohol levy	

Table A2.1. *(Continued)*

Country	Tobacco	Alcohol	Other
Brazil	Tobacco	Beverages	
Bulgaria	Tobacco products	Beer and other alcoholic beverages	
Colombia	Tobacco	Beer; liquors	
Costa Rica	Tobacco	Alcoholic beverages	Non-alcoholic beverages
Dominican Republic	Tobacco products	Alcoholic beverages	
Ecuador	Cigarettes	Beer	Fizzy drinks
Guatemala	Tobacco and derivatives	Beer; alcoholic beverages	Soft drinks; other beverages
Kazakhstan	Tobacco	Alcohol	
Mauritius	Tobacco products	Spirits, liquors and alcoholic beverages	Sugar content of soft drinks; sugar brokerage
Lower-middle-income countries			
Côte d'Ivoire	Ad valorem tax on tobacco; Tax on tobacco for sports development; Tax on tobacco	Tax on drinks	
Egypt	Tobacco and cigarettes		
El Salvador	Cigarettes	Beer	Soft drinks; special contributions sugar
Honduras	Cigarettes	Beer; liquors	Soft drinks
Kenya			Sugar levy
Nicaragua	Cigarettes	Beer; alcoholic beverages	Soft drinks
Philippines	Tobacco	Alcohol	
Senegal	Taxes on tobacco	Taxes on alcohols	Taxes on fats; tax on colas; tax on teas; tax on coffee
Solomon Islands	Tobacco	Beer; spirits	
Tunisia	Tobacco	Alcoholic drinks	
Low-income countries			
Burkina Faso	Tax on tobacco and matches	Drinks	Taxes on coffee, tea and cola nuts
Congo, Democratic Republic	Domestic excises and excises on imports – tobacco and matches	Domestic excises and excises on imports – beverages	

(Continued)

Table A2.1. *(Continued)*

Country	Tobacco	Alcohol	Other
Mali	Local taxes on tobacco	Taxes on alcoholic beverages	Special tax on drinks
Niger	Domestic tobacco and cigarette tax	Alcoholic beverages tax	
Uganda	Excise tax on cigarettes	Excise tax on beer; excise tax on spirits/waragi	Excise tax on soft drinks; excise tax on sugar

Source: OECD Global Revenue Statistics database.

References

1. OECD. *Revenue Statistics Interpretative Guide;* 2018a. https://www.oecd.org/tax/tax-policy/oecd-classification-taxes-interpretative-guide.pdf.
2. OECD. *Consumption Tax Trends 2018: VAT/GST and Excise Rates, Trends and Policy Issues.* Paris: OECD Publishing; 2018b.
3. OECD. *Revenue Statistics 2019.* Paris: OECD Publishing; 2019.
4. World Health Organization. *Using Price Policies to Promote Healthier Diets,* 2015, https://www.euro.who.int/__data/assets/pdf_file/0008/273662/Using-price-policies-to-promote-healthier-diets.pdf?ua=1 (accessed on 11 June 2020).
5. OECD. *The Heavy Burden of Obesity: The Economics of Prevention, OECD Health Policy Studies.* Paris: OECD Publishing; 2019.
6. Bittschi B, et al. *Price Elasticities and Implied Tax Revenue for Alcoholic Beverages Evidence from Poland, France and Spain,* 2019. http://www.wifo.ac.at/wwa/pubid/61732.
7. Nelson J. Meta-analysis of alcohol price and income elasticities – With corrections for publication bias. *Health Economics Review.* 2013; 3(1). DOI: 10.1186/2191-1991-3-17.
8. Goodchild M, Sandoval R, Belausteguigoitia I. Generating revenue by raising tobacco taxes in Latin America and the Caribbean. *Revista Panamericana de Salud Pública.* 2017; 1–7. DOI: 10.26633/rpsp.2017.151.
9. Chelwa G, Van Walbeek C. *Does Cigarette Demand Respond to Price Increases in Uganda? Price Elasticity Estimates using the Uganda National Panel Survey and Deaton's method,* BMJ Publishing Group, 2019. https://bmjopen.bmj.com/content/9/3/e026150.
10. Ahsan A. Impact of increasing tobacco tax on government revenue and tobacco consumption. 2014. DOI: 10.13140/RG.2.1.3350.2563.
11. Andreyeva T, Long M, Brownell K. The impact of food prices on consumption: A systematic review of research on the price elasticity of demand for food. *American Journal of Public Health.* 2010; 100(2): 216–222.
12. Allcott H, Lockwood B, Taubinsky D. Regressive sin taxes, with an application to the optimal soda tax. *The Quarterly Journal of Economics.* 2019; 134(3): 1557–1626.

13. Cawley J, et al. The economics of taxes on sugar-sweetened beverages: A review of the effects on prices, sales, cross-border shopping, and consumption. *Annual Review of Nutrition*. 2019; 39(1): 317–338.
14. Slemrod J, Gillitzer C. *Insights from a Tax Systems Perspective.* CESifo Economic Studies; 2014. https://academic.oup.com/cesifo/article/60/1/1/380383?login=true
15. Levell PB. *Redistribution from a Lifetime Perspective;* 2015.
16. Brys B, et al. Tax design for inclusive economic growth. *OECD Taxation Working Papers,* No. 26, OECD Publishing, Paris; 2016. DOI: 10.1787/5jlv74ggk0g7-en.
17. Sassi F, Belloni A, Capobianco C. *The Role of Fiscal Policies in Health Promotion,* OECD Health Working Papers, No. 66; 2013.
18. Marron DM. *Should We Tax Unhealthy Foods and Drinks?* Urban-Brookings Tax Policy Centre Working Paper, December; 2015.
19. Wang C, Coxson P, Shen Y, Goldman L, Bibbins-Domingo K. A Penny-Per-Ounce Tax on Sugar-Sweetened Beverages Would Cut Health and Cost Burdens of Diabetes. *Health Affairs*. 2012; 31(1): 199–207.
20. Long M, et al. Cost effectiveness of a sugar-sweetened beverage excise tax in the U.S. *American Journal of Preventive Medicine*. 2015; 49(1): 112–123.
21. Allcott H, Lockwood B, Taubinsky D. Should we tax sugar-sweetened beverages? An overview of theory and evidence. *Journal of Economic Perspectives*. 2019; 33(3): 202–227.
22. Briggs A, Mytton O, Kehlbacher A, Tiffin R, Elhussein A, Rayner MS, Jebb T. Health impact assessment of the UK soft drinks industry levy: A comparative risk assessment modelling study. *Lancet Public Health* 2017; 2: e15–e22.
23. Chaloupka F, et al. *NBER Working Paper Series. Cigarette Excise Taxation: The Impact of Tax Structure on Prices, Revenues, and Cigarette Smoking,* 2010, http://www.nber.org/papers/w16287.
24. Crawford IA. The Fat Tax. London: Institute of Fiscal Studies; 2004.
25. OECD/KIPF. *The Distributional Effects of Consumption Taxes in OECD Countries,* OECD Tax Policy Studies, No. 22, OECD Publishing, Paris; 2014. DOI: 10.1787/9789264224520-en.
26. Gruber J, Koszegi B. Tax incidence when individuals are time-inconsistent: The case of cigarette excise taxes. *Journal of Public Economics*. 2004; 88(9–10): 1959–1987.
27. Fuchs A, González Icaza F, Paz D. *Distributional Effects of Tobacco Taxation: A Comparative Analysis;* 2019.
28. Mytton OD. Taxing unhealthy food and drinks to improve health. *British Medical Journal,* 2012; 344.
29. Jeff C, Sarah H. *Structure and Tactics of the Tobacco, Alcohol, and Sugary Beverage Industries.* Edinburgh: University of Edinburgh; 2019.
30. Heady C. *The Effect of Ageing on the Financing of Social Health Provision,* OECD, Fiscal Sustainability of Health Systems; 2015.
31. Iglesias R. Increasing excise taxes in the presence of ilegal cigarette market: The 2011 Brazil tobacco reform. *Rev Panam Salud Publica*. 2016; 40(4): 243–249.

https://doi.org/10.1142/9781800612396_0003

Chapter 3

Protecting and Promoting Health Through Taxation: Evidence and Gaps

Lisa M Powell* **and Frank J Chaloupka***

We provide evidence of the extent to which health taxes on tobacco, alcoholic beverages, sugar-sweetened beverages (SSBs) and other food and nutrients reduce demand for these products. We open with a conceptual framework that outlines the mechanisms through which health taxes impact consumption and health outcomes, and how substitution and tax avoidance behaviours may affect the net impact of the taxes. We then review empirical evidence on the tax responsiveness of demand based on estimates from both demand models and tax evaluations, showing that higher prices/taxes on products are associated with lower quantity demanded for taxed products. We also evaluate the differential impacts of the health taxes by demographic and socio-economic status (SES), finding that demand for tobacco and sugary beverages is more price sensitive among lower SES populations. Next, we examine the extent to which health taxes may induce substitution to other products and the extent that consumers may undertake explicit tax avoidance behaviours such as cross-border shopping, as these affect the net impact of a given tax. Finally, we review the evidence on the impact of health taxes on health outcomes – i.e., if the taxes translate into improvements in health and reductions in other

* University of Illinois Chicago, USA.

consumption-related risks. We find that while higher tobacco and alcohol prices/taxes are associated with advantageously reduced health and social outcomes (i.e., lowered levels of tobacco-related cancer and respiratory disease and lowered levels of alcohol-related liver cirrhosis, accidents and violent acts), there is less evidence on the effectiveness of taxes on SSBs and other foods on health outcomes. Overall, the evidence shows that health taxes are effective fiscal measures for reducing the harmful consumption of products such as tobacco, alcohol and SSBs and are an important tool that policymakers can implement to achieve goals of reducing the burden of non-communicable diseases and other consumption-related adverse outcomes.

Health taxes are used to promote health and raise revenue. The focus of this chapter is on providing evidence on the goal of health promotion. In this regard, as part of a public health strategy to promote health, health taxes are used as a fiscal policy instrument aimed at reducing individuals' harmful consumption of products such as tobacco, alcohol and sugar-sweetened beverages (SSBs) with the ultimate goal of reducing adverse health and other outcomes linked to the consumption of such products.[1,2] Figure 3.1 depicts the conceptual framework through which health taxes ultimately are expected to impact consumption and health. As discussed in the introduction of this book, the rationale for a health tax is to correct individuals' harmful levels of consumption of certain products, given that these products' prices do not account for their external costs.

The idea is that the fiscal policy instrument of taxation changes relative prices of taxed versus untaxed products which, in turn, impacts behavior related to consumption. The key mechanism through which this occurs is that taxes generally result in higher prices for consumers, known as tax pass-through (see Chapter 4 of this book for a discussion related to factors affecting tax pass-through). According to the law of demand for normal goods, an increase in the price of a given product, all else constant, will reduce the quantity demanded of that product. How large or small the reduction depends on the price elasticity of demand (the percentage change in the quantity demanded resulting from a 1% increase in price). Price elasticity is a function of various factors, including consumer preferences and whether the good is a necessity or a luxury item, how much of a consumer's income is spent on that good and the availability of substitutes. For example, if a consumer has a strong preference for a good or it is a necessity for them then they will tend to be relatively less price responsive; if they spend a large proportion to their income on the product then price matters more to them and they will tend to be more price responsive; and, if there are many non-taxed substitutes available then they will also be more price responsive as they can easily satisfy their demand by substituting to similar non-taxed products. For many years, conventional wisdom held that the demand for addictive products was unresponsive to changes in price. Advances in economic theory and empirical evidence show that this is not necessarily the case, with demand for addictive products somewhat responsive to price in the short run, and more responsive to price in the long run.[3]

Over the past few decades, extensive evidence has accumulated on the impact of prices and taxes on the demand for tobacco products and alcoholic beverages, and, in recent years, similar evidence has emerged on the demand for SSBs. Much of the early evidence on tobacco and alcohol demand came from high-income countries (HICs). Although there has been considerable research on the demand for tobacco products in low- to middle-income countries (LMICs) over the past 15–20 years, similar evidence on alcohol demand is limited. A number of demand models have been estimated for SSBs, mostly based on data from HICs. However, more recently, there is an emerging literature on the impact of SSB taxes on sales/purchases/consumption for both LMICs and HICs.

To fully understand the underpinnings of the net impact on consumption and ultimately health outcomes, as depicted in Figure 3.1, it is also important to understand the extent to which taxes may induce substitution within types of the taxed products (e.g. to cheaper brands) or products taxed at relatively low rates and to non-taxed products (some of which may also be harmful to health) and the extent that consumers may undertake explicit tax avoidance behaviours such as cross-border shopping as these can change the net impact of a given tax. That is, substitution and tax avoidance behaviours influence consumption of taxed and untaxed products and may to some extent offset improvements in health and other outcomes.

Fig. 3.1. Impact of health taxes on consumption and health outcomes.

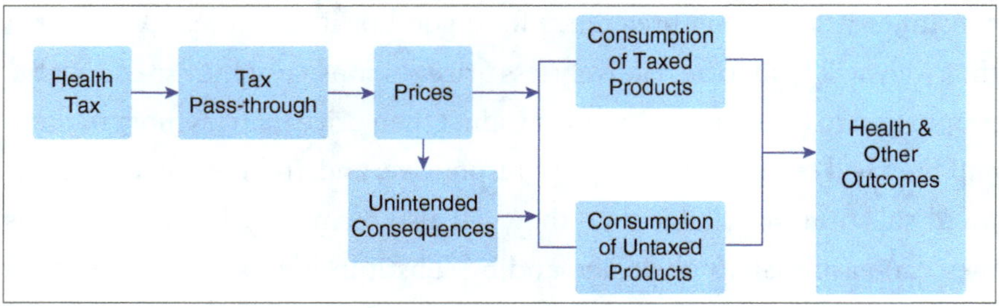

In this chapter, we review evidence on the price and tax responsiveness of the demand for tobacco, alcohol and SSB products and the extent to which such responsiveness varies by demographic and socio-economic characteristics. In terms of assessing health taxes on foods and beverages, we focus our review on SSBs but supplement it with some examples of taxes on other selected food products and nutrients. Next, we assess unintended consequences including the impact of changes in prices on substitution within taxed products and to non-taxed products and unintended tax avoidance behaviours such as cross-border shopping outside of the taxing jurisdiction. Finally, we review available evidence on the extent to which prices/taxes are associated with consumption-related health and other well-being outcomes.

It should be noted that this chapter itself is not a formal systematic review of the evidence; rather, we summarise the evidence based on existing reviews and meta-analyses and we draw on selected papers to provide country-specific examples. There are hundreds of studies on the impact of prices and taxes on demand for tobacco, alcohol and SSBs. These studies are based on a variety of data, including aggregate time-series data for a single jurisdiction, pooled cross-sectional time-series data from multiple jurisdictions (e.g. US states, countries in a given region or at the same income level) and individual-level survey data (including data from repeated cross-sectional surveys and from longitudinal surveys). Similarly, these studies apply a wide variety of econometric and other statistical methods, as well as alternative underlying theoretical and conceptual approaches. While all data, methods and approaches have limitations, the general consistency of the findings from these studies – that higher taxes/prices will lead to reductions in demand for the products and the consequences of consumption – is striking.

3.1. Evidence of impact of prices and taxes on consumption/sales

Numerous studies have estimated the impact of taxes and prices on the consumption or volume sold of various targeted products. Some studies use direct measures of consumption or various aspects of behaviour, including prevalence, frequency of use, intensity of use and cessation, using self-reported individual-level survey data. Other studies use direct measures of volume sold or purchases based on store-level scanner data or household scanner or expenditure survey data. Others use some proxy for consumption, such as tax-paid sales or total production plus imports less exports.

3.1.1. Evidence for tobacco products

An extensive body of research, including for countries at all income levels, has estimated the impact of prices and taxes on the demand for tobacco products.[4,5] Most of this research focuses on the demand for manufactured cigarettes, given that these account for the vast majority of tobacco consumption, but similar evidence exists on the demand for other tobacco products, such as bidis, cigars, pipe tobacco, smokeless tobacco, and, more recently, electronic cigarettes.

Estimates of the price elasticity of cigarette demand from numerous studies from HICs generally fall in the range from −0.25 to −0.5, implying that a 10% increase in price will reduce overall cigarette consumption by between 2.5% and 5%.[5] Estimates from LMICs are more variable, mostly falling in the range from −0.2 to −0.8, indicating that a 10% increase in price will reduce consumption by 2–8%.[4,5] Figure 3.2 illustrates this based on recent experiences in Brazil, where cigarette taxes and prices were increased significantly since 2000.

Fig. 3.2. Per capita cigarette sales and cigarette prices in Brazil, inflation adjusted, 2003–2013.

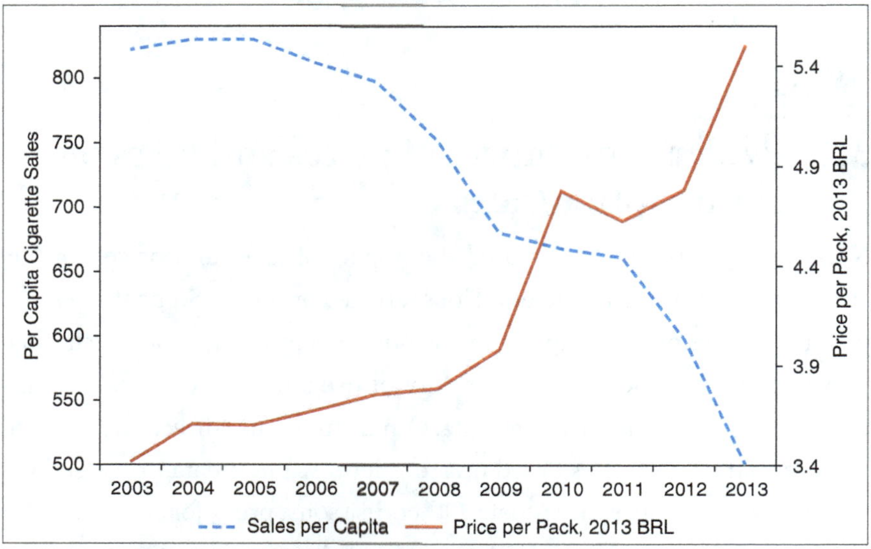

Source: Ministry of Health, Brazil; EIU; World Bank; and authors' calculations.

The wider range of elasticity of demand estimates in LMICs results from a variety of factors, including lower incomes, complex tobacco tax structures, trends in cigarette affordability, the availability of other tobacco products and the extent of illicit cigarette trade.[4]

More limited evidence for other tobacco products generally finds estimates of price elasticity greater than those for cigarette demand.[6] One recent study from Bangladesh, for example, found that a 10% increase in prices would reduce bidi smoking by just over 10%, while reducing smokeless tobacco consumption by almost 4%.[7] Emerging evidence for new nicotine products, such as e-cigarettes, suggests that the demand for these products is more responsive to price than demand for cigarettes.[8,9]

In general, estimates indicate that price responsiveness of tobacco use is greater among youth and falls with age, with smoking initiation, particularly initiation of daily or regular smoking, highly responsive to price.[4,5] With respect to cessation, it is estimated for the United States that a 10% price increase induces almost 2% of smokers to quit smoking.[4]

Estimates based on survey data indicate that roughly half of the impact of price on tobacco use comes through changes in prevalence, mostly the result of current users quitting, with the other half the result of continuing users reducing their consumption.[4,5] Tobacco use is a highly addictive behaviour and economic models of addiction imply that the effects of price will grow over time. Estimates indicate that the long-run effect of price is about double the short-run impact.[4,5]

Numerous studies have assessed the impact of tax and price changes on tobacco use. One study, for example, found that the largely tax-induced cigarette price increases in Brazil accounted for 46% of the decline in adult smoking prevalence, which was halved from 1989 to 2010.[10] The 2018 World Bank report *Tobacco Tax Reform at the Crossroads of Health and Development* includes multiple case studies from a wide range of countries illustrating the success of significant tobacco tax increases in reducing tobacco use, including in the Philippines, Ukraine, Colombia, South Africa and France.[11]

3.1.2. Evidence for alcoholic beverages

Similar evidence exists on the impact of taxes and prices on the demand for alcoholic beverages. Research from HICs has produced generally consistent findings about the impact of taxes and prices on overall demand for alcoholic beverages (beer, wine and spirits).[12,13] Systematic reviews and/or meta-analyses find that estimates of the overall price elasticity for alcohol from HIC studies are in the range from −0.51 to −0.77.[14,15] In general, estimates show that the demand for spirits is most responsive to price, while demand for beer is least responsive.[14–17] For example, one comprehensive review of estimates from HICs found that a 10% price increase would reduce beer consumption by between 1.7% and 4.6%, wine consumption by between 3.0% and 6.9% and spirits consumption by between 2.9% and 8.0%.[14] One systematic review and meta-analysis of the limited research from LMICs concluded that the price elasticity of alcohol demand in LMICs is similar to that found in studies from HICs with the available estimates producing an average elasticity of −0.64.[16]

Many studies from HICs use survey data to examine the impact of taxes and prices on different aspects of drinking behaviour, such as the frequency and intensity of drinking and drinking prevalence.[14,15] In general, these studies find that all aspects of drinking are responsive to changes in the prices of alcoholic beverages, including various measures of excessive drinking, such as binge drinking.[14,15] Some studies have also found that price responsiveness differs based on how much drinkers consume, with light and moderate drinkers more responsive to price than heavy drinkers.[14,18]

A number of studies have assessed the impact of tax increases or decreases on alcohol use. For example, a recent evaluation of the increase in the sales tax on alcoholic beverages from 6% to 9% in the US state of Maryland found that overall alcohol sales were 3.8% lower than they would have been in the absence of the tax increase.[19] Another study from Switzerland found that the significant reduction in import duties on distilled spirits, which led to a drop in imported spirits' prices of between 30% and 50%, led to a 30% increase in spirits consumption in the 3 months after the change.[20]

3.1.3. Evidence for SSBs and selected other foods and nutrients

Studies on the impact of prices on the demand for sweetened beverages (e.g. carbonated beverages, fruit drinks, sports drinks, ready-to-drink teas and coffees, energy drinks and flavored waters including both SSBs and non-sugar sweetened beverages [NSSBs]) find that the elasticity is around −0.8, based largely on evidence from HICs.[21] Studies that focus on SSB demand only find that demand is more responsive to price, with the elasticity around −1.2, with the greater elasticity reflecting the opportunity to substitute from SSBs to other NSSBs in response to an increase in sugary drink prices.[22,23] Recent studies of SSB demand from LMICs produce similar or greater elasticity estimates. For example, recent studies from LMICs in the region of the Americas for Brazil, Mexico, Ecuador, Chile and Guatemala estimated price elasticities of SSB demand of −0.85, −1.06, −1.20, −1.37

and −1.39, respectively.[24–28] Similarly, a recent study from South Africa estimated elasticities of −1.18 and −1.17 for carbonated soft drinks and fruit juice concentrates, respectively.[29] A study from India estimated a price elasticity of SSB consumption of −0.94 which is slightly lower than the −1.2 SSB estimate.[30] Evidence from demand models for other selected foods that are considered high in nutrients recommended to limit (i.e. high in sugars, saturated fats and sodium) have generally been found to be price inelastic (i.e. price elasticity in absolute value < 1). For example, a comprehensive review provides the following mean prices elasticities: sweets/sugars (−0.34); fats/oils (−0.48); and, food away from home (−0.81).[21]

Based on a recent systematic review, a meta-analysis found that a 10% increase in an SSB tax is associated with a 10% decline in SSB purchases and dietary intake, corresponding to a tax elasticity of demand of −1.0.[31] Indeed, as SSB taxes have increasingly been implemented worldwide over the last decade, a number of evaluations have been undertaken to assess the impact of these taxes on sales, purchases and consumption of taxed beverages. A substantial body of evidence has been produced assessing the impact of Mexico's 1 peso per litre SSB tax, the first of the recent SSB taxes to be implemented based on a public health rationale. Evaluations of this tax found declines of approximately 6–8% in sales and purchases of the taxed beverages and the evidence shows that this impact was sustained two years post-tax implementation.[32–34] A recent evaluation of the 10% ad valorem SSB excise tax in Barbados found a 4.3% reduction in SSB sales volume.[35] Evaluations of Chile's 2014 tiered beverage tax structure that increased the tax rate from 13% to 18% on high-SSBs and lowered it 13% to 10% on low-sugar sweetened beverages (including NSSBs), found reductions in purchases of high-sugar sweetened beverages with either no change or an increase in purchases for low-sugar sweetened beverages.[36,37] Both the Barbados and Chile taxes are ad valorem (based on a percentage of price) rather than specific (based on the unit of the product) excise taxes, and as noted in Chapter 8, when comparing the impact of statutory rates for ad valorem excise taxes, one must consider where they are applied in the value chain. For example, in Barbados, the ad valorem excise tax is applied to the producer price, which is a lower base value, whereas in Chile, the ad valorem excise taxes are applied to the retail price excluding VAT. Therefore, even in cases where statutory ad valorem excise tax rates may be the same across countries, if they are applied at different points in the value distribution chain, their effective impact on prices (and, hence demand) may be different.

The 2012 increase in the Danish SSB tax and the subsequent 2014 repeal of the tax were associated, respectively, with significant decreases and then increases in household purchases of taxed beverages with similar levels of response estimated for the tax increase and decrease equivalent to a price elasticity of −1.3.[38] Evidence from an evaluation of the 2012 French sweetened beverage tax on purchases finds that the tax was associated with a reduction in soft drink purchases for heavy consumers but not for consumers generally; however, this is not surprising given the low tax rate which only raised prices by about 5%.[39] Following public health calls for industry to reduce sugar content in food and beverages along with the 2016 announcement of the introduction of the 2018 UK tiered soft drink industry levy (SDIL) tax (24 pence/L for beverages with >8 g sugars per 100 mL and 18 pence/L for beverages with 5–8 g/L), a recent study found that between 2015 and 2018, sales of soft drinks in the top sugars tier (>8g/L) fell by 41%, sales in the mid-sugars tier (5–8 g/L) fell by 73% and sales in the low-sugars tier (0.1–4.9 g/L) increased by 41%; and, the net reduction in the volume sold of sugars per day from soft drinks was 4.6 g per capita per day (equivalent to a 30% reduction).[40]

In the United States, evidence from the 1-cent per ounce tax in Berkeley, CA, the first of the recent local jurisdictions to impose SSB excise taxes, found that SSB consumption fell 21% compared to a 4% increase in comparison cities, while relative water consumption increased 63% compared to 19% in the same comparison cities.[41] Another study found that Berkeley supermarket volume sold of taxed beverages fell 9.6% compared to an increase of 6.9% in non-Berkeley stores and that sales of untaxed beverages rose 3.5% in Berkeley versus 0.5% in non-Berkeley stores; but found no significant changes in SSB intake when using individual-level data.[42] Yet another Berkeley study, based on individual-level data three years post-tax, found that SSB consumption fell by 0.55 times per day while water consumption increased by 0.85 times per day – both relative to changes in comparison cities.[43] A study for Oakland's penny per ounce SSB tax found no statistically significant effects for either purchases (except for soda) or consumption of taxed SSBs.[44] A study of the Seattle, Washington, 1.75-cent per ounce SSB tax found that in the first year post-tax implementation volume sold of taxed SSBs fell by 22% and there was no evidence of this impact being offset by cross-border shopping.[45] Two US local jurisdictions imposed excise taxes that applied to both SSB and NSSBs. Regarding the 1.5-cent per ounce tax on SSBs and NSSBs implemented in Philadelphia, Pennsylvania, a study based on repeated cross-sectional random-digit-dial phone surveys found a reduction in the odds of daily regular soda (−40%) and energy drink (−64%) consumption as well as an increase in daily bottled water consumption (+58%).[46] Using store scanner data, a recent Philadelphia study found a 51% reduction in volume of taxed beverages in the taxed jurisdiction with a net decrease of 38% when accounting for cross-border shopping.[47] A study of the Cook County, Illinois, 1-cent per ounce tax on SSBs and NSSBs (repealed after 4 months) found a 27% reduction in sales volume of taxed beverages with a net reduction of 21% after accounting for increased sales volume in Cook County's 2-mile border area.[48]

There is also some limited evidence available from evaluations of taxes that have focused on other food categories or nutrients. For example, an evaluation of the impact of the 2011 Danish tax on saturated fat on the purchases of food product categories such as butter, butter blends, margarine and oils found that the tax was associated with a decrease in purchases in the range of 10–15%.[49] Several studies have evaluated the impact of Mexico's 8% tax on non-essential energy-dense foods and have found that household purchases of taxed foods were 4.8–5.1% lower 1-year following the implementation of the tax and that this impact was slightly larger 2 years post-tax (−7.4% at 2 years' post-tax).[50,51]

3.2. Evidence of differential impacts on demand

Many studies of tobacco use based on survey data have assessed the differential effects of taxes and prices on different population subgroups, including those defined by age, gender and socio-economic status (SES). In contrast, relatively fewer studies have done this for alcohol and SSB demand.

3.2.1. Differential impacts for tobacco products

Studies generally find that younger and/or lower SES groups are relatively more responsive to price.[4,5] Estimates of price elasticity for youth smoking prevalence from LMICs and HICs, for example, tend to be two to three times greater than those for adults, while a few studies from HICs estimate that a 10% price increase would reduce youth smoking initiation by 4% or more (the average impact across ages), with larger reductions in the transition from experimental smoking to regular smoking.[4,5] One recent study from Chile similarly found that a 10% increase in price reduced the likelihood of smoking initiation by 4%.[52] Also, studies find greater price effects on cessation among young smokers. Most studies assessing differences by SES find that high-SES populations are largely unresponsive to cigarette prices, while low-SES population are highly responsive.[4,5] Consistent with this, studies that have assessed differences by educational attainment generally find that more educated populations are less sensitive to price than less-educated populations.[5] In contrast, no consistent patterns are seen in the relatively few studies that have assessed gender differences in price responsiveness of tobacco use.[53] Finally, little evidence exists about differences in price responsiveness by smoking intensity; one study from the United States found that heavier smokers reduced consumption by more than lighter smokers when cigarette prices increased.[54]

3.2.2. Differential impacts for alcoholic beverages

Several studies have explored differences in elasticities by age and gender, producing some evidence that drinking and excessive drinking among young men are more responsive to price than drinking among older men and among women.[15] However, there does not appear to be a consistent pattern on the extent of price responsiveness among young consumers, particularly across drinking intensity levels.[2] In contrast to the evidence for tobacco, estimates of price elasticities for alcoholic beverages appear similar across countries of different income levels, while there is some limited evidence that within a given country, drinking in lower SES populations is more responsive to price than drinking in higher income populations.[55]

3.2.3. Differential impacts for SSBs and selected other foods and nutrients

Findings from several studies indicate that SSB demand among lower income populations responds more to price than demand among higher income populations.[56–58] A tax evaluation from Mexico found that lower SES households responded more to the SSB tax than higher SES households.[32,59] In terms of differences by consumption level, another evaluation of the Mexico SSB tax found differences based on household purchase levels, with larger reductions (16.1–20.0%) among households that initially had higher purchases of taxed beverages compared to slight increases (0.6–1.9%) among households who initially had lower purchases of taxed beverages.[60] Additionally, this same study found that the reduction in purchases among the high purchasers of taxed beverages was greater for those who were low SES.[60]

An evaluation of Mexico's tax on non-essential energy-dense foods found that the decline in purchases of taxed foods was greater for low-SES (−10.2%) and middle-SES (−5.8%) households, whereas purchases were unchanged among high-SES households.[50]

A meta-analysis of food price elasticities globally found that changes in prices have the greatest impact on demand in low-income countries: for example, the estimated elasticity of demand for low-income country, middle-income country and HIC, respectively, was −0.74, −0.68 and −0.56 for sweets and −0.60, −0.54 and −0.42 for fats and oils.[61]

3.3. Evidence on substitution and tax avoidance

It is important to understand the extent to which taxes may induce substitution and toward which types of products and the extent that consumers may undertake explicit tax avoidance behaviours as these can change the net impact of a given tax. That is, substitution and tax avoidance behaviours will to some extent offset the purpose of the tax.

Consumers will substitute away from taxed products towards untaxed products as a result of the change in relative prices introduced by the tax. If the tax base of the product category being taxed captures the full range of targeted products then substitution from say taxed SSBs to untaxed water or milk would not be an unintended consequence and, hence, would not offset the health aim of the tax. But if a tax was placed, for example, on beer and not wine and as a result some substitution occurred to wine then this would offset the intended outcome of reducing alcohol intake. Similar unintended consequences can exist if, for example, only cigarettes, but not other forms of tobacco products are taxed. Additionally, there may be cross-price/tax substitution to products outside of the taxed product category that may be an unintended consequence. For example, a tax on SSBs may induce substitution to more sweets if the consumer is looking to obtain sugar in another form. Tax avoidance may also take the form of substitution within taxed product categories. For example, in the presence of an ad valorem excise tax, to minimise the impact of a tax, consumers may substitute down to cheaper brands or cheaper (per volume) package sizes of taxed products.

Additionally, in the cases of local-level taxes, or national taxes in places without hard borders, consumer proximity to the border of an untaxed jurisdiction will allow for relatively easy tax avoidance in the form of cross-border shopping, which may dampen the net impact on consumption of a given tax. Additionally, although not discussed below as part of cross-border shopping, it should be noted that tax pass-through (the extent to which taxes raise consumer prices) within local tax jurisdictions may be lower in retail outlets located closer to an untaxed border area which, for example, has recently been found in a study for SSB tax pass-through.[62]

Finally, firms in the taxed industry and their allies often argue that new or higher taxes will result in extensive tax evasion, including unrecorded manufacturing, large-scale smuggling of untaxed products, purchases from low-tax jurisdictions for resale in higher tax jurisdictions, sale of counterfeit products and other activities. Evidence for cigarettes shows that other factors, such as high levels of corruption, ineffective customs and tax administration and weak governance are as or more important than tax and price differentials in explaining tax evasion.[5] Issues related to illicit trade and enforcement mechanisms are addressed comprehensively in Chapter 9 of this book.

3.3.1. Evidence for tobacco products

Most studies of demand for multiple tobacco products find evidence of substitution among products in response to changes in relative prices, particularly among more 'like' products (e.g. roll-your-own tobacco, little cigars and cigarettes), while increases in income lead users to 'trade up' to products they perceive as higher quality (e.g. switching from local cigarette brands to international brands or switching from bidis to manufactured cigarettes).[6] In Lebanon, for example, increases in cigarette prices relative to water pipe tobacco prices led some cigarette smokers to switch to water pipe.[63] One recent study based on US sales data found that cigarettes were substitutes for a variety of other combustible tobacco products, including roll-your-own tobacco, little cigars and cigarillos, as well as for e-cigarettes.[64]

Several cigarette demand studies based on tax-paid sales data from US states have included measures of the incentives for cross-border activity, reflecting a mix of both individual smokers crossing state lines to purchase cigarettes in nearby lower tax states, as well as more organised larger scale purchases of cigarettes in lower tax states for resale in higher tax states.[65,66] Others have used a similar approach to capture cross-border activity in the European Union.[67] These studies generally find that the greater the difference in prices across borders, the larger the extent of cross-border activity. Additionally, some tobacco use surveys that include questions about purchase behaviours report that the likelihood of cross-border purchases rises as respondents are nearer borders with lower prices and as the price differences across borders are larger.[68,69]

3.3.2. Evidence for alcoholic beverages

A limited literature from HICs has assessed the substitutability of alcoholic beverages, generally finding consistent evidence of substitution between alcoholic beverages in the same category, but more mixed evidence of substitution across categories. One comprehensive study from Australia, for example, found relatively consistent evidence of substitution among different varieties of beer (premium, full strength, mid strength and low alcohol), as well as between red and white wines and light and dark spirits, but found less consistent evidence of substitution across beverage categories.[70] Similarly, one US study produced inconsistent and mostly statistically insignificant estimates for the effects of wine and spirits prices on beer consumption, suggesting little cross-category substitution.[71]

Similarly, albeit fewer, studies have assessed cross-border shopping for alcohol beverages. One study based on US state-level tax-paid alcoholic beverage sales, for example, concluded that cross-border shopping accounted for between 20% and 40% of the price elasticity of distilled spirits sales.[72] Another study based on sales data from Swedish municipalities concluded that there was considerable cross-border price elasticity and that this elasticity increased as municipalities were closer to the border.[73] Concerns about cross-border shopping led Denmark, Finland and Sweden to lower alcoholic beverage taxes when they joined the European Union.[74]

3.3.3. Evidence for SSBs and selected other foods and nutrients

There is generally consistent evidence of substitution among different types of non-alcoholic beverages in response to changes in relative prices, such as substituting to bottled water and milk in response to higher SSB prices.[75] Indeed, several tax evaluations have found increases in sales/purchases/consumption of untaxed beverages, particularly bottled water, following the introduction of SSB taxes.[32,35,41,45] For example, a recent evaluation of the 10% ad valorem SSB excise tax in Barbados found a 5.2% increase in sales volume for untaxed beverages.[35] However, recent evaluations of the Cook County, IL, and Philadelphia, PA, sweetened beverage taxes found no significant increases in volume sold of untaxed beverages.[47,48] A recent meta-analysis of SSB taxes found mixed results on substitution with significant increases in untaxed beverage consumption in three of four jurisdictions assessed but no significant change in one of the jurisdictions (Chile).[31] It should be noted that most of the recently implemented SSB taxes even with health goals provide exemptions to 100% fruit juice which contain free sugars and to milk products including those with added sugars such as flavoured milk and thereby can lead to substitution to untaxed products containing sugars, which may offset the intended health benefits of the tax.

A few modelling studies have estimated substitution between beverages and other sources of calories, concluding that increases in beverage prices can lead to some substitution to various foods, partially offsetting the reductions in added sugar and/or caloric intake from reduced consumption of the higher priced beverages.[76,77]

Tax evaluations to date have generally used data that are aggregated by beverage category and while scanner data have distinguished formats, individual-level consumption data have not, and hence we do not have a clear understanding on the extent to which consumers may be brand switching to lower cost brands or switching to different formats. Further, tax evaluations on the extent to which consumers may be substituting to other forms of 'sugars' such as purchasing more sweets or other vices such as salty snacks or alcohol are lacking. Substitution to other forms of discretionary (foods and beverages not necessary for the provision of nutrients) calories may offset the intended health benefits of SSB taxes and evaluations are needed to understand these tax avoidance behaviors and potential unintended consequences.

Several evaluations of the local-level sweetened beverage taxes in the United States have examined the extent of cross-border shopping associated with those taxes. A study of the Philadelphia, PA, tax found that cross-border shopping in the neighbouring zip codes offset the decrease in volume sold of taxed beverages in Philadelphia by 24%.[47] Similarly, a study of the Cook County, IL, sweetened beverage tax found significant cross-border shopping in the 2-mile border area of Cook County which offset the reduction in volume sold of taxed beverages by 22%.[48] However, unlike the local taxes in Philadelphia and Cook County, a recent study of the local SSB tax in Seattle found no significant change in volume sold of taxed beverages in the 2-mile border area.[45] These mixed results suggest when cross-border shopping does occur it somewhat offsets the tax impact but does not fully wipe it out and that geographic context and the proximity with which the population lives to the borders are important considerations for whether in fact it will occur and by how much.

At the national level, it has been reported that the Danish SSB tax was associated with Danish-German cross-border shopping (with a reported estimate of 23% of soft Danish drink purchases) and, in turn, was a significant concern related to the repeal of that tax.[78]

3.4. Evidence on health and other consumption-related outcomes

It is important to understand the extent to which taxes that are intended to change health behaviors actually translate into improvements in health and reductions in other consumption-related risks. For example, do tobacco taxes reduce lung cancer? Do taxes on alcohol reduce cirrhosis of the liver, drinking and driving, alcohol-related violence incidents? Do SSB taxes reduce the prevalence of type 2 diabetes and obesity?

3.4.1. Evidence for tobacco products

Evidence shows increases in cigarette taxes and prices are associated with reductions in the diseases and premature deaths caused by smoking. One US study, for example, found that higher state cigarette taxes reduced overall mortality at the state level, as well as deaths from throat, lung and other cancers and respiratory diseases.[79] Another recent US study using county-level data concluded that higher cigarette taxes would increase life expectancy, with a one-dollar tax increase raising life expectancy by one year.[80] Other studies find that higher cigarette taxes lower hospitalisations for heart failure and reduce the severity of childhood asthma.[81,82] Estimates show that smoking among pregnant women is particularly responsive to price, with prevalence elasticities two to three times greater than for adults.[83] As a result, higher taxes and prices reduce low-birthweight births, sudden infant death syndrome and overall infant mortality.[84,85] One recent study using country-level data from the EU estimated that a one euro increase in the price of a pack of cigarettes was associated with a drop of 0.23 deaths per 1,000 live births in the same year, and an additional drop of 0.16 deaths per 1,000 live births in the following year.[86] The positive impact of cigarette taxes and price on health is illustrated in Figure 3.3, showing that the increases in the French cigarette tax in the 1990s and early 2000s were associated with immediate reductions in cigarette consumption, followed soon after by reductions in lung cancer deaths among young men.[87]

3.4.2. Evidence for alcoholic beverages

More consistent evidence for the impact of taxes and prices on excessive drinking comes from the relatively large evidence base, again limited almost entirely to studies from HICs, on various harms from excessive drinking. Researchers have studied a variety of outcomes, including motor vehicle crashes and fatalities; deaths from liver cirrhosis, alcohol dependence and various other diseases caused by excessive drinking; incidence of sexually

Fig. 3.3. Smoking, tax and male lung cancer, France, 1980–2010.

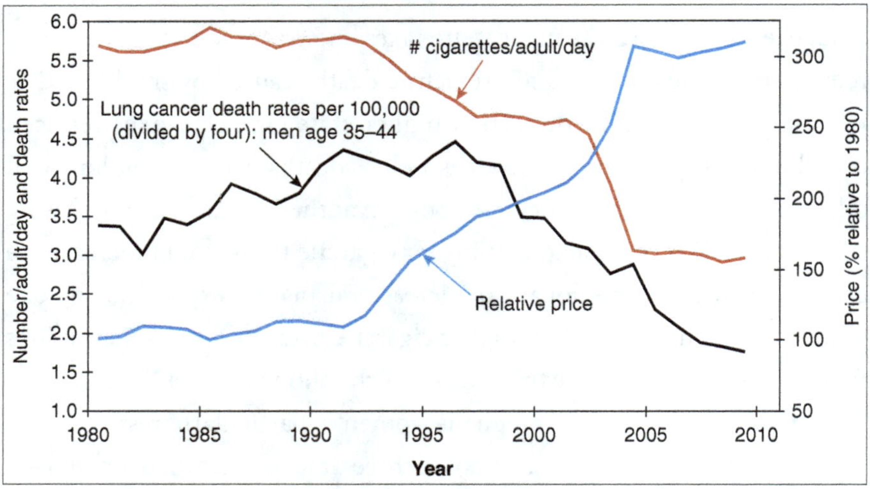

Source: Jha P. Death and taxes: Epidemiological and economic evidence on smoking. *Global Heart*. 2012; 7(2): 139–142.

transmitted diseases; crime and violence, including homicides, rape, robbery, child abuse and spousal abuse; and, workplace accidents. A number of comprehensive reviews of the evidence on the impact of alcohol consumption on these adverse outcomes demonstrate generally consistent evidence that higher taxes and prices lead to reductions in the consequences of excessive drinking.[14–16] Another review of 50 studies examining the impact of taxes and prices on various harms caused by alcohol, concluded that the tax elasticity for all alcohol-related disease and injury outcomes was −0.35.[88] The authors further estimated that a doubling of alcohol taxes would reduce fatalities from traffic crashes by 11%, sexually transmitted diseases by 6% and violence by 2%.

3.4.3. Evidence for SSBs and selected other foods and nutrients

Evidence has yet to emerge based on evaluations that directly assess the impact of recent SSB taxes on health outcomes. Limited evidence exists on the impact of prices or sales taxes of carbonated beverages (i.e. soda). For example, a longitudinal study that examined carbonated beverage prices found that higher prices were related to lower body mass index (BMI) among

US children in kindergarten through eighth grade.[89] Based on US sales tax data, mixed evidence exists on the association of state-level sales taxes and body weight outcomes among adolescents and adults; however, these were relatively small sales taxes.[22]

A number of recent simulation studies have provided evidence on the expected impact of SSB taxes on health outcomes and have found associations with reduced health risks related to type 2 diabetes,[30,90–93] dental carries,[94,95] cardiovascular disease[93,94] and obesity.[30,91,94,96,97] For example, one recent study assessed the expected impact of the SSB tax in Mexico on diabetes and obesity based on changes in volume in SSB consumption associated with the tax and estimated that 10 years post-tax implementation body weight would fall, on average by 0.15 kg/m^2 per person, equivalent to a 2.54% reduction in the prevalence of obesity and that by 2030 there would be 86,000–134,000 fewer cases of diabetes.[91]

A number of studies have examined the association between 'fast-food' prices and body weight outcomes in the United States among both adults and children. A review[22] of this literature reveals that, for adults, the results generally found no associations. However, one study found that among lower income (proxied by food assistance eligibility) adults higher fast-food prices were significantly associated with lower BMI. Similarly, while there were no significant associations found for younger children generally, higher fast-food prices were found to be statistically significantly associated with lower BMI among low-SES children. For adolescents, however, there was consistent evidence that higher fast-food prices were significantly associated with lower weight outcomes, particularly among those who were low to middle SES and among those adolescents who were in the upper tail of the BMI distribution.

3.5. Conclusion

Health taxes are intended to reduce the consumption of products that are associated with health risks and other adverse outcomes. Governments worldwide have a long history of using tobacco and alcohol taxes and are increasingly using taxes on SSBs and other selected foods and nutrients as policy tools for the prevention of non-communicable diseases. This chapter provided evidence from both demand models and tax evaluations that showed that higher prices and taxes on products such as tobacco, alcoholic beverages, SSBs and other selected foods are associated with lower demand. The evidence for tobacco and alcohol, along with other selected foods, reveals that demand is price responsive but generally inelastic (price elasticity less than 1), whereas the demand for SSBs is, on average, more price responsive (price elasticity equal to or greater than 1). However, with regard to the demand for tobacco, it should be noted that there is limited evidence for emerging products such as electronic cigarettes and no evidence to date for heated tobacco products. For tobacco, SSBs and other selected foods, the evidence suggests that lower income populations are relatively more price sensitive compared to their higher income counterparts, whereas for alcohol there does not appear to be a consistent differential pattern in price sensitivity by SES. Additionally, there is limited available evidence for alcohol from low- and middle-income countries. Further, there is consistent evidence that youth smoking is more sensitive to higher prices, and tobacco taxes have been shown to be effective in reducing smoking initiation.

This chapter also highlighted the importance of understanding potential substitution and tax avoidance from taxes that may dampen the intended effects and ultimate effectiveness in improving health outcomes. For example, it was shown that in the face of higher prices individuals may substitute to lower priced brands of the taxed products. And, that it is important that taxes are comprehensive in the coverage of alternative forms of the given products otherwise individuals are likely to substitute across product types. Evidence was also presented on the presence of tax avoidance measures such as cross-border shopping and it was shown to potentially dampen the impact of the tax, but it is only of particular relevance where taxes are implemented at the local level or in nations with soft borders.

The body of evidence linking prices/taxes to health and other outcomes is not as extensive as that for demand of the taxed products and it tends to be more widely available for HICs. For tobacco, there are numerous studies that show that higher cigarette taxes and prices are associated with reduced disease, premature deaths and other smoking-related adverse outcomes such as low-birth weight. A substantial and robust body of literature demonstrates that higher alcohol taxes and prices are associated with reduced disease and death (such as from liver cirrhosis) and a host of other adverse outcomes related to excessive drinking such as motor vehicle crashes, sexually transmitted diseases, crime, violence and workplace accidents. Although simulation estimates suggest that SSB taxes will reduce outcomes such as type 2 diabetes and obesity, and policy evaluations show a reduction in demand, the direct link between SSB taxes and prices and health outcomes has not yet been established; in part, because SSB taxes that raise prices by a significant amount are only recently beginning to emerge.

Overall, the evidence shows that health taxes reduce the harmful consumption of products such as tobacco, alcohol and SSBs and are an important tool that policymakers can implement to achieve goals of reducing the burden of non-communicable diseases and other consumption-related adverse outcomes.

Key messages

- Evidence from both demand models and tax evaluations show that higher prices/taxes on products such as tobacco, alcoholic beverages, non-alcoholic sugar-sweetened beverages (SSBs) and other selected foods reduce the consumption of these products.
- Compared to the demand for sugary beverages, which is generally more price sensitive and suggests a price elasticity greater to or equal to one, the demand for tobacco, alcohol and other selected foods, is generally inelastic with a price elasticity less than one.

- The extent to which demand responds to prices/taxes varies by demographic and socioeconomic characteristics, with lower-income populations and younger populations generally more price sensitive.
- Evidence shows that it is important for policymakers to be aware of tax avoidance behaviors as health taxes are associated with some degree of cross-border shopping.
- While tobacco and alcohol taxes are associated with advantageously reduced health ans social outcomes (e.g. lowered respiratory diseases, liver cirrhosis and accidents), there is less evidence on the effectiveness of taxes on sugary beverages and other foods on health outcomes.
- In terms of gaps in the literature, with regard to tobacco, there is limited evidence on emerging products such as electronic-cigarettes and no evidence to date for heated tobacco products. Further, there is limited available evidence on the effects of alcohol taxes in low and middle-income countries, as well as limited evidence that links sugary beverage prices/taxes to health outcomes.

References

1. Chaloupka FJ, Powell LM, Warner KE. The use of excise taxes to reduce tobacco, alcohol, and sugary beverage consumption. *Annual Review of Public Health.* 2019; 40: 187–201.
2. Sassi F, Belloni A, Capobianco C. The Role of Fiscal Policies in Health Promotion. OECD Health Working Paper No. 66; 2013. DOI: 10.1787/5k3twr94kvzx-en.
3. Grossman M. The economic approach to addictive behavior. In Tommasi M, Ierulli K (eds) *The New Economics of Human Behaviour.* Cambridge: Cambridge University Press; 1995.
4. International Agency for Research on Cancer. *Effectiveness of Tax and Price Policies for Tobacco Control – IARC Handbooks of Cancer Prevention,* Tobacco Control, Volume 14. Lyon France: International Agency for Research on Cancer; 2011.
5. National Cancer Institute and World Health Organization. The Economics of Tobacco and Tobacco Control, NCI Tobacco Control Monograph Series 21. Bethesda, MD and Geneva, Switzerland: National Cancer Institute and World Health Organization; 2016.
6. Jawad M, Leet JT, Glantz S, Millett C. Price elasticity of demand for non-cigarette tobacco products: A systematic review and meta-analysis. *Tobacco Control.* 2018; 27(6): 689–695.

7. Ahmed N, Hossain J, Huque R, Hassan MT, Mozumder TA. *The Economics of Tobacco Taxation in Bangladesh.* Dhaka, Bangladesh: Brac University, Brac Institute of Governance and Development; 2019.
8. Stoklosa MA, Drope J, Chaloupka FJ. Prices and e-cigarette demand: Evidence from the European Union. *Nicotine & Tobacco Research.* 2016; 18(10): 1973–1980.
9. Huang J, Gwarnicki C, Xu X, Caraballo RS, Wada R, Chaloupka FJ. A comprehensive examination of own- and cross-price-elasticities of tobacco and nicotine replacement products in the US Preventive Medicine. *Preventive Medicine.* 2018; 117: 107–114.
10. Levy D, de Almeida LM, Szklo A. The Brazil SimSmoke policy simulation model: The effect of strong tobacco control policies on smoking prevalence and smoking-attributable deaths in a middle income nation. *PLoS Medicine.* 2012; 9(11): e1001336.
11. Márquez V, Patricio Y, Moreno-Dodson B. *Tobacco Tax Reform at the Crossroads of Health and Development: Technical Report of the World Bank Group Global Tobacco Control Program (Portuguese).* Washington, DC: World Bank Group; 2018.
12. Sornpaisarn B, Shield KD, Österberg E, Rehm J (eds). *Resource Tool on Alcohol Taxation and Pricing Policies.* Geneva: World Health Organization; 2017.
13. World Health Organization Regional Office for Europe. *Alcohol Pricing in the WHO European Region: Update Report on the Evidence and Recommended Policy Actions.* Copenhagen: WHO Regional Office for Europe; 2020.
14. Wagenaar AC, Salois MJ, Komro KA. Effects of beverage alcohol price and tax levels on drinking: A meta-analysis of 1003 estimates from 112 studies. *Addiction.* 2009; 104(2): 179–190.
15. Elder RW, Lawrence B, Ferguson A, Naimi TS, Brewer RD, Chattopadhyay SK, Toomey TL, Fielding JE and the Task Force on Community Preventive Services. The effectiveness of tax policy interventions for reducing excessive alcohol consumption and related harms. *American Journal of Preventive Medicine.* 2010; 38(2): 217–229.
16. Sornpaisarn B, Shield K, Cohen J, Schwartz R, Rehm J. Elasticity of alcohol consumption, alcohol-related harms, and drinking initiation in low-and middle-income countries: A systematic review and meta-analysis. *International Journal of Drug and Alcohol Research.* 2013; 2(1): 45–58.
17. Gallet CA. The demand for alcohol: A meta-analysis of elasticities. *Australian Journal of Agricultural and Resource Economics.* 2007; 51: 121–135.
18. Ayyagari P, Deb P, Fletcher J, Gallo W, Sindelar JL. Understanding heterogeneity in price elasticities in the demand for alcohol for older individuals. *Health Economics.* 2013; 22: 89–105.
19. Esser MB, Waters H, Smart M, Jernigan DJ. Impact of Maryland's 2011 alcohol sales tax increase on alcoholic beverage sales. *The American Journal of Drug and Alcohol Abuse.* 2016; 42(4): 404–411.
20. Heeb J, Gmel G, Zurbrügg C, Kuo M, Rehm J. Changes in alcohol consumption following a reduction inprice of spirits: A natural experiment in Switzerland. *Addiction.* 2003; 98(10): 1433–1446.
21. Andreyeva T, Long MW, Brownell KD. The impact of food prices on consumption: A systematic review of research on the price elasticity of demand for food. *American Journal of Public Health.* 2010; 100(2): 216–222.

22. Powell L, Chriqui JF, Khan T, Wada R, Chaloupka FJ. Assessing the potential effectiveness of food and beverage taxes and subsidies for improving public health: A systematic review of prices, demand, and body weight outcomes. *Obesity Reviews.* 2013; 14(2): 110–128.
23. Cabrera Escobar MA, Veerman JL, Tollman SM, Bertram MY, Hofman KJ. Evidence that a tax on sugar sweetened beverages reduces the obesity rate: A meta-analysis. *BMC Public Health.* 2013; 13(1): 1072.
24. Claro RM, Levy RB, Popkin BM, Monteiro CA. Sugar-sweetened beverage taxes in Brazil. *American Journal of Public Health.* 2012; 102(1): 178–183.
25. Colchero MA, Salgado JC, Unar-Munguía M, Hernández-Ávila M, Rivera-Donmarco JA. Price elasticity of the demand for sugar sweetened beverages and soft drinks in Mexico. *Economics & Human Biology.* 2015; 19: 129–137.
26. Paraje G. The effect of prices and socio-economic level on the consumption of sugar-sweetened beverages (SSBs): The case of Ecuador. *PLoS One.* 2016; 11(3): e0152260.
27. Guerrero-López CM, Unar-Munguía M, Colchero MA. Price elasticity of the demand for soft drinks, other sugar-sweetened beverages and energy dense food in Chile. *BMC Public Health.* 2017; 17(1): 180.
28. Chaco V, Paraje G, Barnoya J, Chaloupka FJ. Own-price, cross-price, and income elasticities on milk and soft drinks in Guatemala. *PloS One.* 2018; 13(10): e0205931.
29. Stacey N, Tugendhaft A, Hofman K. Sugary beverage taxation in South Africa: Household expenditure, demand system elasticities, and policy implications. *Preventive Medicine.* 2017; 105: S26–S31.
30. Basu S, Vellakkal S, Agrawal S, Stuckler D, Popkin B, Ebrahim S. Averting obesity and Type 2 diabetes in India through sugar-sweetened beverage taxation: An economic-epidemiologic modeling study. *PLoS Med.* 2014; 11(1): e1001582.
31. Teng AM, Jones AC, Mizdrak A, Signal L, Genç M, Wilson N. Impact of sugar-sweetened beverage taxes on purchases and dietary intake: Systematic review and meta-analysis. *Obesity Reviews.* 2019; 20(9): 1187–1204.
32. Colchero MA, Guerrero-López CM, Molina M, Rivera JA. Beverage sales in Mexico before and after the implementation of a sugar sweetened beverage tax. *PLoS One.* 2016; 11(9): e0163463.
33. Colchero MA, Popkin BM, Rivera JA, Ng SW. Beverage purchases from stores in Mexico under the excise tax on sugar sweetened beverages: Observational study. *BMJ.* 2016; 352: h6704.
34. Colchero MA, Rivera-Donmarco J, Popkin BM, Ng SW. In Mexico, evidence of sustained consumer response two years after implementing a sugar-sweetened beverage tax. *Health Affairs (Millwood).* 2017; 36(3): 564–571.
35. Alvarado M, Unwin N, Sharp SJ, Hambleton I, Murphy MM, Samuels TA, Suhrcke M, Adams J. Assessing the impact of the Barbados sugar-sweetened beverage tax on beverage sales: An observational study. *International Journal of Behavioral Nutrition and Physical Activity.* 2019; 16(1): 13.
36. Caro JC, Corvalán C, Reyes M, Silva A, Popkin B, Taillie LS. Chile's 2014 sugar-sweetened beverage tax and changes in prices and purchases of sugar-sweetened

beverages: An observational study in an urban environment. *PLoS Med.* 2018; 15(7): e1002597.

37. Nakamura R, Mirelman A, Cuadrado C, Silva N, Dunstan J, Suhrcke ME. Evaluating the 2014 sugar-sweetened beverage tax in Chile: An observational study in urban areas. *PLoS Med.* 2018; 15(7): e1002596.
38. Schmacker R, Smed S. Do prices and purchases respond similarly to soft drink tax increases and cuts? *Economics and Human Biology.* 2020; 37: 100864.
39. Capacci S, Allais O, Bonnet C, Mazzocchi M. The impact of the French soda tax on prices and purchases. An ex post evaluation. *PLoS One.* 2019; 14(10): e0223196.
40. Bandy LK, Scarborough P, Harrington RA, Rayner M, Jebb SA. Reductions in sugar sales from soft drinks in the UK from 2015 to 2018. *BMC Medicine.* 2020; 18(1): 20.
41. Falbe J, Thompson HR, Becker CM, Rojas N, McCulloch CE, Madsen KA. Impact of the Berkeley excise tax on sugar-sweetened beverage consumption. *American Journal of Public Health.* 2016; 106(10): 1865–1871.
42. Silver LD, Ng SW, Ryan-Ibarra S, Taillie LS, Induni M, Miles DR, Poti JM, Popkin BM. Changes in prices, sales, consumer spending, and beverage consumption one year after a tax on sugar-sweetened beverages in Berkeley, California, US: A before-and-after study. *PLoS Med.* 2017; 14(4): e1002283.
43. Lee MM, Falbe J, Schillinger D, Basu S, McCulloch CE, Madsen KA. Sugar-sweetened beverage consumption 3 years after the Berkeley, California, sugar-sweetened beverage Tax. *American Journal of Public Health.* 2019; 109(4): 637–639.
44. Cawley J, Frisvold D, Hill A, Jones D. Oakland's sugar-sweetened beverage tax: Impacts on prices, purchases and consumption by adults and children. *Economics and Human Biology.* 2020; 37: 100865.
45. Powell LM, Leider J. The impact of Seattle's sweetened beverage tax on beverage prices and volume sold. *Economics and Human Biology.* 2020; 37: 100856.
46. Zhong Y, Auchincloss AH, Lee BK, Kanter GP. The short-term impacts of the Philadelphia beverage tax on beverage consumption. *American Journal of Preventive Medicine.* 2018; 55(1): 26–34.
47. Roberto CA, Lawman HG, LeVasseur MT, Mitra N, Peterhans A, Herring B, Bleich SN. Association of a beverage tax on sugar-sweetened and artificially sweetened beverages with changes in beverage prices and sales at chain retailers in a large urban setting. *JAMA.* 2019; 321(18): 1799–1810.
48. Powell LM, Leider J, Leger PT. Impact of a sweetened beverage tax on beverage volume sold in Cook County, IL, and its border area. *Annals of Internal Medicine.* 2020; 172: 390–397.
49. Jensen JD, Smed S. The Danish tax on saturated fat – Short run effects on consumption, substitution patterns and consumer prices of fats. *Food Policy.* 2013; 42: 18–31.
50. Batis C, Rivera JA, Popkin BM, Taillie LS. First-year evaluation of Mexico's tax on nonessential energy-dense foods: An observational study. *PLoS Med.* 2016; 13: 1–14.
51. Taillie LS, Rivera JA, Popkin BM, Batis C. Do high vs. low purchasers respond differently to a nonessential energy-dense food tax? Two-year evaluation of Mexico's 8% nonessential food tax. *Preventive Medicine.* 2017; 105: S37–S42.

52. Guindon GE, Paraje GR, Chaloupka FJ. Association of tobacco control policies with youth smoking onset in Chile. JAMA Pediatrics. 2019; 173(8): 754–762.
53. World Health Organization. *Gender, Women, and the Tobacco Epidemic*. Geneva: World Health Organization; 2010.
54. Cavazos-Rehg PA, Krauss MJ, Spitznagel EL, et al. Differential effects of cigarette price changes on adult smoking behaviours. *Tobacco Control.* 2014; 23: 113–118.
55. Sassi F, Belloni A, Mirelman AJ, et al. Equity impacts of price policies to promote healthy behaviours. *Lancet.* 2018; 391(10134): 2059–2070.
56. Finkelstein E, Zhen C, Nonnemaker J, Todd JE. Impact of targeted beverage taxes on higher- and lower-income households. *Archives of Internal Medicine.* 2010; 170(22): 2028–2034.
57. Wada R, Han E, Powell LM. Associations between soda prices and intake: Evidence from 24-h dietary recall data. *Food Policy.* 2015; 55: 54–60.
58. López-Olmedo N, Popkin BM, Taillie LS. The socioeconomic disparities in intakes and purchases of less-healthy foods and beverages have changed over time in urban Mexico. *Journal of Nutrition.* 2018; 148(1): 109–116.
59. Colchero MA, Molina M, Guerrero-Lopez CM. After Mexico implemented a tax, purchases of sugar-sweetened beverages decreased and water increased: Difference by place of residence, household composition, and income level. *Journal of Nutrition.* 2017; 147(8): 1552–1557.
60. Ng SW, Rivera J, Popkin B, Colchero MA. Did high purchasers respond differently to the excise tax on sugar-sweetened beverages in Mexico? *Public Health Nutrition.* 2019; 22(4): 750–756.
61. Cornelsen L, Green R, Turner R, Dangour AD, Shankar B, Mazzocchi M, Smith MD. What happens to patterns of food consumption when food prices change? Evidence from a systematic review and meta-analysis of food price elasticities globally. *Health Economics.* 2015; 24: 1548–1559.
62. Cawley J, Frisvold D. The pass-through of taxes on sugar-sweetened beverages to retail prices: The case of Berkeley, California. *Journal of Policy Analysis and Management.* 2017; 36(2): 303–326.
63. Salti N, Chaaban J, Nakkash R, Alaouie H. The effect of taxation on tobacco consumption and public revenues in Lebanon. *Tobacco Control.* 2015; 24(1): 77–81.
64. Huang J, Gwarnicki C, Xu X, Caraballo RS, Wada R, Chaloupka FJ. A comprehensive examination of own- and cross-price elasticities of tobacco and nicotine replacement products in the US Preventive Medicine. *Preventive Medicine.* 2018; 117: 107–114.
65. Farrelly MC, Pechacek TF, Chaloupka FJ. The impact of tobacco control program expenditures on aggregate cigarette sales: 1981–2000. *Journal of Health Economics.* 2003; 22(5): 843–859.
66. Becker GS, Grossman M, Murphy KM. An empirical analysis of cigarette addiction. *American Economics Review.* 1994; 84(3): 396–418.
67. Merriman D, Yurekli A, Chaloupka FJ. How big is the worldwide cigarette-smuggling problem? In Jha P, Chaloupka FJ (eds). *Tobacco Control in Developing Countries.* Oxford, UK: Oxford University Press; 365–392, 200.

68. Nagelhout GE, van den Putte B, Allwright S, Mons U, McNeill A, Guignard R, Beck F, Siahpush M, Joossens L, Fong GT, de Vries H. Socioeconomic and country variations in cross-border cigarette purchasing as a tobacco tax avoidance strategy. Findings from the ITC Europe Surveys. *Tobacco Control.* 2014; 23(Suppl. 1): i30–i38.
69. Driezen P, Thompson ME, Fong GT, Demjen T, Tountas Y, Trofor AC, Przewozniak K, Zatonski WA, Fernandez E, Mons U, Vardavas CI. Cross-border purchasing of cigarettes among smokers in Six Countries of the EUREST-PLUS ITC Surveys. *Tobacco Induced Diseases.* 2018; 16(Suppl. 2): A13.
70. Srivastava P, McLaren KR, Wohlgenant M, Zhao X. Disaggregated econometric estimation of consumer demand response by alcoholic beverage types. *Australian Journal of Agricultural and Resource Economics.* 2015; 59(3): 412–432.
71. Ruhm CJ, Snow Jones A, McGeary KA, Kerr WC, Terza JV, Greenfield TK, Pandian RS. What US data should be used to estimate the price elasticity of demand for alcohol? *Journal of Health Economics.* 2012; 31: 851–862.
72. Stehr M. The effect of Sunday sales bans and excise taxes on drinking and cross-border shopping for alcoholic beverages. *National Tax Journal.* 2007; 60(1): 85–105.
73. Asplund M, Friberg R, Wilander F. Demand and distance: Evidence on cross-border shopping. *Journal of Public Economics.* 2007; 91(1–2): 141–157.
74. Nordlund S, Osterberg E. Unrecorded alcohol consumption: Its economics and its effects on alcohol control in the Nordic countries. *Addiction.* 2000; 95: S551–S564.
75. Smith TA, Lin BH, Lee JY. *Taxing Caloric Sweetened Beverages: Potential Effects on Beverage Consumption, Calorie Intake, and Obesity.* Washington, DC: DIANE Publishing, United States Department of Agriculture; 2010.
76. Finkelstein EA, Zhen C, Bilger M, Nonnemaker J, Farooqui AM, Todd JE. Implications of a sugar-sweetened beverage (SSB) tax when substitutions to non-beverage items are considered. *Journal of Health Economics.* 2013; 32(1): 219–239.
77. Zhen C, Finkelstein EA, Nonnemaker JM, Karns SA, Todd JE. Predicting the effects of sugar-sweetened beverage taxes on food and beverage demand in large demand systems. *American Journal of Agricultural Economics.* 2014; 96(1): 1–25.
78. Schmacker R, Smed S. Do prices and purchases respond similarly to soft drink tax increases and cuts? *Economics and Human Biology.* 2020; 37: 100864.
79. Bowser D, Canning D, Okunogbe A. The impact of tobacco taxes on mortality in the USA, 1970-2005. *Tobacco Control.* 2016; 25(1): 52–59.
80. Baum A, Aguilar-Gomez S, Lightwood J, Bruzelius E, Glantz SA, Basu S. Estimating the long-run relationship between state cigarette taxes and county life expectancy. *Tobacco Control.* 2020; 29(1): 81–88.
81. Ho V, Ross JS, Steiner CA, Mandawat A, Short M, Ku-Goto MH, Krumholz HM. A nationwide assessment of the association of smoking bans and cigarette taxes with hospitalizations for acute myocardial infarction, heart failure, and pneumonia. *Medical Care Research and Review.* 2017; 74(6): 687–704.
82. Hatoun J, Davis-Plourde K, Penti B, Cabral H, Kazis L. Tobacco control laws and pediatric asthma. *Pediatrics.* 2018; 141: S130–S135.

83. Ringel JS, Evans WN. Cigarette taxes and smoking during pregnancy. *American Journal of Public Health.* 2001; 91(11): 1851–1856.
84. Evans WN, Ringel JS. Can higher cigarette taxes improve birth outcomes? *Journal of Public Economics.* 1999; 72(1): 135–154.
85. Markowitz S. The effectiveness of cigarette regulations in reducing cases of Sudden Infant Death Syndrome. *Journal of Health Economics.* 2008; 27(1): 106–133.
86. Filippidis FT, Laverty AA, Hone T. Association of cigarette price differentials with infant mortality in 23 European Union countries. *JAMA Pediatrics.* 2017; 171(11): 1100–1106.
87. Jha P. Death and taxes: Epidemiological and economic evidence on smoking. *Global Heart.* 2012; 7(2): 139–142.
88. Wagenaar AC, Tobler AL, Komro KA. Effects of alcohol tax and price policies on morbidity and mortality. *American Journal of Public Health.* 2010; 100(11): 2270–2278.
89. Wendt M, Todd JE. The effect of food and beverage prices on children's weights. Economic Research Service Report No. 118. US Department of Agriculture, Economic Research Service; 2001.
90. Barrientos-Gutierrez, T, Zepeda-Tello R, Rodrigues ER, Colchero MA, Rojas-Martinez R, Lazcano-Ponce E, Hernandez-Avila M, Rivera-Dommarco J, Meza R. Expected population weight and diabetes impact of the 1-peso-per-litre tax to sugar sweetened beverages in Mexico. *PloS One.* 2017; 12(5): e0176336.
91. Saxena A, Stacey N, Puech PDR, Mudara C, Hofman K, Verguet S. The distributional impact of taxing sugar-sweetened beverages: Findings from an extended cost-effectiveness analysis in South Africa. *BMJ Global Health.* 2019; 4(4): e001317.
92. Saxena A, Koon AD, Lagrada-Rombaua L, Angeles-Agdeppa I, Johns B, Capanzana M. Modelling the impact of a tax on sweetened beverages in the Philippines: An extended cost-effectiveness analysis. *Bulletin of the World Health Organization.* 2019; 97(2): 97.
93. Basto-Abreu A, Barrientos-Gutiérrez T, Vidaña-Pérez D, Colchero MA, Hernández-F M, Hernández-Ávila, M, Ward ZJ, Long MW, Gortmaker SL. Cost-effectiveness of the sugar-sweetened beverage excise tax in Mexico. *Health Affairs.* 2019; 38(11): 1824–1831.
94. Sowa PM, Keller E, Stormon N, Lalloo R, Ford PJ. The impact of a sugar-sweetened beverages tax on oral health and costs of dental care in Australia. *European Journal of Public Health.* 2019; 29(1): 173–177.
95. Jevdjevic M, Trescher AL, Rovers M, Listl S. The caries-related cost and effects of a tax on sugar-sweetened beverages. *Public Health.* 2019; 169: 125–132.
96. Long MW, Gortmaker SL, Ward ZJ, Resch SR, Moodie, Sacks G, Swinburn BA, Carter RC, Wang YC. Cost effectiveness of a sugar-sweetened beverage excise tax in the US *American Journal of Preventive Medicine.* 2015; 49(1): 112–123.
97. Vecino-Ortiz AI, Arroyo-Ariza D. A tax on sugar sweetened beverages in Colombia: Estimating the impact on overweight and obesity prevalence across socio economic levels. *Social Science & Medicine.* 2018; 209: 111–116.

https://doi.org/10.1142/9781800612396_0004

Chapter 4

Supply-Side Responses to Health Taxes

Annalisa Belloni* and Franco Sassi†

Health taxes are typically levied on manufacturers. The impact of health taxes on consumption, and ultimately on health, depends on the extent of which taxes are transferred from manufacturers onto the prices faced by consumers, referred to as tax pass-through. We discuss the theoretical economic arguments and the empirical evidence on key factors influencing tax pass-through for tobacco, alcohol, and sugar-sweetened beverage (SSB) products, and provide general conclusions and recommendations for government policy. Key drivers of tax pass-through include strategic behaviours of manufacturers and retailers (production and marketing strategies, particularly for multi-product firms), market structure (especially the degree of concentration of a market), and supply and demand price elasticities. Based on empirical observations, taxes on tobacco, alcohol and SSBs are usually passed on to consumers through increases in market prices, sometimes exceeding the amount of the tax. The extent of tax pass-through can vary widely, depending on type of product, package size, brand characteristics, store type, etc. Furthermore, strategic firm behaviours may be triggered by features of tax design. For instance, ad valorem, or mixed specific

* World Health Organization, Switzerland.

† Imperial College London, UK.

and ad valorem tax structures may incentivise manufacturers to differentiate their brands and price levels, while specific excise taxes tend to reduce relative price differences between products, stifling potential substitutions. Moreover, specific taxes based on ingredients (e.g. grams of alcohol, or sugar), may incentivise manufacturers to reformulate their products, or to increase the promotion of products with a lower concentration of the taxed ingredient. The evidence presented underscores the importance for policymakers to carefully adjust the design, and closely monitor the impacts, of health taxes, to ensure that health benefits are not hindered by firms' strategic responses.

4.1. Introduction

Health taxes alter the conditions in which the markets for the taxed products operate. Markets adjust to the introduction of health taxes through changes on both the demand and the supply sides. Although we discuss changes, or responses, on the two sides separately in this book (demand-side responses are discussed in Chapter 3), they are closely interdependent. In this chapter, we discuss supply-side responses, limiting the focus on the actions undertaken by manufacturers and retailers to safeguard the profitability and sustainability of their businesses in the jurisdictions in which health taxes are introduced. The responses discussed in this chapter are purely the economic responses, involving aspects of the production and marketing of the products concerned, and strategic industrial decisions regarding aspects of the firms' core business. These are distinct from, but often complementary to, the political responses examined in Chapter 12, and they exclude illicit responses.

In theoretical economic models assuming perfectly competitive market dynamics, demand and supply adjustments following the introduction of consumption taxes are largely automatic. In these markets, individual firms are price takers and there is little scope, if any, for discretional action. In real-life circumstances, and especially in the markets for the products that are typically targeted by health taxes, competition is far from perfect (see Chapter 12 for an assessment of market concentration). In fact, a significant scope exists for supply-side players to act strategically in response to the introduction of health taxes in order to mitigate any adverse consequences on their businesses.

Health taxes, as other excise duties, are usually levied on manufacturers and not on final consumers. Taxing manufacturers reduces the administrative burden and the risk of non-compliance. However, this also increases opportunities for suppliers to shape the market impacts of health taxes, potentially undermining the effectiveness of a tax in the pursuit of public health goals. The impact of health taxes on consumption, and thus health, is dependent on the degree to which market prices for the taxed products are increased. A key determinant of the effect of health taxes is the degree to which taxes, or tax increases, are transferred onto the prices faced by consumers, which is often referred to as tax pass-through. When the pass-through rate is greater than 1, there is overshift of the tax (i.e., prices rise above the tax increase) while if it is lower than 1, the tax is under-shifted (i.e., prices rise below the tax increase). The final tax pass-through rate is determined as the ratio between the price increase faced by consumers and the amount paid for the tax at the relevant tax point. Intermediate pass-through rates can also be calculated — e.g. at the manufacturer's level — but what matters the most in the case of health taxes is the final pass-through rate. When health taxes are ad valorem (see Chapter 8 for a detailed discussion of ad valorem versus specific excise taxes), the pass-through rate is still calculated as a proportion of the amount paid for the tax. The percentage increase in prices faced by consumers should not be expected to match the tax rate in the case of ad valorem taxes. Health taxes are in fact typically levied on manufacturers (i.e., on ex-factory or ex-customs prices) and the prices paid by manufacturers do not reflect the prices faced by consumers, as they typically exclude transport and distribution costs and retail mark-ups. It is important to note that retail mark-ups may be set as a percentage of manufacturer prices, so they may inflate pass-through rates. In this case, a portion of the price increase faced by consumers is paid to retailers, independently of manufacturers' pass-through strategies.

Industry pricing policies in response to health taxes are to some extent predictable because they are driven, or at least influenced, by market forces and by tax design. However, the markets in which health taxes may be applied vary widely. The specific characteristics of those markets may influence the responses of commercial players to a degree that could significantly impact the ability of the tax to fulfill its public health purpose. The planning of effective health taxes requires full consideration of possible responses from the industries concerned as well as from consumers (discussed in Chapter 3) and requires careful design (discussed in Chapter 8).

In this chapter, we discuss the theoretical economic arguments and the empirical evidence on key factors influencing the degree to which taxes are passed on to consumers. We also discuss the extent to which these factors vary across products, countries or other relevant dimensions.

Basic economic theory suggests that prices are set at the level at which demand and supply meet. In competitive markets, taxes are passed through to consumers (up to full pass-through, depending on the underlying demand and supply price elasticities) when there is a constant marginal cost of production. However, the markets in which most tobacco, alcoholic and non-alcoholic beverages are sold tend to have levels of concentration that set them apart from competitive markets. In more concentrated markets, suppliers have market power and therefore more scope for exercising their discretion in responding to health taxes. In practice, this often translates into an over-shifting of taxes onto consumers. However, suppliers may decide to adopt different strategies leading to different levels of pass-through. Suppliers decision will depend on the characteristics of the demand they face, on their production costs, on their product portfolio and on the competitive environment in which they operate. This is because in less competitive markets prices are set above marginal cost. Therefore, manufacturers can under-shift the tax and still have positive margins or over-shift the tax to maintain revenues in the face of declining sales volume.

In addition to market structure, other factors potentially affecting the effectiveness of a tax are strategic behaviours of manufacturers and retailers (e.g. production and marketing strategies, particularly for multi-product firms), supply and demand elasticities, the characteristics of the jurisdiction in which the tax is applied and the design of the tax (e.g. specific or ad valorem; tiered rates, etc.). In the next section, we illustrate several considerations concerning the above elements that are of general value and can be applied to all categories of products that are typically targeted by health taxes. In the following sections, we present more specific considerations that apply to specific product categories.

While some industry responses can hinder the effectiveness of health taxes, others can align with price incentives. This happens, for instance, when health taxes lead to product reformulation that may mitigate the detrimental health impacts of the products concerned. A special focus by White et al. associated with this chapter focuses on the use of taxation as an incentive to product reformulation, using the example of the Soft Drinks Industry Levy in the United Kingdom. Health taxes can also create an incentive for producers to shift advertising and promotion to non-taxed (or lower taxed) products. This is another example of alignment between industry responses and price incentives when taxes are designed in a way that penalise less healthy products (e.g. taxes targeting alcohol or sugar level).[1]

In the final section of this chapter, we draw some general conclusions and recommendations for government policy highlighting the similarities and differences between the markets for the three main product categories targeted by health taxes.

4.2. Factors affecting supply-side responses to health taxes

While supply-side responses largely translate into different degrees of pass-through of health taxes, firms' decisions on pass-through are driven by a large and complex set of factors and strategic considerations. Whoever design and implement health taxes must be aware of those in order to ensure taxes are effective in the pursuit of health goals. Firms will aim at safeguarding the profitability of their businesses against risks that may derive from changes in competitors' and consumers' behaviours following the introduction of health taxes.

In perfectly competitive markets, individual firms are price takers and face a perfectly elastic demand curve. They will only be able to sell their products at one price, the market-determined price. Tax pass-through in those settings is also determined at the market level and individual suppliers can only adapt to the new price level and sell whatever quantity of the product they are able and willing to sell at that price. As previously mentioned, however, many of the markets for products typically targeted by health taxes are characterised by a reduced level of competition and this of course is not merely incidental. Reduced levels of competition are typically the result of specific features of a market, such as barriers to entry or product heterogeneity, which limit opportunities for existing and potential competitors to contest other firms' market position. Heavy regulation of an industrial sector, unless specifically aimed at preventing firms from acquiring dominant positions, contributes to creating barriers to entry into the markets in which firms in that industry operate. In such markets, firms strive to acquire a critical mass and critical assets (especially intangible assets such as knowledge and, arguably, lobbying and influence capacity) to operate in a regulated environment and withstand the burden of regulation. Health taxes can also create an incentive for increasing levels of concentration (i.e., reducing levels of competition) in the markets in which they are applied. As we discuss below, this type of development is also in keeping with the strategies that firms are likely to adopt to minimise risk from consumer responses to health taxes.

4.2.1. Health taxes and the firm's competitive environment

Competitors' responses to health taxes may jeopardise a firm's business. One example in which a firm's business can be threatened by competitors' responses to health taxes is when a competitor has the capacity to influence the design of the tax in a direction that particularly suits their business (e.g. by setting the tax base in a way that excludes some of their products or setting tax rate thresholds at convenient levels). Another example is when competitors are in a better position to reformulate their products (e.g. because of a technological advantage) and mitigate the impact of taxation on their sales and customer base. In the situations described here, larger players have an advantage over smaller ones. In fact, firms that enjoy a competitive advantage are able to contain price increases following the implementation of health taxes. On the other hand, other firms will either lose market shares because their prices are no longer competitive, or be forced to reduce their pass-through rates in order to remain competitive, but most likely with detrimental consequences on the profitability of their business.

An alternative scenario may occur in situations in which no competitors are able to enjoy meaningful technological or market advantages and relatively few larger firms operate in the market. In this scenario, cooperation between larger firms, effectively operating as a cartel, may lead to higher degrees of pass-through. This will translate to higher prices for consumers in the presence of a relatively inelastic demand.

4.2.2. Health taxes and firms' expectations of consumer response

The behaviour of competitors is only one of the factors taken into consideration by firms in their response to health taxes. Consumer behaviour is at least as important, and demand-side responses to health taxes can be even more nuanced than competitors' responses. It is legitimate to expect that firms possess information on the price elasticity of the demand for their products. However, price elasticity is a simple number that summarises the outcomes of a relatively complex array of behaviours triggered by price changes. Every product has its own market, but consumers make their consumption choices considering the prices of different products and making trade-offs between different types of consumption, based on their cross-price elasticities. This creates a dynamic equilibrium in which choices are constantly adapted following price fluctuations and preference changes, and the introduction of health taxes causes further adaptation in consumer choices. Trade-offs made by consumers translate into substitutions between products and types of consumption. A price hike for a given product category due to the introduction of a health tax may trigger at least three different types of substitutions,[2] as follows:

a. a switch to cheaper products in the same product category, often termed 'trading-down';
b. a switch to alternative products that are close substitutes for the products originally consumed (examples may include artificially sweetened beverages for sugar-sweetened ones, different types of alcoholic beverages or tobacco products, etc.);
c. a switch to different and unrelated types of consumption.

The higher the price elasticity for a particular product, the more likely consumers are to engage in substitutions when the price of that product increases. An inelastic demand (elasticity between 0 and 1, in absolute value) means that after a price increase, consumers will end up spending more on the product in question and consuming less of it (the reduction in quantity is not large enough to offset the impact of the price increase). Therefore, consumers will be left with less available income after purchasing the product in question and will be unlikely to increase the consumption of other products. On the other hand, an elastic demand (elasticity larger than 1, in absolute value) for a product whose price is increased will be associated with a decreased spend on that product (in this case the reduction in quantity does offset the impact of the price increase). This means that consumers will increase their demand for other products, effectively engaging in substitutions. Price elasticity is partly determined by the inherent preferences of consumers, but it is also largely influenced by market characteristics, chiefly, the availability and prices of close substitutes on the market. Other things being equal, an inelastic demand constitutes an incentive for firms to pass taxes through to consumers. By doing so, firms increase their revenues and maximise their profits with a limited risk of seeing consumers switch to alternative products. The opposite is true when firms face an elastic demand.

4.2.3. Health taxes, firm size and market structure

As describe previously, the price elasticity of demand may be a sufficient guide for determining pass-through rates in the short term. However, when health taxes are applied over a long period of time and become a structural feature of a given market (as in the case of markets for tobacco products and alcoholic beverages) firms are likely to develop strategies to ensure the sustainability of their business in the face of future tax hikes. There will be a push towards market concentration and product differentiation that will enable firms to capture consumers engaging at least in the types of substitutions described in (a) and (b) in Section 4.2.2. Multi-product firms operating in dominant market positions are common in markets for products targeted by health taxes. These firms are typically in a position to offer similar products under different brands with different market profiles and prices, as well as close and not-so-close substitutes to taxed products. Therefore, a large part of the substitutions triggered by health taxes will occur within the firm's product portfolio, with reduced or no loss of revenue for the firm. In established markets such as those for tobacco and alcohol products, portfolio diversification has been pushed to include new product concepts, such as electronic cigarettes or non-alcoholic beer or wine. Firms with diversified product portfolios are likely to favour high pass-through rates even in the presence of a less inelastic demand, because they have less to fear from consumer substitutions than smaller, single-product firms. Similarly, at the retail level, there is evidence that larger retailers pass through more of the tax than independent retailers.[3]

4.2.4. Health taxes and tax pass-through patterns

Evidence shows that health taxes are usually passed onto consumers as price increases and are sometimes over-shifted (specific examples by product category are provided in the sections below). This can occur across all products or just in specific segments of the market, for example higher price products and private labels, as the demand for those is usually less price-sensitive[4–7] or smaller package sizes compared to large package sizes.[8–12] This might reflect producer's strategies to keep the level of consumption high without discouraging the consumption of large package beverages, which are more penalised by the excise tax[9] and have a more price-sensitive demand.[8]

Moreover, due to the imperfect competitive nature of the market, we observe asymmetric pass-through, which tends to be higher after a tax increase than after a tax cut. For example, pass-through rates for beer of 1.34 (over-shift) for tax increases and 0.27 (under-shift) for tax reductions have been reported,[13] as well as pass-through rates for sugar-sweetened beverages (SSB) taxes of between 1.6 and 1.8 after a tax increase and between 0.9 and 1.2 after a tax reduction.[14]

Pass-through is reduced when more opportunities exist for tax avoidance, both for consumers and producers. For instance, when substitutes for taxed products are available and consumer demand is price-sensitive or when it is easy to buy products outside the taxing jurisdictions. Evidence shows that a lower pass-through is observed for tobacco,[15] alcohol[16,17] and SSBs[13,18,19] sold in stores near borders with low-tax jurisdictions and for products like cigarettes sold by the carton, for which cross-border avoidance is greatest.[15] To avoid this strategic behavior, in Catalonia, a regional jurisdiction in Spain where a tax was applied on SSBs, the legislation included a mandatory requirement of complete pass-through to consumers.[20]

The elasticity of supply, which is based on the amount of competition among manufacturers and retailers, has also an impact on pass-through.[19] When competition is higher and the margins are lower, pass-through is also lower and this happens, for example, in smaller jurisdictions.[21]

Finally, the presence of a more complex tax structure (e.g. ad valorem or mixed specific and ad valorem taxes) can provide more opportunities for manufacturers for a strategic differentiation of brands and price levels.[5]

4.2.5. Health taxes and state monopolies

In many countries, the markets for tobacco and alcohol products are dominated by state monopolies. When the first edition of the WHO Tobacco Atlas was published in 2002, an estimated 40% of cigarettes worldwide were being consumed in countries that had state monopolies,[22] but the number of countries with monopolies had been on a long-term declining trend. State monopolies remain mostly in countries in North Africa and the Middle East, China, South-East Asia and in some eastern European countries. However, given the increasing prominence of the Chinese tobacco market, the share of the global cigarette market they account for has not declined. Tobacco monopolies have different characteristics in different countries and may cover production and imports as well as sales of tobacco products. A smaller number of countries have state monopolies for alcohol products, especially in North America, northern and central Europe. These monopolies today mostly control the sale of alcohol products for off-trade consumption.[23]

Commercial responses triggered by health taxes in countries where state monopolies exist can be significantly different from those described elsewhere in this chapter. Governments that set taxes in markets in which they have monopolies also have the power to determine, or largely influence, the way taxes affect the businesses involved and the consumers of the taxed products. There is at least some evidence that state monopolies operate differently from private monopolies when taxes are introduced or raised. Tax pass-through to consumers ranges from low levels in instances of tobacco tax increases in China[24] to higher levels (e.g. in Egypt, Ref.[25]) but with no reported evidence of over-shifting, which would be expected in a private monopoly or highly concentrated market.

Alcohol monopolies were often established to control the social externalities of alcohol consumption, so their pricing policies tend to be consistently geared towards that overarching goal, independently of taxation. In line with this, price promotions and discounts are uncommon in sales monopolies.[26] Evidence from Finland shows that tax pass-through rates have been higher in the off-trade sector (covered by the state monopoly) than in the on-trade sector, but differences in pass-through between beverages in the off-trade sector have been even larger than differences between on-trade and off-trade rates, ranging from 0.77 (for beer) to 1.44 (for spirits), on average, between 2002 and 2011.[26]

In a larger number of countries, governments exercise monopolistic powers by reserving the right to license the production or sale of tobacco and alcohol products to independent commercial entities. These arrangements, however, confer a more limited degree of control to the state compared to the production and sale monopolies discussed earlier. Their impact on business responses to health taxes is mainly through the increased levels of concentration they produce in the relevant markets.

4.3. Supply-side responses to the introduction of tobacco taxes

Tobacco companies, as other oligopoly industries, use a number of strategies to respond to tax increases and other tobacco control efforts by governments and in the US smokers bear approximately 52% of cigarette excise taxes.[27]

Evidence from countries with different level of income shows that, across the tobacco market as a whole, taxes are usually passed through to consumers and can be over-shifted in high-income countries.[28] Keeler et al.[29] estimated that a 1 cent increase in cigarette taxes would increase retail prices by 1.1 cents, on average, in the United States.

However, industries adopt differential *pricing strategies* and while taxes on low-price brands are not always fully passed onto consumers (under-shifting), taxes on higher-price brands are over-shifted (i.e., consumer price increase more than the tax).[4,28,30–32]

The tobacco market tends to be concentrated in the low-price and the mid-price segments.[4,33] As the demand is less inelastic in this segment of the market, price is usually not increased after a tax increase, while it is over-shifted in higher price market segment where demand is less price sensitive. Manufacturers adopt this strategy to cross-subsidise low-price brands with excess profit earned from high-price brands. By attracting more price-sensitive smokers to buy cheaper products, they keep or even expand overall market, thus undermining the intended public health impact of the tax policy.

In South Africa, for example, there is evidence that taxes were over-shifted before 2010 but seem to have been under-shifted since then. The high margins created by the over-shifting before 2010 attracted new businesses to the market which competed largely on price. The presence of lower price cigarettes in the market in more recent years and the increased level of competition made it more difficult for industries to pass tax increases onto the consumers.[30]

A study based on an extensive literature review and analysis of survey and commercial data in the United Kingdom found that industries over-shifted taxes by an average of more than 4.00 pence per annum on all brand segments, but price increases were higher for more expensive brands.[4] More recent evidence from the United Kingdom shows that despite regular tax increases, prices for the cheapest tobacco products (like factory-made and roll-your-own) remained steady from 2013 while sales increased.[34]

Conversely, data from China show that after the 2015 tax increase, the State Tobacco Monopoly Administration also raised cigarette prices on average by 11%, with the cheapest products increasing by 20% and the more expensive ones by less than 10%.[24]

Sometimes tobacco companies can decide to under-shift tax increases as a temporary strategy to limit reduction in demand and retain price-sensitive consumers. For example, in Ukraine prices of cigarettes fell by 11% between

2007 and 2008 while excise taxes rose by 6% in the same period of time, while they rose by more than the tax after 2009.[35]

When considering the prices effectively paid by consumers, after accounting for strategic consumer behaviours such as trading down (e.g. brand down-switching) or cross-border shopping, there is some evidence that light and occasional smokers end up facing slightly larger price increases following tax increases.[36]

4.3.1. Impact of tax structures on prices

Simple tax structures like a uniform specific tax *(i.e., monetary value per quantity)* reduce industries strategic behaviours compared to multi-tiers or ad valorem taxes *(set as a percentage of the value of the product, e.g. as a percentage of the price)*[37–39] leading to higher tax pass-through.[40] Specific excise taxes are therefore more effective than ad valorem taxes in reducing price variability and the potential switching between products and thus at reducing overall consumption.[5] On the other hand, ad valorem taxes can have little impact on prices if the tobacco industry lowers the ex-factory price as in the case of Vietnam.[41]

A study looking at all European countries has found that northern European countries apply mostly specific taxes, while southern European countries prefer ad valorem taxes favouring the production/selling of domestic products. The study shows that specific taxes always have a greater effect on prices than ad valorem taxes.[37]

When differential tax increases are introduced (e.g. for premium versus economy brands) companies can apply pricing strategies to maintain their market share. For example, they can reduce the price of their products to avoid the tax increases, or, in the case of multi-product firms, they can use portfolio pricing strategies to optimise revenues by accounting for likely substitutions across products. The tobacco industry can also change the tobacco attributes (e.g. weight, length) or tobacco processes relabelling products to avoid tax.[35] Where multi-tiered tax based on price level is in place, for example, in Egypt and Pakistan, prices of tobacco products tend to cluster near the top of each tier.[33]

4.3.2. Introducing cheap products or lowering prices

Tobacco manufacturers have used a variety of price-related marketing strategies like multi-pack discounts, or couponing, to counter the effects of tax increases. Similar pricing strategies became widely used in the United States in the 1980s and 1990s in response to competitive pressures following a series of federal tax increases.[27] A large US tobacco manufacturer offered coupons to some of its most price-sensitive consumers (e.g. women, youth) allowing them to buy cigarettes at discounted prices just before an excise tax increase in 2009.[35] Evidence has shown that these practices have been successful in increasing tobacco use (e.g. Ref.[42]).

In response to actual or foreseen tax increases, tobacco manufacturers have also introduced new low-price or ultra-low-price products in the relevant markets, or reduced pack size for some of their products to ensure the availability of cheap options to consumers. In the United Kingdom, ultra-low-price products were introduced in 2006 and their market share doubled in 3 years.[4] In the United States, the market share of 'branded generics' — cigarettes combining value attributes with an association to a reputable brand — increased threefold after a tax increase in 1983[27] and branded generics came to dominate the discount cigarette market from the 1980s onwards.

4.4. Supply-side responses to the introduction of alcohol taxes

As in the case of tobacco, the alcohol market is highly concentrated. The oligopoly status, which is mainly within a specific sector, i.e., beer and spirits, allows industries more freedom to set their prices and avoid high tax burdens and allows them to spend considerably in marketing creating significant barriers to entry for new companies.[43]

The alcohol market is more diverse and segmented than tobacco with different types of beverages (e.g. beers, spirits and wine) as well as different brands and consumption location (i.e. off premise versus on premise). Moreover, alcohol taxes account for a smaller proportion of the alcohol prices (7% on average in the United States) when compared with tobacco. However, this proportion varies substantially between location (from 3.65% to 10.2% in different US states) and across beverage types from 4.7% for scotch to 10.2% for whiskey.[44]

Many studies show that alcohol taxes are more than fully passed-through to consumer prices.[10,45,46] However, there is heterogeneity in tax pass-through across types of beverages, product size, packaging, brands, stores, size of tax change and border effects.[10] Tax pass-through varies also across products based on their price and point of sale, with lower pass-through in the off-trade sector[44] and for cheaper alcoholic beverages.[6,47,48]

A recent systematic review and meta-analysis of alcohol tax pass-through conclude that beer taxes are over-shifted and wine-spirits taxes are fully shifted, however, full-shifting of taxes cannot be rejected based on bias-corrected meta-regressions for any beverage and all alcohol.[17] The study also found that the effect of tax changes on price occurs within a few months and can vary considerably at borders.[16,17]

For beer, there is a strong border effect, with stores far from the border over-shifting taxes to consumer prices and stores closer to borders under-shifting them,[13,16] while this is not the case for spirits.[13]

A modelling study using data for 27 OECD countries from 2003 to 2016 shows that taxes for wine, cognac and the liqueur 'Cointreau' are over-shifted being respectively 2.51, 1.71 and 1.14; while there is more variation in the degree of pass-through for other alcoholic beverages, including beer, gin and Scotch whisky.[48] In South Africa, the excise tax on beer is over-shifted to consumers. The pass-through coefficient is estimated at 4.83 (95% CI: 4.02; 5.64) for lager, and at 4.77 (95% CI: 4.04; 5.50) for all beer (which includes dark beer).[10]

The large differences in tax pass-through across different types of alcoholic beverages and brands reflect different demand elasticities for different products. There is evidence that pass-through is higher for higher priced products[6,48,49] and higher income consumers.[16] For example, evidence from the United Kingdom shows that alcohol retailers appear to respond to increases in alcohol tax by under-shifting their cheaper products and over-shifting their more expensive products for all types of alcoholic beverages. In the off-trade sector, the under-shift for the cheapest products is larger for beer (0.85) and spirits (0.86) and it is seen for the cheapest 5% of products for beer and for the cheapest 15% of products for spirits.[6] In the on-trade sector, the under-shift is larger for wine and sparkling wine (respectively 0.55 and 0.75 at the lowest quintile) and the over-shift is evident only for the most expensive beverages in the top quintile.[49]

In terms of sales volume, cheap alcohol represents the majority of the units in the market, 67% and 31% respectively for beer and spirits in the United Kingdom[6] and it is vastly consumed by high-risk groups with low income. Therefore, the under-shift of the tax for these products is likely to produce smaller consumption reductions and implementing other policies like minimum price or restriction on price promotions may increase the effectiveness of the tax policy.

Evidence from the United States shows that the burden of beer taxation increases across the income distribution. Higher income consumers are more affected by increase in beer tax rates than lower income consumers. While the prices paid by low-income households do not change after the tax increase, the pass-through increases with income, from 0.125 for middle-income households to 0.265 for high-income households. The negative changes in prices paid by low-income consumers can sometimes be explained by drinkers downgrading to lower quality products.[16]

The level of pass-through may also vary according to the location of consumption, but the evidence is quite mixed. In Alaska, average pass-through rates were found to be around 2 for off-premises spirit sales and close to 4 for on-premises sales while pass-through is around 2 for both on-premises and off-premises sales of beers.[45]

Beer excise duties are under-shifted in Ireland (0.5 off-trade, 0 on-trade) and Finland (0.8 off-trade, 0.7 on-trade), and over-shifted in off-trade sales in Latvia (1.9) and Slovenia (2.5).[26] For spirits, excise duties are under-shifted in on-trade sales in Finland (0.8) and Ireland (0.1), but over-shifted in off-trade sales in Finland (1.4) and Latvia (1.3), while they are under-shifted in off-trade sales in Ireland (0.7) and Slovenia (0.7).[26]

4.4.1. Impacts of tax structures on prices

Excise tax structure has an impact on alcohol tax pass-through and a combination of specific and ad valorem taxes has more predictive power for prices, than a single type of tax. Similarly to tobacco, a more complex tax structure is associated with greater price variability giving more opportunities to companies and consumers for tax avoidance. A recent study found that a mixed beer excise tax structure was associated with 38% greater beer price variability, whereas a mixed liquor excise tax structure was associated with 60–77% greater liquor price variability. However, wine excise tax structure was not significantly associated with price variability. This may be because the pricing strategy for wine is different from that of other alcoholic beverages; as the origin of the wine, instead of the quality, plays an important role in pricing.[50]

Specific taxes applied to all alcohol products would make alcohol less affordable and would decrease the volume of alcoholic beverages consumed, but not necessarily reduce the volume of alcohol consumed (as consumers may switch to stronger alcohol products). On the other hand, a tax based on alcohol content would be more effective at reducing alcohol consumption. A dose-tax system can also incentivise producers to reformulate their products reducing the alcohol content and/or to increase the advertising from higher to lower alcohol products. For example in South Africa, beer advertising has been moving towards lower alcohol beers coinciding with the increased incentive towards producing lower alcohol beer.[1]

4.5. Supply-side responses to the introduction of food and non-alcoholic beverages taxes

The non-alcoholic beverages market is also highly concentrated. Usually, food and beverage manufacturers pass the full or near to full amount of taxes onto consumers[19,21] or they increase the price by an even bigger amount.[12,51–53]

For example, there is evidence of over-shifting for excise taxes on soft drinks in Denmark where the three largest grocery chains account for 85% of total sales[13,14] and in Saudi Arabia where two companies account for 92% of the sales.[53] Similarly, the pass-through for the SSB tax implemented in Mexico in 2014 was between 0.96 and 1.20 for carbonated soft drinks (where two firms are responsible for 85% of the sales) compared to a value between 0.53 and 0.74 for non-carbonated soft drinks. The latter has a lower market share compared to soft drinks and higher price elasticity of demand which can explain the reduced level of pass-through of the tax.[54]

In line with the theory presented previously, the pass-through is lower for products sold in larger containers[8,12] as well as when the competition is higher and the margins are lower.[21] For example, in smaller jurisdictions like in Berkeley, California, the estimated pass-through of the tax varied by products and was on average between 43.1% and 47% across all SSBs, brands and sizes.[18,55] The pass-through increased by between 25.8% (for cases of cans) and 33.3% (for 2-liter bottles) for each mile of distance from the closest rival store selling untaxed SSBs.[18] The SSB tax implemented in Seattle provides another example of a tax applied in a small jurisdiction. After the first year of implementation, the pass-through rate was 59% ranging from 55% for family-size products to 66% for individual-size products.[11]

Non-alcoholic beverages can be considered highly differentiated products (i.e., differentiating from each other in terms of taste and quality) and multi-product firms use portfolio pricing strategies to optimise revenues by accounting for likely substitutions across products.[56,57]

A post hoc study after the introduction of the French soda tax in January 2012, estimated that consumer prices increased gradually. Six months after its introduction, the tax was fully shifted to soda prices (representing the vast majority — 75% — of the total supermarket sales of non-alcoholic beverages) while about 94% and 62% of the tax was passed through to consumers for fruit drinks and flavoured waters, respectively, but with a high degree of heterogeneity across retailers and brands. Taxes on private labels and small producers' brands were generally over-shifted while they were under-shifted for large producers' brands.[7] Private label products generally have lower prices and combining this with the higher pass-through, suggest that the low-income households might be impacted the most by the soda tax in France.[7]

These results (not over-shifting) can be explained by the elasticity of demand for non-alcoholic beverages which is estimated to be significantly larger than 1 (see Chapter 3 for more evidence on price elasticity of demand). Products with the larger price elasticity and easier to substitute (i.e., water), have the lowest level of pass-through. While it is more difficult to substitute fruit drinks as pure fruit juices are significantly more expensive than taxed fruit drinks and no real substitute exists for sodas.

The rate of pass-through can also vary across different types of retailers. In France, there are two main retailing groups and there is fierce price competition between them based on low price, which can explain the low pass-through rate in big retailers versus smaller ones.[7]

Differences in tax pass-through across different types of retailers have also been shown after the introduction of a fat tax in Denmark[58] and the pass-through of SSB taxes was higher for products sold in stores than those sold in restaurants in Boulder, Colorado.[59]

There is not much evidence available on the changes in **marketing strategies** after the introduction or increase of SSB taxes, but it is likely that firms use advertising strategies or increase the frequency of sale prices (coupons, discounts) in order to increase consumption or keep it at the same level after changes in prices as shown in the case of alcohol taxes.[1] One example from Mexico shows that after the implementation of the soda tax, industries responded with aggressive in-store promotions and marketing.[54]

4.5.1. Impact of tax structures on prices

Taxes on food and non-alcoholic beverages can be structured as either specific, volume-based taxes (e.g. per litre), or content-based taxes (e.g. per gram of sugar) or value-based taxes (i.e. as a % of the price). The level of pass-through varies based on the size and structure of the tax and some tax designs can also incentivise product reformulation.

Ad valorem taxes may incentivise consumers to switch to cheaper alternatives (brand down-switching) as in the case of the Barbados SSB tax. Evidence shows that the Mexico SSB tax (specific) was more fully passed on to price than the Barbados tax (ad valorem).[60]

In France, a modelling study preceding the implementation of the soda tax, predicted an over-shift of 7% to 33% for a specific duty on soft drinks, while an equivalent ad valorem tax would be under-shifted by 10–40%.[57] The same was shown for a possible tax on saturated fat in the United Kingdom, leading to the conclusion that a specific rate excise tax would reduce saturated fat purchases more, and generate more substitution, than an ad valorem tax.[56]

Specific taxes based on the ingredients rather than whole products incentivise producers to reformulate their products to reduce the concentration of the taxed ingredient. Therefore, the overall impact of ingredient-specific taxes, like sugar-based taxes, is more difficult to predict, as firms simultaneously must decide how to change the product content as well as pricing. The level of tax pass-through may incentivise consumers to shift to lower sugar products, but sugar intake reductions may also occur regardless of consumers changing their beverage intake if industries reformulate their products.

As recommended by WHO, several countries have introduced SSB taxes based on their sugar content.[61]

Recently implemented taxes in the United Kingdom and in the Republic of Ireland are two-tier taxes, with a lower tax for less caloric beverages and a higher rate for more caloric ones. This design incentivises consumers to substitute less caloric drinks for more caloric ones and incentivises manufacturers to decrease the calorie content of their beverages to move to a lower tax band as explained in the case study associated to this chapter.

Another example of products reformulation after the implementation of a health tax comes from Hungary. In 2011, Hungary introduced the public health product tax — a tax levied on food products containing unhealthy levels of sugar, salt and other ingredients. This led many manufacturers to reduce or eliminate those ingredients in their products and consumers to switch to healthier substitutes. After one year from the implementation, approximately 40% of food manufacturers changed their product formulas to either reduce or eliminate the taxed ingredients (28% and 12%, respectively).[62]

South Africa also implemented an SSB tax based on sugar content at a rate of around 0.15 US cents for each gram of sugar over an initial threshold of 4 g/100 mL. While the sugar content remained unchanged for prominent brands and was accompanied by less than full pass-through, other industries responded to the tax increase by reformulating their products as well as increasing their price.[8]

4.6. Conclusion

In this chapter, we have presented theoretical arguments and empirical evidence to illustrate the types of responses that businesses most directly affected by health taxes can be expected to deploy. Those responses are of great importance for fiscal and health policymakers in the planning and management of new and existing taxes. Business responses have the potential to augment or hinder the effect of taxes on the consumption of taxed products, and ultimately on health, while they have a more limited influence on tax revenues.

A key dimension of business responses to health taxes is the degree to which taxes are transferred onto the prices faced by consumers or tax pass-through. If pass-through is limited or null, consumer behaviours are unlikely to be swayed by the tax. If, on the other hand, pass-through is high, full or even greater than one (price increase larger than the tax) consumers are likely to respond to the tax by reducing their consumption of the taxed products, even when their price sensitivity (elasticity) is low.

The evidence presented in this chapter shows that key drivers of pass-through include strategic behaviours of manufacturers and retailers (production and marketing strategies, particularly for multi-product firms), market structure (especially the degree of concentration of a market) and relative supply and demand elasticities.[52,57] However, we have also emphasised that the systematic application of health taxes on specific products causes the markets for those products to adapt and evolve in directions that are not neutral to the health impact of taxes.

Some of the market characteristics that are conducive to high pass-through rates, namely a price-inelastic demand and high levels of market concentration, are common in the markets typically targeted by health taxes. In this chapter, we discuss how applying health taxes pushes those markets towards even higher levels of concentration and often towards product differentiation. The latter is a strategy that serves several purposes. It is a way for firms to segment a market, expand their customer base but also sometimes increase their market power in specific segments. When this happens, firms can be expected to behave as if they were operating in a concentrated market, passing taxes through to consumers to a large extent. Product differentiation also allows firms to avoid losing customers who engage in product substitutions because of price increases, by offering substitutes to taxed products in addition to the taxed products themselves. This too goes in the direction of increasing tax pass-through. However, firms that have a differentiated portfolio of products have the option of redistributing price increases across a range of products, taxed and not taxed, if this proves to be the best way to optimise their profit margins.[56,57] A similar behaviour may make the tax less effective in reducing the consumption of the taxed products. To prevent the adverse consequences of such portfolio pricing strategies on the effectiveness of health taxes, governments need to carefully consider the nature of the firms that operate in the relevant markets, and they need to set the tax base (range of products subject to the tax) to include, if possible, products that those firms might use in a strategic pricing response.

Strategic firm behaviours may also be driven by features of tax design and by the type of jurisdiction to which they apply. In this chapter, we have discussed, for instance, how specific and ad valorem excise taxes create different incentives for tax pass-through, and how a tiered rate structure may lead to changes in product characteristics,[40] including product reformulation, also discussed in a special focus associated with this chapter. Taxes applied in small jurisdictions, where they can more easily be avoided by consumers, lead to competitive pressures to keep prices low and to reduced levels of tax pass-through. These considerations underscore the importance of a careful tax design (discussed in detail in Chapter 8), as well as wider control over marketing strategies (advertising and promotions), and potentially price regulation measures in addition to health taxes, to maximise the health benefits of taxes. An appropriate tax design has the potential to prevent, or counter the effects of, most unwarranted firm responses to health taxes. However, fiscal policymakers need to avoid designs that would unduly increase the complexity of tax administration and enforcement.

Governments cannot be expected to comprehensively predict responses by business players at the tax design stage. But it is of paramount importance that governments are aware of the range of possible responses and monitor closely the impacts of taxes as well as the characteristics of the markets in which they are applied. Regularly adjusting the design of health taxes is important to ensure their effectiveness is not hindered by changes in market structure and strategic responses.

Key messages

- Strategic behaviour of industry affects how health taxes are passed on to consumers. Depending on how the tax is designed, the impact can either hinder or promote health (e.g. through changes in product formulation and marketing).
- Health taxes are usually passed on to consumers in three fundamental ways: (a) full pass-through where the tax hike translates into an equivalent price increase; (b) undershifted where the price increase is less than the tax increase and (c) overshifted where the price increase is more than the tax increase.
- The degree of pass-through depends on the industry structure. The degree of pass-through is higher in more concentrated markets and for products with a very price-inelastic demand. Pass-through is reduced when more opportunities exist for tax avoidance.
- Multi-product firms operating in dominant market positions as well as larger retailers are likely to favour high pass-through rates even in the presence of a less inelastic demand as they can offer substitute products to consumers.
- Features of tax design can have a major influence on industry responses, including tax pass-through. A thorough understanding and clear foresight of possible responses are necessary for the design of effective health taxes.

References

1. Blecher E. Taxes on tobacco, alcohol and sugar sweetened beverages: Linkages and lessons learned. *Social Science & Medicine*. 2015; 136–137: 175–179.
2. White JS, Ross H. Smokers' strategic responses to sin taxes: Evidence from panel data in Thailand. *Health Economics*. 2015; 24(2): 127–141.
3. Cawley J, Frisvold D, Hill A, Jones D. Oakland's sugar-sweetened beverage tax: Impacts on prices, purchases and consumption by adults and children. *Economics and Human Biology*. 2020; 37: 100865.

4. Gilmore AB, Tavakoly B, Taylor G, Reed H. Understanding tobacco industry pricing strategy and whether it undermines tobacco tax policy: The example of the UK cigarette market. *Addiction.* 2013; 108(7): 1317–1326.
5. Shang C, Lee HM, Chaloupka FJ, et al. Association between tax structure and cigarette consumption: Findings from the International Tobacco Control Policy Evaluation (ITC) Project. *Tobacco Control.* 2019; 28: s31–s36.
6. Ally AK, et al. Alcohol tax pass-through across the product and price range: Do retailers treat cheap alcohol differently? *Addiction.* 2014; 109(12): 1994–2002.
7. Berardi N, et al. The impact of a 'Soda tax' on prices. Evidence from French micro data. *Applied Economics.* 2016; 48(41): 3976–3994.
8. Stacey N, Mudara C, Ng SW, van Walbeek C, Hofman K, Edoka I. Sugar-based beverage taxes and beverage prices: Evidence from South Africa's Health Promotion Levy. *Social Science & Medicine.* 2019; 238: 112465.
9. Colchero MA, Salgado JC, Unar-Munguía M, Molina M, Ng S, Rivera-Dommarco JA. Changes in prices after an excise tax to sweetened sugar beverages was implemented in Mexico: Evidence from urban areas. *PLoS One.* 2015; 10(12): e0144408.
10. Russell C, van Walbeek C. How does a change in the excise tax on beer impact beer retail prices in South Africa? *South African Journal of Economics.* 2016; 84: 555–573.
11. Powell LM, Leider J. The impact of Seattle's sweetened beverage tax on beverage prices and volume sold. *Economics and Human Biology.* 2020; 37: 100856.
12. Powell LM, Leider J, Léger PT. The impact of the Cook County, IL, sweetened beverage tax on beverage prices. *Economics and Human Biology.* 2020; 37: 100855.
13. Bergman UM, Hansen NL. Are excise taxes on beverages fully passed through to prices? The Danish evidence. *Finanzarchiv.* 2019; 75(4): 323–356.
14. Schmacker R, Smed S. Do prices and purchases respond similarly to soft drink tax increases and cuts? *Economics and Human Biology.* 2020; 37: 100864.
15. Chiou L, Muehlegger EJ. Consumer response to cigarette excise tax changes. HKS Faculty Research Working Paper Series, RWP10-020, John F. Kennedy School of Government, Harvard University, Cambridge; 2010.
16. Harding M, Leibtag E, Lovenheim MF. "The heterogeneous geographic and socioeconomic incidence of cigarette taxes: Evidence from Nielsen Homescan data." *American Economic Journal: Economic Policy.* 2012; 4(4): 169–198.
17. Nelson JP, Moran JR. Effects of alcohol taxation on prices: A systematic review and meta-analysis of pass-through rates. *The B.E. Journal of Economic Analysis & Policy.* 2019; 20(1): 1–21.
18. Cawley J, Frisvold D. The pass-through of taxes on sugar-sweetened beverages to retail prices: The case of Berkeley, California. *Journal of Policy Analysis and Management.* 2017; 36: 303–326.
19. Cawley J, Thow AM, Wen K, Frisvold D. The economics of taxes on sugar-sweetened beverages: A review of the effects on prices, sales, cross-border shopping, and consumption. *Annual Review of Nutrition.* 2019; 39: 317–338.

20. Castelló JV, Casasnovas GJ. Impact of SSB taxes on sales. *Economics and Human Biology.* 2020; 36: 100821.
21. Griffith R, O'Connell M, Smith K, Stroud R. "The evidence on the effects of soft drink taxes." IFS Briefing Note BN255, The Institute for Fiscal Studies; 2019, https://ifs.org.uk/uploads/BN255-the-evidence-on-the-effects-of-soft-drink-taxes.pdf.
22. Mackay JL, Eriksen MP. The tobacco atlas. World Health Organization; 2002, https://apps.who.int/iris/handle/10665/42580.
23. Cisneros Örnberg J, Ólafsdóttir H. How to sell alcohol? Nordic alcohol monopolies in a changing epoch. *Nordic Studies on Alcohol and Drugs.* 2008; 25(2): 129–153.
24. Goodchild M, Zheng R. Early assessment of China's 2015 tobacco tax increase. *Bulletin of the World Health Organization.* 2018; 96(7): 506–512.
25. Hanafy K, Saleh ASE, Elmallah MEBE, Omar HMA, Bakr D, Chaloupka FJ. *The Economics of Tobacco and Tobacco Taxation in Egypt.* Paris: International Union Against Tuberculosis and Lung Disease; 2010.
26. Rabinovich L, et al. *Further Study on the Affordability of Alcoholic Beverages in the EU.* Cambridge, RAND Europe; 2012.
27. Chaloupka FJ, et al. "Tax, price and cigarette smoking: Evidence from the tobacco documents and implications for tobacco company marketing strategies." *Tobacco Control.* 2002; 11(Suppl. I): i62–i72.
28. Brock B, et al. Tobacco product prices before and after a state wide tobacco tax increase. *Tobacco Control.* 2016; 25(2): 166–173.
29. Keeler TE, et al. "Do cigarette producers price-discriminate by state? An empirical analysis of local cigarette pricing and taxation." *Journal of Health Economics.* 1996; 15(4): 499–512.
30. Linegar DJ, van Walbeek C. The effect of excise tax increases on cigarette prices in South Africa. *Tobacco Control.* 2018; 27(1): 65–71.
31. Nargis N, et al. Tobacco industry pricing undermines tobacco tax policy: A tale from Bangladesh. *Preventive Medicine.* 2020; 132: 105991.
32. Juárez B, Thrasher JF, Reynales Shigematsu LM, Hernández Ávila M, Chaloupka FJ. Tax, price and cigarette brand preferences: A longitudinal study of adult smokers from the ITC Mexico Survey. *Tobacco Control.* 2014; 23 Suppl 1(01): i80–i85.
33. WHO (World Health Organization). *WHO Technical Manual on Tobacco Tax Administration.* World Health Organization; 2010. https://apps.who.int/iris/handle/10665/44316.
34. Hiscock R, Branston JR, McNeill A, et al. Tobacco industry strategies undermine government tax policy: Evidence from commercial data. *Tobacco Control.* 2018; 27: 488–497.
35. Ross H, Tesche J, Vellios N. Undermining government tax policies: Common legal strategies employed by the tobacco industry in response to tobacco tax increases. *Preventive Medicine.* 2017; 105S: S19–S22.

36. DeCicca P, Kenkel D, Liu F. "Who pays cigarette taxes? The impact of consumer price search." NBER Working Paper, March; 2010.
37. Delipalla S, O'Donnell D. Estimating tax incidence, market power and market conduct: The European cigarette industry. *International Journal of Industrial Organization.* 2001; 19: 885–908.
38. Chaloupka FJ, Kostova D, Shang C. Cigarette excise tax structure and cigarette prices: Evidence from the global adult tobacco survey and the U.S. National Adult Tobacco Survey. *Nicotine & Tobacco Research.* 2014; 16(1): 1–6.
39. Shang C, Chaloupka FJ, Fong GT, et al. The association between tax structure and cigarette price variability: Findings from the ITC Project. *Tobacco Control.* 2015; 24 (Suppl. 3): iii88–iii93.
40. Prasetyo BW, Adrison V. Cigarette prices in a complex cigarette tax system: Empirical evidence from Indonesia. *Tobacco Control.* 2019; 29(6): 618–623.
41. Tobacconomics. *Vietnam Country Factsheet: Tobacco Tax Structures.* Chicago: Tobacconomics; 2018.
42. Slater SJ, Chaloupka FJ, Wakefield M, Johnston LD, O'Malley PM. The impact of retail cigarette marketing practices on youth smoking uptake. *Archives of Pediatrics and Adolescent Medicine.* 2007; 161(5): 440–445.
43. Jernigan D, Ross CS. The alcohol marketing landscape: Alcohol industry size, structure, strategies, and public health responses. *Journal of Studies on Alcohol and Drugs.* 2020; Suppl. 19: 13–25.
44. Siegel M, et al. State-specific liquor excise taxes and retail prices in 8 US states. *Substance Abuse.* 2013; 34(4): 415–421.
45. Kenkel DS. Are alcohol tax hikes fully passed through to prices? Evidence from Alaska. *The American Economic Review.* 2005; 95(2): 273–277.
46. Young DJ, Bielinska-Kwapisz A. Alcohol taxes and beverage prices. *National Tax Journal* 2002; 55(1): 57–74.
47. Hunt P, Rabinovich L, and Baumberg B, Preliminary assessment of economic impacts of alcohol pricing policy options in the UK. Santa Monica, CA: RAND Corporation, 2011. https://www.rand.org/pubs/technical_reports/TR858-1.html.
48. Shang C, Ngo A, Chaloupka FJ. The pass-through of alcohol excise taxes to prices in OECD countries. *The European Journal of Health Economics.* 2020; 21(6): 855–867.
49. Wilson LB, Pryce R, Angus C, Hiscock R, Brennan A, Gillespie D. The effect of alcohol tax changes on retail prices: How do on-trade alcohol retailers pass through tax changes to consumers? *The European Journal of Health Economics.* 2021; 22(3): 381–392.
50. Shang C, Wang X, Chaloupka FJ. The association between excise tax structures and the price variability of alcoholic beverages in the United States. *PLoS One.* 2018; 13(12): e0208509.
51. Miao Z, Beghin JC, Jensen HH. "Taxing sweets: Sweetener input tax or final consumption tax?" *Contemporary Economic Policy.* 2012; 30(3): 344–361.

52. Andreyeva T, Chaloupka FJ, Brownell KD. "Estimating the potential of taxes on sugar-sweetened beverages to reduce consumption and generate revenue." *Preventive Medicine.* 2011; 52(6): 413–416.
53. Alsukait R, Wilde P, Bleich SN, Singh G, Folta SC. Evaluating Saudi Arabia's 50% carbonated drink excise tax: Changes in prices and volume sales. *Economics & Human Biology.* 2020; 38: 100868.
54. Colchero MA, Popkin BM, Rivera JA, Ng SW. Beverage purchases from stores in Mexico under the excise tax on sugar sweetened beverages: Observational study. *BMJ.* 2016; 352: h6704.
55. Falbe J, Rojas N, Grummon AH, Madsen KA. Higher retail prices of sugar-sweetened beverages 3 months after implementation of an excise tax in Berkeley, California. *American Journal of Public Health.* 2015; 105: 2194–2201.
56. Griffith R, Nesheim L, O'Connell M. "Sin taxes in differentiated product oligopoly: An application to the butter and margarine market." Working paper, November 30, 2010.
57. Bonnet C, Requillart V. "Sugar policy reform, tax policy and price transmission in the soft drink industry." Working Paper No. 4, Transparency of Food Pricing, TRANSFOP; 2012.
58. Jensen JD, Smed S. The Danish tax on saturated fat – Short run effects on consumption, substitution patterns and consumer prices of fats. *Food Policy.* 2013; 42(C): 18–31.
59. Cawley J, Crain C, Frisvold D, Jones D. The pass-through of the largest tax on sugar-sweetened beverages: The case of Boulder, Colorado NBER Working Paper No. 25050 September 2018.
60. Alvarado M, et al. Assessing the impact of the Barbados sugar-sweetened beverage tax on beverage sales: An observational study. *International Journal of Behavioral Nutrition and Physical Activity.* 2019; 16: 13.
61. WHO (World Health Organisation). *Fiscal Policies for Diet and the Prevention of Noncommunicable Diseases.* Geneva: World Health Organization; 2016.
62. WHO (World Health Organisation). *Public Health Product Tax in Hungary: An Example of Successful Intersectoral Action Using a Fiscal Tool to Promote Healthier Food Choices and Raise Revenues for Public Health; 2015.* https://www.euro.who.int/__data/assets/pdf_file/0004/287095/Good-practice-brief-public-health-product-tax-in-hungary.pdf.
63. Anderson SP, de Palma A, Kreider B. "Tax incidence in differentiated product oligopoly." *Journal of Public Economics.* 2001; 81(2): 173–192.

https://doi.org/10.1142/9781800612396_0005

Special Focus 1

The UK Soft Drinks Industry Levy as an Incentive for Beverage Reformulation

Martin White*, Jean Adams*, Cherry Law†, and Peter Scarborough‡,
On behalf of the SDIL Evaluation team[a]

SF 1.1. Background, design and implementation of the SDIL

A tax on sugar-sweetened non-alcoholic beverages (soft drinks) was announced by the UK Treasury on 16th March 2016. The explicit aim of the Soft Drinks Industry Levy (SDIL) is to stimulate changes in industry behaviour and to reduce the sugar content of soft drinks through innovation and reformulation. The SDIL is a tax on manufacturers and importers of soft

* University of Cambridge, UK.

† London School of Hygiene & Tropical Medicine, UK.

‡ University of Oxford, UK.

[a] The evaluation of the SDIL reported in this chapter has been funded by the UK National Institute of Health Research, Public Health Research Programme (Grant numbers PHR 16/49/01 and 16/130/01). Martin White and Jean Adams were also supported by the Medical Research Council (grant numbers grant Nos MC_UU_12015/6 and MC_UU_00006/7). The team comprises Martin White (chief investigator); Jean Adams, Adam Briggs, Steven Cummins, Richard Harrington, Oliver Mytton, Michael Rayner, Harry Rutter, Peter Scarborough, Richard Smith (co-investigators); Linda Cobiac, Marcus Keogh-Brown, Cherry Law, David Pell, Catrin Penn-Jones, Tarra Penney, Nina Rodgers, Henning Tarp-Jensen, Dolly Theis (project staff).

Table SF1.1. Structure of the UK Soft Drinks Industry Levy.

	Sugar concentration (g/100 mL)	**Levy rate (£/L)**
Higher levy tier	≥8	0.24
Lower levy tier	≥5 and <8	0.18
No levy tier	<5	0.00 (no levy)

drinks in tiers according to the sugar concentration of drinks (Table SF1.1). Companies manufacturing or importing <1 million litres of eligible drinks per year are exempt from the levy, as are milk-based drinks, pure fruit juices, drinks sold as powders and drinks containing >0.5% alcohol by volume.

The SDIL was implemented on 1st April 2018. The 2-year delay between announcement and implementation allowed time for businesses to respond. From June 2016, there was a period of public consultation, after which the levy design was finalised and then passed into law in the Finance Bill of May 2017.[1]

The introduction of the SDIL followed a lengthy period of growing concern among government, civil society and professionals about the extent and continuing rise of excess body weight and poor diet among the British population. The emergence of a national obesity epidemic from the late 1980s onwards led to a series of government obesity strategies (13 in total from 1992 to 2015),[2] the establishment of a National Obesity Observatory, which later became part of Public Health England, a government agency established in 2013 and a number of government enquiries.

These actions were increasingly encouraged by a growing and vocal advocacy coalition, which latterly found a celebrity champion in Jamie Oliver (television chef and entrepreneur). Oliver's September 2015 television documentary 'Sugar Rush' called for a tax on sugary drinks and Oliver successfully introduced a 10 pence levy on soft drinks in 37 of his own restaurants.[3]

In May 2015, the World Health Organization (WHO) recommended taxation of SSBs to reduce sugar consumption as an effective intervention to curtail the modifiable risk factors for non-communicable diseases

(NCDs).[4,5] This recommendation was endorsed by the UK government's Scientific Advisory Committee on Nutrition (SACN) (July 2015),[6] the House of Commons Health Select Committee (October 2015)[7] and Public Health England's Sugar Reduction: the evidence for action (October 2015).[8]

Excess consumption of calorie-dense foods and beverages containing high levels of free sugars contributes to the burden of NCDs. Further, epidemiological evidence increasingly shows that sugar in liquid form is uniquely dangerous for health, given its association with obesity and incidence of type 2 diabetes.[9,10] Simulation studies have strengthened arguments for reducing sugar consumption by modelling the impacts of SSB taxes.[11–13] Nevertheless, the announcement of the SDIL in early 2016 came as a surprise to many, given repeated indications by senior representatives of the UK Government that such a measure would not be considered.

Following the announcement of the SDIL in 2016, there was an immediate negative reaction from the UK soft drinks industry in the public media and trade press. This rhetoric played out over the year as the public consultation continued and Government prepared to legislate, with warnings of severe economic impacts forecasted. Once the SDIL became law, the tone of the media discourse changed, appearing instead to reassure industry stakeholders that any damage or repercussions for industry resulting from the SDIL could be mitigated and that industry was supportive of government efforts to improve health.[14]

SF 1.2. Planning an evaluation

An independent evaluation of the SDIL was funded by the UK National Institute for Health Research (NIHR). The evaluation considered the SDIL as a series of events within a complex adaptive system. It sought to assess how the SDIL might affect a wide range of potential economic, social and health-related outcomes and to model potential future impacts. Initial theorisation of the potential impacts across sectors drew on established theory in relation to economics, population interventions and systems thinking and by reviewing evidence from evaluation and modelling studies of other SSB taxes. This led to the development of an initial conceptual map of the system, including potential impacts and hypothesised causal pathways. Consensus on this was sought through dialogue with key stakeholders in interviews and an online Delphi study, leading to a final concept map.[15] This enabled the development of hypotheses concerning multiple potential impacts of the SDIL, both intended and unintended, and their pathways of action. Identification of the data available to test these hypotheses then led to the design of a pragmatic set of evaluative studies, mostly using routinely available data and natural experimental designs.[16]

SF 1.3. Impacts on sugar content, price and package sizes of soft drinks

A key initial analysis explored the effects of the SDIL on sugar concentration in drinks. The study analysed data on the full range of soft drinks on offer in UK supermarkets from 2015 to 2019, exploring changes in formulation, distinguishing independent branded and supermarket branded drinks. A controlled interrupted time series design assessed changes in levy-eligible (intervention) compared to ineligible (control) drinks in a total of 209,637 observations of soft drinks available on UK supermarket shelves over 85 weekly time points between September 2015 and February 2019. Observed trends in sugar concentration were compared with the counterfactual of predicted proportion of drinks over the lower levy threshold, modelled from pre-intervention trends.[17]

From the announcement in 2016 there was a gradual, but accelerating trend in reduction of the proportion of drinks on sale that were over the lower levy threshold (5 g/100 mL sugar). There was then a substantial step change in this proportion at the time of implementation, followed by a continuing downward trend, such that by 11 months post-implementation (February 2019) the proportion of intervention drinks over the lower levy sugar threshold had reduced from 51.7 (95% confidence interval: 50.9 to 52.6%) pre-announcement to 15.4% (14.8 to 15.9%), a fall of 33.8 (33.3 to 34.4) percentage points. There was little evidence of any impact of the announcement or implementation of the SDIL on the proportion of

Fig. SF1.1. Changes in proportion of soft drinks over the lower levy sugar threshold, September 2015–February 2019.

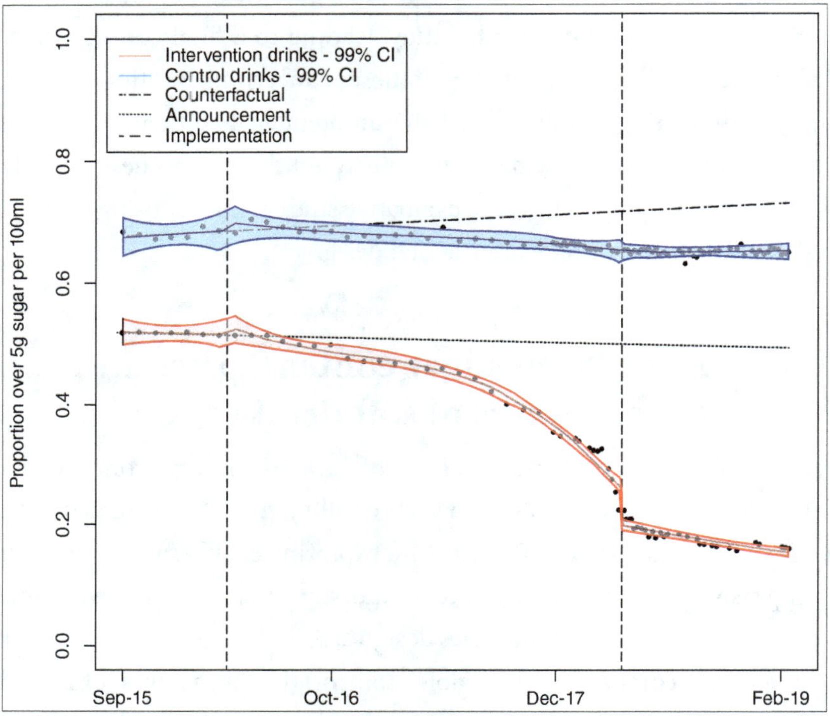

control category (non-eligible) drinks with sugar concentrations over the lower levy threshold (Figure SF1.1).[17]

Figure SF1.2 shows how the distribution of the sugar concentration of soft drinks on supermarket shelves changed from before the announcement of the SDIL to after implementation. Drinks are colour-coded by levy tier. Pre-announcement, there were peaks in the distribution at 0 and 11 g/100 mL, representing sugar-free and market leading higher levy tier drinks, respectively. After implementation, the zero sugar category grew by about 20%, new peaks appeared just below the 5 g/100 mL and 8 g/100 mL levy thresholds and the proportion of drinks in the higher levy tier decreased substantially, albeit with a peak remaining at 11 g/100 mL.[17]

The SDIL was not primarily designed to be a tax on consumers, with manufacturers and importers expected either to pay the levy or produce

Fig. SF1.2. Distribution of SDIL-eligible soft drinks available in UK supermarkets by sugar concentration, pre-announcement and post-implementation of the SDIL.

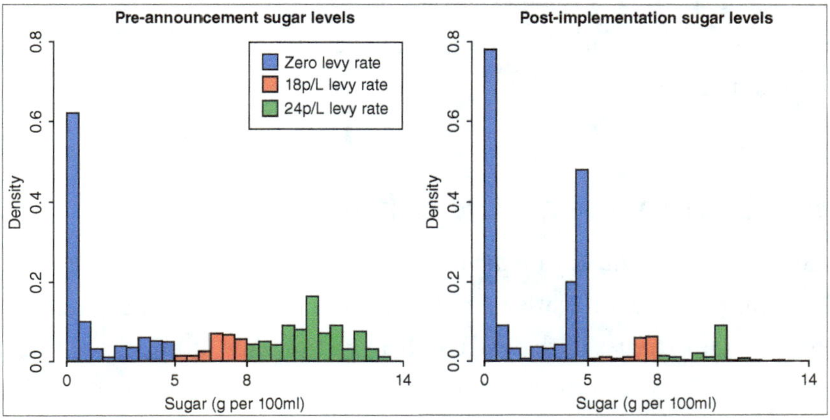

drinks with a lower sugar content to avoid paying the levy. However, it was hypothesised that some manufacturers would not reformulate or introduce new lower sugar alternatives, but seek other ways to mitigate the cost of the tax to their business. We hypothesised they may do this by, for example, passing on some or all of the cost of the levy to consumers, innovating and diversifying their market offer to increase profits, or by changing package sizes and prices of their existing offerings, or by additional marketing or a combination of this diverse range of tactics.

Higher levy tier drinks had an average pre-implementation price of £2.51/L (2.403 to 2.622), which increased by £0.075/L post-implementation, representing a +31 (+15 to +48) % pass-through rate for the tax in this category of drinks. In contrast, lower levy tier drinks had an average pre-implementation price of £3.193/L (3.058 to 3.334) and this reduced by £0.107 (0.06 to 0.153) post-implementation, representing a pass-through rate of −50 (−85 to −33) %.

Higher levy tier drinks increased in package volume by an average of only 1 (−15 to 17) mL from before to after implementation of the tax. Lower levy tier drinks, however, increased in volume by an average of 13 (3 to 23) mL.

Underlying these average changes in sugar concentration, price and package sizes of soft drinks lay some differences in individual brands, and independent versus supermarket products, which suggest strategies specific to different market niches were adopted that require further detailed investigation.[17]

SF 1.4. Impacts on the soft drinks industry

Analysis of early industry media discourse concerning the SDIL suggested that it might have a negative impact on industry and thus the national economy. Our studies of the SDIL to date have looked at business impacts in two ways. First, a study examined the effects of the announcement of the SDIL, and subsequent events, on the share prices of the soft drink companies listed on the London Stock Exchange using event study methodology.[18] This found that, although there were some small, daily abnormal stock market returns[b] on the day of the announcement (16th March 2018) and the following day — less than a 4% loss of value altogether — share prices quickly returned to normal such that overall, share prices continued to rise over the following year. Thus, while the SDIL announcement was initially perceived as detrimental news by the market, negative stock returns were short-lived, indicating a lack of major concern by shareholders. There was no evidence of a negative stock market reaction to the two subsequent announcements: release of draft legislation on 5th December 2016 and confirmation of the tax rates on 8th March 2017.[18]

The second study looked at the value of soft drinks manufactured in the United Kingdom that is for domestic sales. Using interrupted time series methods, the analysis examined whether and how domestic turnover of UK soft drinks manufacturers changed after the announcement and the implementation of the SDIL, using data from 2010 to 2019.[19] Overall,

[b] Percentage change in daily share price — the difference between actual % changes in daily share price minus the predicted % change in share price under normal fluctuation.

there was a statistically significant impact on both the level (−5.6%) and trend (−0.5%) of domestic turnover in the 2-year period between the SDIL announcement and implementation (2016–2018). The results thus showed evidence of a short-term, negative impact of the SDIL announcement, but this effect did not continue post-implementation. The findings suggest that manufacturers were, to a large extent, able to mitigate the effects of the levy before it came into effect. Thus, downturns in soft drink manufacturers' domestic sales likely reflected inward investment in reformulation and other activities in response to the levy.[19]

SF 1.5. Conclusions and implications

The SDIL was designed as a fiscal policy aiming to change industry behaviour by bringing about reduction in the sugar content of soft drinks to improve population health. Although evaluation of health impacts is forthcoming (further studies of impacts on purchasing and dietary consumption of soft drinks, dental caries and obesity, as well as modelling longer term impacts on morbidity and mortality, quality of life and costs-effectiveness are in progress),[16] findings to date suggest that the levy is achieving the intended aim.

Despite bleak forecasts by the soft drinks industry at the time of the announcement of the SDIL, the announcement and implementation of the SDIL do not appear to have had substantial or lasting negative impacts on businesses, albeit companies appear to have had to invest to change their offers to consumers in order to successfully mitigate the effects of the tax. This suggests the SDIL is beneficial for population health and neutral for industry.

Consideration of the SDIL as a series of events in a complex system (or set of interrelated complex systems) has enabled evaluators to hypothesise a wide range of potential impacts of the levy across sectors. From this, an evaluation that captures these diverse impacts has been designed in order to gain a balanced understanding of the health and economic effects associated with the SDIL. This provides a promising approach to evaluation that may be useful to assess the impacts of future health taxes and other public health interventions.

References

1. HM Treasury. The Soft Drinks Industry Levy Regulations 2018. London: HM Treasury; 2018. http://www.legislation.gov.uk/uksi/2018/41/contents/made (accessed 31/07/2020). [Available from: http://www.legislation.gov.uk/uksi/2018/41/contents/made accessed 18th May 2018.]
2. Theis DRZ, White M. Is obesity policy in England fit for purpose? Analysis of government strategies and policies, 1992–2020. *The Milbank Quarterly*. DOI: https://doi.org/10.1111/1468-0009.12498.
3. Cornelsen L, Mytton OT, Adams J, et al. Change in non-alcoholic beverage sales following a 10-pence levy on sugar-sweetened beverages within a national chain of restaurants in the UK: Interrupted time series analysis of a natural experiment. *Journal of Epidemiology and Community Health*. 2017; 71(11): 1107–1112.
4. World Health Organisation. Tackling NCDs: 'Best buys' and other recommended interventions for the prevention and control of noncommunicable diseases, 2017. https://apps.who.int/iris/handle/10665/259232.
5. Waqanivalu T, Nederveen L, Oppong D, et al. Fiscal Policies for Diet and Prevention of Noncommunicable Diseases. Technical Meeting Report, 5–6 May 2015. Geneva, Switzerland: World Health Organization; 2016.
6. Scientific Advisory Committee on Nutrition. Carbohydrates and Health. London: Public Health England; 2015.
7. House of Commons Health Committee. Childhood Obesity – Brave and Bold Action. London: House of Commons; 2015.
8. Tedstone A, Targett V, Allen R. Sugar Reduction: The Evidence for Action. London: Public Health England; 2015.
9. Imamura F, O'Connor L, Ye Z, et al. Consumption of sugar sweetened beverages, artificially sweetened beverages, and fruit juice and incidence of type 2 diabetes: Systematic review, meta-analysis, and estimation of population attributable fraction. *BMJ*. 2015; 351. https://www.bmj.com/content/351/bmj.h3576. DOI: https://doi.org/10.1136/bmj.h3576.
10. Xi B, Huang Y, Reilly KH, et al. Sugar-sweetened beverages and risk of hypertension and CVD: A dose-response meta-analysis. *The British Journal of Nutrition*. 2015; 113(5): 709–717.
11. Briggs ADM, Mytton OT, Madden D, et al. The potential impact on obesity of a 10% tax on sugar-sweetened beverages in Ireland, an effect assessment modelling study. *BMC Public Health 13*, 2013; 860. https://doi.org/10.1186/1471-2458-13-860.
12. Briggs ADM, Mytton OT, Tiffin R, et al. Overall and income specific effect on prevalence of overweight and obesity of 20% sugar sweetened drink tax in UK:

Econometric and comparative risk assessment modelling study. *BMJ.* 2013; 347(October): 1–17.

13. Mytton O. Time for a sugary drinks tax in the UK? *Journal of Public Health.* 2015; 37(1): 24–25. https://doi.org/10.1093/pubmed/fdu033.
14. Penney T, Adams J, White M. LB4 Industry reactions to the UK soft drinks industry levy: unpacking the evolving discourse from announcement to implementation. *J Epidemiol Community Health,* 2018; 72: A43. https://jech.bmj.com/content/72/Suppl_1/A43.1.info.
15. Penney TP, Adams JM, Briggs ADM, Cummins SJ, Harrington R, Monsivais P, Mytton O, Rayner M, Rutter H, Scarborough P, Smith R, White M. Evaluation of the impacts on health of the proposed UK industry levy on sugar sweetened beverages: developing a systems map and data platform, and collection of baseline and early impact data. NIHR Public Health Research Programme – Rapid Review Report. *Southampton: National Institute for Health Research,* 2017. (https://njl-admin.nihr.ac.uk/document/download/2010910). *PLoS One (Under Review).*
16. White M, Cummins S, Rayner M, et al. Evaluation of the health impacts of the UK Treasury Soft Drinks Industry Levy (SDIL). Protocol. [ISRCTN: 18042742]. Southampton: NIHR Public Health Research Programme. https://njl-admin.nihr.ac.uk/document/download/2010886 (accessed 13th July 2018); 2017.
17. Scarborough P, Adhikari V, Harrington RA, et al. Impact of the announcement and implementation of the UK Soft Drinks Industry Levy on sugar content, price, product size and number of available soft drinks in the UK, 2015-19: Controlled interrupted time series analysis [ISRCTN18042742]. *PLoS Med.* 2019; 17(2): e1003025.
18. Law C, Cornelsen L, Adams J, et al. An analysis of the stock market reaction to the announcements of the UK Soft Drinks Industry Levy. *Economics and Human Biology.* 2020b; 38: 100834.
19. Law C, Cornelsen L, Adams J, et al. The impact of UK soft drinks industry levy on manufacturers' domestic turnover. *Economics and Human Biology.* 2020a; 37: 100866.

https://doi.org/10.1142/9781800612396_0006

Chapter 5

The Labour Market Impact of Health Taxes

Sarah Mounsey*, Lisa M Powell†, and Frank J Chaloupka†

Health taxes are used worldwide to reduce unhealthy consumption of specified products. However, policymakers can be hesitant to introduce or increase health taxes due to claims from industry of negative labour impacts and economic downturn, particularly in lower-income contexts. We provide an in-depth synthesis of the global literature to evaluate these claims across the labour market spectrum. We ground the evidence around a comprehensive conceptual framework and describe the foundation from which labour market characteristics drive direct and indirect industry employment and how health taxes interact with these features. We draw on empirical and modelled evidence to critically illustrate the labour impact outcomes of these interactions across the affected sectors. We first focus on employment impacts of health taxes, describing limitations inherent in these study methodologies. Next, we explore productivity impacts of health taxes including the losses and costs incurred from consumption of the taxed products and productivity gains from pricing policies aimed to reduce consumption of unhealthful products. The evidence suggests that affected industries can expect job losses from reduced consumption, and the economy will incur transient restructuring costs; however, consumer spending on

* University of Sydney, Australia.

† University of Illinois Chicago, USA.

other goods and services and spending of increased government tax revenue drives a sectoral shift resulting in either minimal, neutral job losses or even gains. Furthermore, the implementation of health taxes can help reverse the indirect costs to an economy from productivity losses attributable to morbidity and mortality from consumption of targeted products. It should be noted that most of the labour impacts of health taxes evidence were from industry-reported studies, which utilised inappropriate methodology showing partial, gross impacts, while the more robust studies provide no evidence of significant negative labour impacts. Further evaluations should include the potential unintended consequences of health taxes including labour market impacts.

5.1. Introduction

In this chapter, we discuss the labour impacts of health taxes in the global context. Specifically, we provide a description of general labour market features and provide the reader with a conceptual framework to navigate how health taxes are expected to interact with the labour market features for employment and productivity changes. To illustrate these mechanisms, we then draw from empirical evidence on the employment effects of health taxes and productivity changes associated with consumption of tobacco, alcohol and SSBs/energy-dense foods. Finally, we discuss health taxes and their relationship with the attainment of the sustainable development goals (SDGs).

Globally, health taxes have proved a popular and effective intervention for reducing non-communicable disease (NCD). The *WHO Report on the Global Tobacco Epidemic, 2017*[1] indicates 38 countries have endorsed and implemented tobacco taxes at the recommended level of 75% of the retail price of a pack of cigarettes; a further 62 countries have levy taxes of between 50% and 75% of the retail price and 61 countries have levy taxes between 25% and 50%.[2] The *WHO Global Status Report on Alcohol and Health (2018)*[3] indicated 95% of member countries have various excise alcohol taxes in an attempt to improve the health, social and economic harm alcohol abuse incurs. The World Bank[4,5] reported that, as of January 2020, more than 50 SSB taxes were in effect and more than 40 countries have adopted various SSB taxes nationally (also recognised as a WHO 'best buy' intervention at 20% or greater).[6] In response to tax implementation, concerns have been raised repeatedly, often by industry actors, regarding the potential negative labour impacts.[7,8] In order to determine the validity of these concerns, we describe the foundation from which labour market characteristics drive industry employment and how health taxes interact with these features.

Jobs in tobacco, alcohol and sugar industries may be created *directly* (e.g. agricultural – farming of tobacco, vineyards or sugar) – and with immediate effect – or *indirectly*. That is, indirectly by other sectors providing input to the manufacturing component of the products' supply chain (e.g. chemicals, machinery), the value-add of the raw product (e.g. cigarettes, alcoholic beverages or SSBs/energy-dense foods), or selling the end products (e.g. retail, hospitability, trade).[9] *Indirect* employment can also be generated through service sectors impacted by the direct consumption of the final product (e.g. health, pharmaceuticals, dental) and its unintended consequences (e.g. cancer, liver failure, NCDs). In the case of tobacco, this can be expanded for indirect consumption (i.e. second-hand smoking and its negative health consequences). These *indirect* sectoral effects can also be immediate, but are generally considered medium-to-long term.[10] Figure 5.1 is a diagrammatic representation of the framework in which health taxes interact with employment and productivity.

Simply, increased taxes (with at least some tax pass-through to the consumer) will, depending on the price elasticity of demand of the good, lead to lower demand and therefore consumption of the taxed good. The overall impact on demand is an empirical question and depends on both the size of the tax in the given industry and the level of consumer responsiveness for a given product and context. For instance, consumer responsiveness to SSBs shows greater price elasticity than for tobacco or alcohol, which is more price inelastic. However, generally, the taxed industry will see decreased *gross*

Fig. 5.1. Assumed interactions of health taxes on overall employment and productivity.

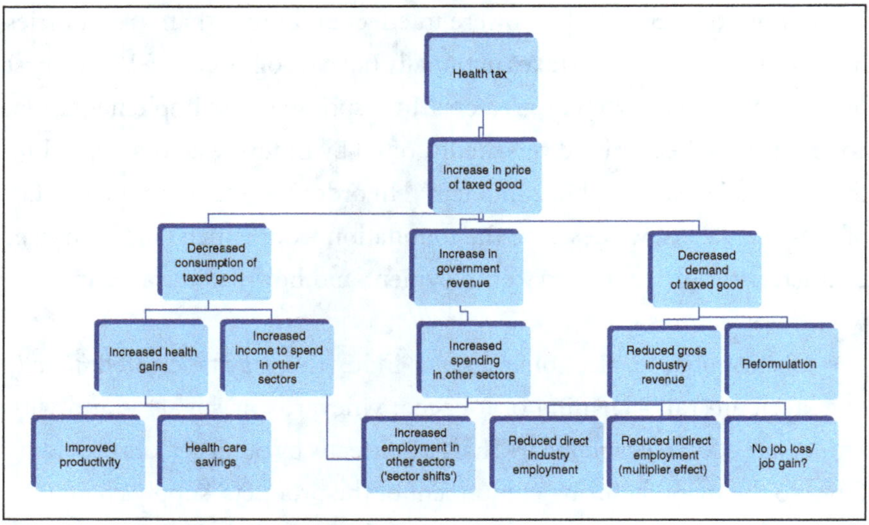

Source: Author's own (2020).

revenue and *direct* job loss. *Indirect* employment will also decrease (known as the multiplier effect, see Box 5.1). However, individuals will substitute their spending to other products and hence generate increased demand and a new revenue stream for those products. Sometimes this may be within the same industry such as in the beverage and alcohol industries through substitution to non-taxed beverages (i.e. water or low alcohol products) often produced by the same companies producing the taxed beverages and/ or through product reformulation efforts towards non-taxed lower sugar or lower alcohol beverages, thereby minimising overall reduced demand. Also, the government will generate tax revenue, introducing new spending in other sectors which will add to the increased consumer spending on other products and services. Together, this new spending creates extra demand and new employment in other sectors. As overall consumption of the taxed products decreases, revenue generated may also decrease; however, as Chaloupka et al.[11] highlight, this, for most countries, this remains a long way off. In summary, instead of employment losses and economic decline as industry suggests, the balance of spending and employment ultimately – albeit with transient restructuring costs – will shift across sectors.

In addition, and separately to the employment impacts, within this framework we can also expect health taxes to improve productivity across sectors, largely through improved health, reduced absenteeism (i.e. days absent from the workplace), reduced presenteeism (unproductive time at the workplace), reduced disability, increased life expectancy and more years of working life. With sufficiently high tax levels that induce behaviour change, these indirect benefits can offset the negative income losses caused by the taxes, particularly for low-income households, and have a largely progressive impact.[12]

Furthermore, the practice of 'earmarking' or 'hypothecation' a proportion of the revenue generated in several countries (e.g. Ecuador, Egypt, Estonia, Finland, Iceland, India, Korea, Nepal and Thailand) is a popular complementary intervention to address any potential taxation-related impacts and tobacco health-related issues. The potential to fund complementary policy mechanisms targeting alternative livelihoods for farmers, public awareness and community education programmes under such scenarios is promising and aligns with WHO recommendations of a comprehensive package of policy instruments to achieve maximum impact. In the Philippines, the 2013 reform of the tobacco tax structure saw a significant increase in the tobacco tax and consequently, the revenue generated. Included in this reform, and aligning with WHO's FCTC articles 17 and 18 (promoting alternative livelihoods for tobacco farmers), 15% of the generated revenue was 'earmarked' to 'assist tobacco farmers in planting alternative crops or implementing other livelihood projects.'[13] With nearly 40,000 tobacco farmers in the Philippines this is important, particular as nearly 20% of these farmers believe it is the only viable crop for their land.[13]

Similarly, tax revenue from SSB taxes could be used to help transition sugar farmers dependent on sugarcane farming to alternative crops or activities for income generation. We refer the reader to Chapter 9 on 'How to maximise resources for health and bolster support' for more information on earmarking of health taxes.

We will now draw on empirical evidence to illustrate the labour impact outcomes of these interactions across the affected sectors.

Box 5.1. Understanding the evidence

Employment and productivity impacts of health taxes rely largely on studies using econometric modelling methodologies which can be – and often are – separate components of a bigger analysis. For example, when determining productivity impacts, it may be necessary to first estimate the impact of multiple morbidities on mortality averted (MSLT) before a cost-effectiveness analysis (CEA) can be done; similarly, it may be necessary to analyse an input-output matrix (IOA) before extending the analysis to include multiplier effects (ME) or to extend the analysis with models like CGE or REMI which use IOA as their basis for their analysis. Below, we provide a brief overview of employment- and productivity-related methodologies.

Employment-related methodology

- **Input-output analysis (IOA)**
  IOA is a well-established economic tool comprising all production, consumption and monetary flows to (inputs) and from (outputs) discrete economic sectors for all traditional economic activity in a nation's economy. In other words, as a result of input of materials from other sectors, the (beverage) industry can sell its output, as an intermediate input product to another industry, or as a final product to families, to the government or to the external sector.[14]
  Note: IOS methodology is limited for modelling the impact of a

pricing policy as it does not incorporate consumer response (i.e. substitution to other goods and services).

- **Multiplier effects (ME)**
  A benefit of IOA is the ability to calculate employment multiplier effects (ME) or in other words, to quantify the employment impact of a pricing policy (e.g. from a health tax) on the taxed industry (e.g. tobacco) and across all industries in an economy (e.g. trade, services, agriculture).[14] For example, if an increased tobacco tax of 10% decreases employment by 2 jobs for every $150,000 lost directly through decreased tobacco production, the indirect impact on other industries related to the production of the tobacco may also decrease by say, 1 job per $150,000 lost. This makes the ME for a 10% tobacco tax 3 jobs.
- **Computable general equilibrium (CGE)**
  CGE combines economic theory with real economic data to quantify the economic impact of a policy change scenario (in this review, an increased price of SSBs). It can take into account a reduction in demand or a substitution between products. Here, comparison between no tax (baseline) and the increased tax (policy simulation) estimated what the effect of this demand change would be on the main macroeconomic variables and its sub-components as well as those on the industry level components of the economy.[15]
- **Regional Economic Models, Inc. (REMI)**
  REMI modelling incorporates IOA as a component of its modelling approach. REMI is useful for addressing what effects policies have on an economy or which project may warrant tax incentives. Impacts assessed are economic (i.e. employment, general and GDP).[15]
- **Interrupted time series analysis (ITSA)**
  ITSA is a statistical method useful for determining the initial effects of an intervention or policy when random controlled

trials (RCTs) are impractical or premature. The process involves taking multiple, repeated observations at regular intervals before and after an intervention (for this chapter, health taxes). Changes in trends after the intervention are then determined through statistical analysis.[16]

Productivity-related methodology

- **Multi-state lifetables (MSLT)**
  Life tables are well established and widely used in Public Health to provide information on life expectancy at different ages for different disease processes and therefore depicts a population's health status. However, to estimate total impact of multiple morbidities (like NCDs) 'multi-state' lifetables become a simple and appropriate methodological approach to incorporate several diseases in a lifetable while factoring in comorbidity affects. With this in mind, public health researchers can look into the effects of a preventative intervention (like health taxes) on an entire population over time.[17]
- **Cost of illness approach (COI)**
  This modelling approach has been used extensively to estimate the economic costs of smoking. Simply, the gross economic cost of an illness is divided into 'direct costs' incurred in a given year (e.g. health costs or non-health costs) and indirect costs (e.g. productivity losses in the current and future years due to disability and mortality). The sum of the direct and indirect is often expressed as a percentage of gross domestic product (GDP).[18]
- **Human capital approach (HCA)**
  Related to the estimation of indirect costs in the COI approach (above), the human capital approach (HCA) calculates the present value of labour productivity loss due to morbidity and mortality.

The HCA is considered best for reflecting the impacts of a health tax from a societal perspective.[7,19]

- **Cost-effective analysis (CEA)**
  Cost-effective analysis can be summarised as an analysis comparing the cost of alternative procedures or interventions (in this case, health taxes) with the actual or expected health gains in units of life year saved, deaths averted, cost per case cured or cost per symptom-free day. In this chapter, CEA has been combined with HCA (above) to determine increased cost-effectiveness of health taxes with productivity gains.[19,20]

5.2. Employment impacts of health taxes

The health and economic benefits of well-designed health taxes are well established. Despite the growing number of countries adopting this administratively feasible policy tool there are still policymakers who hesitate, primarily due to uncertainty around claims of job loss and economic downturn. In this section, we discuss the evidence for employment impacts of taxes on tobacco, alcohol and SSBs.

5.2.1. Effects from tobacco taxes

For decades, the tobacco industry has claimed that they play a vital role in a nation's economy. Losses to employment and income generation as well as to the significant government revenue contributions are used as leverage to influence policymakers and generate concern around the potential negative economic consequences of implementing or increasing tobacco taxes. However, for most countries, the evidence relating to tobacco control policies does not support these claims. Extensive studies dating back to the 1990s have refuted such claims and served as evidence to show the loss to productivity and increased health care costs of premature morbidity and mortality due to tobacco consumption far outweigh the economic contributions made; and, threats to job losses are greatly overstated.[21]

In other words, as the economy transitions to a non-tobacco economy, this transition will, in reality, take place over a significant period of time and therefore the impact of employment loss in the tobacco sector is reduced. Also, as our conceptual framework shows (Figure 5.1), employment would grow in other sectors of the economy, thereby offsetting tobacco-related job losses. Indeed, econometric studies around the world very clearly show that any jobs lost are offset with jobs gained but more country-specific evaluations would contribute to this evidence base.[12]

No evidence better exemplifies this impact of tobacco control policies on driving sectoral shifts than if tobacco consumption was either reduced or totally eliminated. For instance, in primary US tobacco-growing regions, over time, jobs lost through such scenarios of reduced or totally eliminated tobacco consumption would be regained in all eight of the non-tobacco regions for both scenarios (Figures 5.2 and 5.3, respectively).[22] Similar findings of net employment gains across sectors were seen in South Africa. Interestingly, this analysis made the distinction between the types of consumer spending that would occur with totally eliminating tobacco consumption through tobacco control policies: if consumers spent their money as average consumers (i.e. expenditure on day-to-day living), between 9,000 and 34,000 jobs would be created; if instead, consumers spent in a way that resembled ex-smoker's expenditure (i.e. including on luxury goods and services with the extra income), up to 50,000 jobs would be created. Finally, the authors indicated if tobacco consumption was not eliminated but reduced, 3,500 jobs would be created.[23]

Figure 5.4 shows potential net changes to employment in several other countries from reduced or completely eliminated tobacco consumption.[21] This work is particularly interesting because it shows the differences between how a tobacco economy may operate and indicates the effect tobacco control policies may have on employment based on tobacco's labour intensity. The

Fig. 5.2. Potential impact from reduced tobacco consumption in the US.

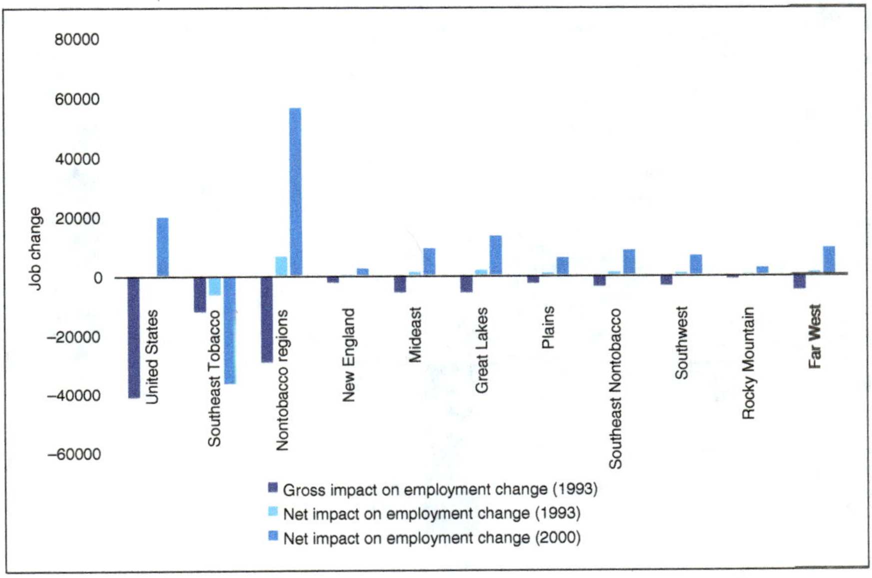

Source: Adapted from Warner et al. (1996).

Fig. 5.3. Potential impact from eliminated tobacco consumption in the US.

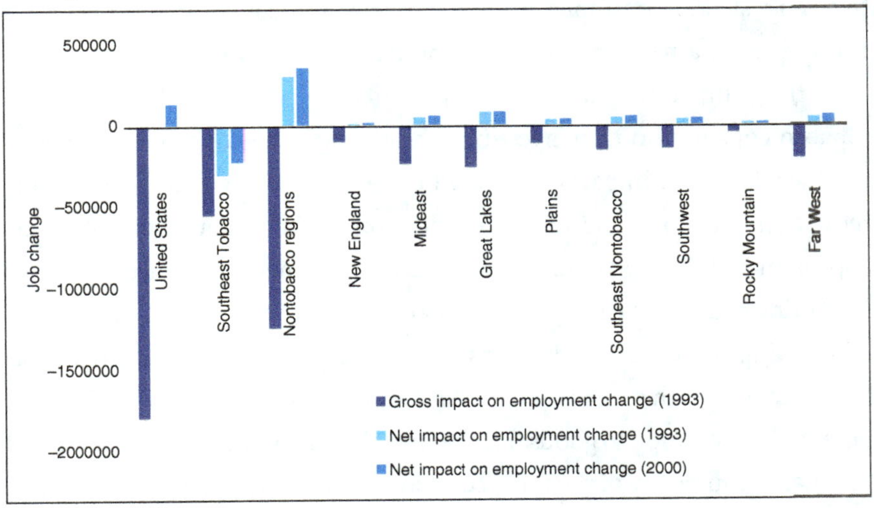

Source: Adapted from Warner et al. (1996).

Fig. 5.4. Potential employment impact from reduced tobacco consumption.

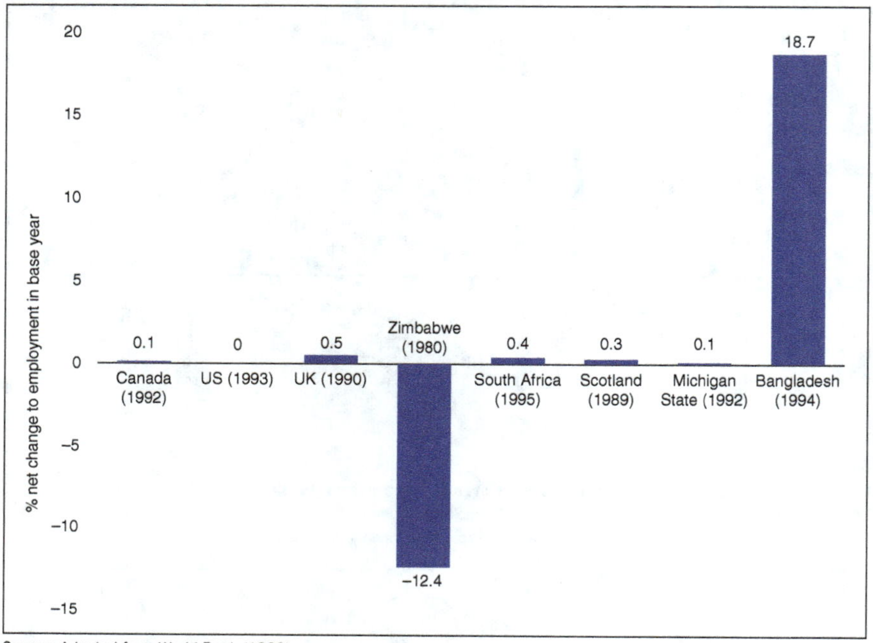

Source: Adapted from World Bank (1999).

two most striking examples in Figure 5.4 are Zimbabwe and Bangladesh. If the former, a net exporter (i.e. produces more raw tobacco for export than they consume), saw markedly reduced or even eliminated global tobacco consumption, changes in domestic cigarette consumption would not have large net impacts on overall employment; however, a significant reduction to exports and related production could potentially result in an approximate 12% drop in tobacco-related employment. In contrast, in a net importing country like Bangladesh, where almost all cigarettes are imported, eliminating domestic cigarette consumption could have an 18% net increase in employment, through income that becomes available for spending on potential substitution to goods from sectors that are produced domestically.[21]

Labour intensity of the tobacco industry (and other industries relating to health taxes) depends on a country's labour market share. Nothing illustrates this clearer than tobacco farming: nearly 90% of global tobacco farming occurs in just 20 countries (predominantly low- and middle-income countries (LMICs)).[9,24] Therefore, tobacco production is a very small part of most other economies. For example, contribution from tobacco industries to overall national employment in other LMICs such as Bangladesh, Pakistan and the Philippines is <0.5%.[25–27] Even countries heavily reliant on tobacco production (see Box 5.2 for a case study on the world's largest tobacco manufacturer), gross job loss estimates from taxation impacts are again, moderate, negligible or show net gains.

Furthermore, and similar to SSBs, the China case study (Box 5.2) and examples of employment levels in top tobacco growing countries in Figure 5.5 illustrate how underlying trends of multinational mergers and technological advances affect the tobacco industry, irrespective of taxes, yet are not incorporated into estimates.[24,25]

Fig. 5.5. Employment trends for major tobacco growing countries.

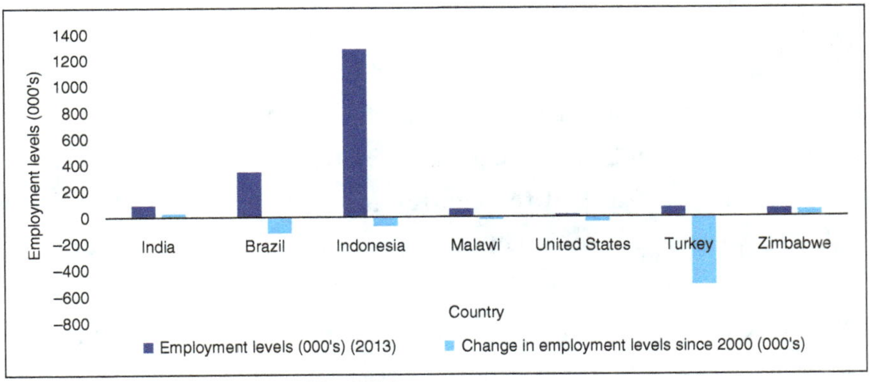

Source: Adapted from International Labour Office (2014).

Box 5.2. Case study: Tobacco tax impact on labour in the world's largest producer and consumer of tobacco[25]

China grows one-third (2.435 million tons of tobacco) of the world's tobacco and consumes one-third (1.7 trillion cigarettes) of the world's cigarettes. In a population of 1.325 billion (2008), there were 300 million smokers. The average age of smoking initiation is decreasing and was 19.7 years in 2002. The health and economic consequences are severe.

In 2020, smoking attributable mortality was expected to rise to 2 million deaths annually. Ten million disability-adjusted life years (DALYs) were reported for tobacco-related morbidity in 2000, ranking it third in NCD risk factors after high blood pressure and alcohol abuse. Nearly another half a million DALYs (approximately 5%) were added for morbidity relating to second-hand smoking.

Smoking attributable disease costs were said to total USD 22.6 billion in 2000. This translated to nearly 2% of China's GDP. Indirect costs due to morbidity and mortality accounted for nearly one-third of this estimate. Put another way and estimated using the human capital approach, the average per person loss of productivity due to premature, tobacco-related deaths would be USD 358 (2000 value).

The tobacco industry has cigarette companies in 24 out of 31 provinces. In 2005, it produced 1.7 trillion cigarettes which contributed to 7.6% of the central government's revenue. The industry employs about a half million people or 0.06% total national employment. Understandably, government is cautious and reluctant with increasing taxes. But how do these concerns stand up to scrutiny?

This case study report indicated that, if tobacco taxation was increased to be 51% of the total retail price, with two price elasticities of −0.15 or −0.50, industry net loss would represent <2% of the USD 12.2 billion revenue gained, a relatively inconsequential amount. Translating this to employment impact, the same price elasticity scenarios (i.e. −0.15 or −0.50), gross estimates of 1,656 or 5,549 job losses, respectively, were suggested.

Considering the industry eliminated nearly 60,000 jobs in an attempt to improve efficiencies through considerable restructuring and merging, this gross job loss from the tax appears minimal. The net effect, after substitution effects and increased government spending, is likely to be even smaller.

5.2.2. Effects from alcohol taxes

Similar to tobacco and SSBs/energy-dense foods, evidence shows taxes on alcohol also have negligible or even positive impacts on employment. For example, estimates of two hypothetical alcohol taxes showed net job creation across five US states: 653–4,583 jobs due to a 5-cent drink excise tax and 621–4,493 jobs due to a 5% sales tax increase.[28] Another study in Maryland, US, proposed the additional spending of USD 1.94 million generated revenue from the 2011 legislated dime per drink excise tax increase would generate jobs in the health sector for additional or scaled-up health programmes.[29] In the UK, a robust (non-industry funded) IOA (see Box 5.1 for definition) study[30] modelled the *net* employment impact of a 10% increase in UK tax rates on all alcohol types. Aligning with evidence from both tobacco and SSB/energy-dense foods industries, the *net* impact showed an increase of employment of 17,000 jobs, with nearly 80% of these occurring through 'sector shifts' (see Figure 5.1) in just four sectors.

Employment increases were also identified in a recent multi-country modelling study by the Organization for Economic Co-operation and Development (OECD).[31] Briefly, this model assumed a rise in taxation leading to a 10% increase in price across all alcohol types and for all 48 modelled OECD countries. Interestingly, the analysis compared taxation with nine other public health interventions to reduce harmful alcohol consumption, including minimum unit pricing, advertising regulations, counselling and so on. On a per-capita basis, taxation was the intervention projected to have the strongest impact on labour market outputs (i.e. the measure of output produced per hour of labour). Indeed, across all countries,

Fig. 5.6. Number of workers added annually per 100,000 people, 2020–2050.

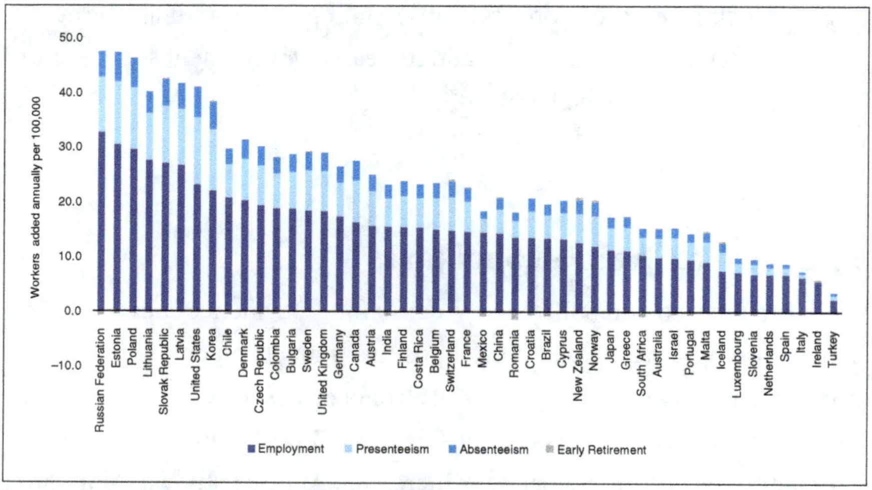

Source: Adapted from OECD Report data, Preventing harmful alcohol use (2021).

estimates indicated up to 809,000 more people would be in employment annually as a result of the increased taxation scenario. Figure 5.6 highlights this potential employment impact of alcohol taxation across the 48 OECD countries modelled over 30 years.

In contrast, and similar to findings on productivity impacts, Dave et al.[32] suggested that alcohol taxes had no systematic relationship with employment; if anything, their estimates showed that larger increases in alcohol taxes decreased employment. The study acknowledged their estimates were large and imprecise, characterised by significant variation in sign and magnitude across samples and types of alcohol taxes, and suggested a non-existent or weak relationship between alcohol taxes and labour market outcomes.

Inherent to all modelling studies are assumptions. These examples are no exception, and the reader must consider the evidence in its entirety when doing any evaluation.

5.2.3. Effects from diet-related taxes

Implementing taxes on SSBs/energy-dense food has significantly increased in the last two decades in countries around the world. With their implementation, several parallels to tobacco and alcohol taxes can be seen. First, these taxes are recommended as part of a comprehensive package of policy tools targeting reduced consumption.[33] Second, they have been largely successful in reducing demand and hence diet-related NCD risk factors and generating significant revenue. Third, similar industry arguments of employment loss and economic decline persist. Finally, the majority of the unfolding evidence of the employment impacts to the SSB industry appear exaggerated and incomplete.[34]

It is critical public health policymakers assess the methodological approach used and the data provided when reviewing the evidence. This is because some methodologies are unable to factor in a critical component of the taxation impact such as substitution and income effects. In particular, among the simulation studies, the analyses are often limited and provide estimates of *gross* direct and indirect job losses only and fail to incorporate redistribution of spending in other areas of the economy.

To illustrate the differences in findings, we draw on a recent global review of the evidence.[34]

All studies in this review were specifically related to taxes on SSBs although one study from Mexico also included taxation of energy-dense food.[16] Among the simulation studies, only one study considered redistribution of consumer and government spending to other goods and services.[35] Indeed, when employment change estimates from different methodological approaches within a country were compared, significantly different results were found.

For example, all industry-funded analyses in the review predicted gross employment losses: in South Africa, the IOA analysis[36] reported substantial gross job losses of approximately 70,000 jobs with the implementation of a hypothetical 20% SSB tax; similarly, two more IOA analyses from Mexico[37] and Philadelphia (US)[38] on actual SSB taxes, reported gross estimates of between 10,000 and 16,000 job losses for Mexico, and nearly 1,200 job losses for Philadelphia; and IOA analyses from Brazil, UK and Maine (US) all reported gross job losses.[39–41] However, non-industry-funded analyses reporting *net* impacts of the same tax in

South Africa indicated less than half the 70,000 value.[42] A comprehensive study in the review came from a REMI analysis of the US jurisdictions of Illinois and California.[35] The study acknowledged job losses in the beverage industry from a hypothetical 20% SSB tax however, reported small net *gains* to employment for both jurisdictions, by incorporating substitution to other goods and services, income effects, as well as increased government spending.

Only three studies to date have assessed pre-post tax impacts on labour market outcomes. As summarised in the systematic review, two analyses from Mexico and Philadelphia utilising interrupted time series analyses (ITSA) with direct observational data of employment and/or overall national unemployment, showed insignificant, negligible impacts.[16,43] That is, no evidence was found to suggest negative labour market impacts following the introduction of these sweetened beverage taxes. More recent empirical evidence,[44] also from Philadelphia, maintains the consensus from more robust studies that an SSB tax does not negatively impact employment. This peer-reviewed synthetic control analysis drew on monthly employment data from 2012 to 2019 to examine changes in total, private sector, limited-service restaurant and convenience store employment, and concluded that the 1.5 cent per ounce Philadelphia excise tax implemented on both caloric and artificially sweetened beverages did not result in job losses up to 2½ years post tax. The authors cited reasons already discussed as the mechanisms for the null effect, including substitution to non-taxed beverages, increased income and revenue spending within the jurisdiction which create jobs in other sectors (sectoral shifts).

Finally, it is worthwhile to note that the systematic review also indicated a lack of analyses addressing external, underlying longer run trends stemming from the industry itself contributing to employment loss in the SSB sector, including leaner production through more sophisticated automation and technology, lower yields from environment and climate change or industry's diversion of investment interests.

5.2.4. Summary of employment impacts of health taxes

Health taxes are widely recognised to decrease NCD burden through decreased consumption of tobacco, alcohol and SSBs/energy-dense foods. However, claims of job losses from these industries have been relentless in their attempts to reverse the tax and continue marketing of their products – particularly in lower income contexts. The use of a simplified conceptual framework of how taxes impact the labour market illustrates clearly the complex interactions involved and the overall net effects. Indeed, affected industries *can* expect job losses from reduced consumption, and the economy *will* incur transient restructuring costs, but consumer spending on other goods and services and spending of increased government tax revenue drive a sectoral shift that results in either minimal, neutral job losses or even gains.

5.3. Productivity impacts of health taxes

As NCD rates rise, the *direct* impact of disease burden on already tight government health care budgets and resources is exacerbated by what is being increasingly recognised as the *indirect* labour impact – particularly, lost productivity. Labour productivity is defined as 'output per unit of labour input' or 'labour market outputs' and is generally measured in GDP per person employed for a given time period.[45]

Against this backdrop, the value of a healthy and productive workforce cannot be underestimated.[45] However, recent global trends indicate rising levels of NCD morbidity and mortality, which undermine labour productivity efforts.[46] Eight million people die each year from tobacco use or exposure (13% of worldwide mortality); almost 3 million people die due to alcohol consumption (5% of worldwide mortality); over 4.5 million people die from being overweight and obesity and 1.6 million people die of diabetes.[47]

Globally, evidence of tobacco-, alcohol- and diet-related productivity loss as well as diet-related tax productivity gains emphasise that reducing consumption of these commodities contributes to reversing productivity loss. From our conceptual framework (Figure 5.1), these occur through the associated health benefits accrued as well as life years gained. For instance, tax-induced reductions in tobacco consumption lead to reductions in premature deaths, including deaths during the ages of 40–60 when smokers would otherwise be employed. Not only would this drive productivity gains but we can expect that, because the risk of death decreases with the years since quitting and the effects occur largely after the age of 40, the effects of the tax could be extended over time.[48] This labour market indicator is a benefit to all taxed industries, *in addition* to the employment impacts of potential job gains described in the previous section.

In this section, we draw on evidence to illustrate the costs incurred and working days lost from tobacco-, alcohol- and diet-related lost productivity together with evidence for diet-related taxes reducing obesity-related productivity losses. However, it is vital that government and public health policymakers understand that due to methodological complexities and data limitations in some countries, studies on these productivity effects must rely on several assumptions – often large and unrealistic. Conclusions must consider relevant, contextual labour market characteristics that will influence the degree to which reduction in consumption of the taxed products actually translate into productivity gains.

5.3.1. Productivity loss associated with tobacco, alcohol and SSB consumption

Costs incurred due to NCDs, tobacco-, alcohol- and SSB/energy-dense food-related productivity losses

Globally, consumption of tobacco, alcohol and SSBs/energy-dense food translates to significant economic loss. A recent US study estimated a total loss of USD 94.9 trillion due to reduced productivity from NCDs over the period 2015–2050 (equivalent to USD 265,000 per capita over the same time period).[49] The authors' rationale for such significant economic loss targeted absenteeism and presenteeism as well as medical expenditure that could otherwise be spent on improving productivity processes.[49]

Similarly, estimates of significant monetary loss from tobacco-related reduced productivity are evident. A UK review[50] reported approximately 50 million working days were lost each year in the UK from smoking-attributable absenteeism, translating to approximately GBP 1.71 billion (USD 2.21 billion). However, a more recent paper in the same review indicated this figure could be closer to GBP 5 billion (USD 6.46 billion) when considering absenteeism and presenteeism together.

There are likely to be large global costs incurred from alcohol-related productivity losses, however, there are considerable challenges of accurately estimating costs, primarily because of the heterogeneity between methodological approaches and data.[51,52] One review of 12 countries including Europe, Australia, Japan, South Korea, Thailand and the US, indicated 16 of the 22 studies showed productivity loss-related costs represented between 23% and 96% of the total costs incurred, translating to the largest proportion of all costs and in nearly half of the studies this cost accounted for the highest proportion of indirect costs (which include productivity loss, premature mortality and 'other' indirect costs) (Figure 5.7).[51] For instance, in Japan, this was equivalent to nearly 80% of

Fig. 5.7. Reduced productivity as a share of total indirect costs attributable to harmful alcohol consumption (%).

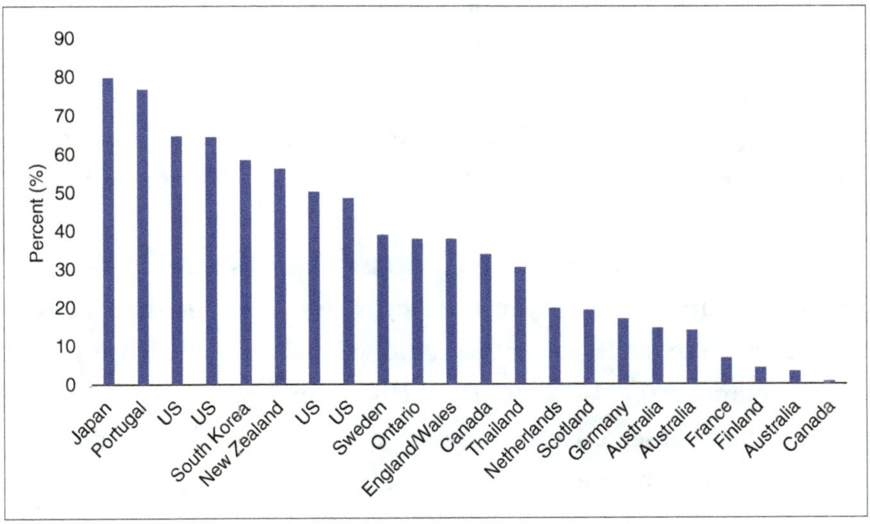

Source: Adapted from Thavorncharoensap, et al. (2009).

Table 5.1. Examples of costs incurred due to alcohol-related productivity loss.

Country	Year of estimate	Cost equivalent in 2020 USD	Cost equivalent in 2020 USD, per capita
UK	1993	2.24 billion	39
China	2008	422 million	422
New Zealand	1995	67 million	28
US	1999	72.2 billion	233

Source: Adapted from Jernigan et al. (2011) and Hu et al. (2008).

the total indirect cost and accounted for both absenteeism and presenteeism. Another review indicated indirect costs were likely to represent between 2.7% and 10.0% of total, global GDP.[52] Table 5.1 provides a summary from a global review of monetary loss associated with lost productivity from alcohol-related illness.[29] This review highlighted that a 25% increase in the US beer tax would prevent 4.6 million workdays lost annually due to workplace injury, equivalent to a reduction of costs from lost productivity of USD 905 million (2020 value).

A Swedish study estimated an increase of 9% absenteeism for male and 15% for female working-age Swedes living near the Finnish borders as a result of the Finnish alcohol tax cut.[53] These findings aligned with an earlier study which showed if taxes in Sweden were reduced to post-2004 Finnish rates, sickness absenteeism would increase by 3–5%.[54] Interestingly, the 2014 study found the higher educated and higher income groups were more affected than the less educated and lower income groups.

Finally, new evidence[55] clearly confirms a link between alcohol-related diseases (e.g. cirrhosis, cancer, dependency, NCDs) and reduced labour force productivity. The modelled analysis indicated that across the 52 modelled OECD countries, 0.11% and 0.24% of labour force productivity was lost annually due to absenteeism and presenteeism, respectively. In addition to the extra healthcare expenditure, this lost labour force productivity across

OECD countries translated to an average loss of USD PPP[a] 351 per capita per year, with Ireland showing the largest loss of almost USD PPP 882 per capita per year and Turkey showing the lowest loss of approximately USD PPP 23 per capita per year. Figure 5.8 shows the non-OECD countries of Cyprus, Indonesia and Saudi Arabia to have even lower losses.

In contrast to this evidence, a previous OECD report[56] showed mixed effects for the impact on labour market productivity in relation to alcohol intake, reflecting the apparent level and pattern of drinking. But this report also suggested nearly 11 million working days were lost in the UK by alcohol-dependent workers in 2001 with a total cost to the UK economy of £1.2 billion (approximately USD 1.9 billion). Similarly, alcohol-related productivity losses cost the European Union €59 billion (approximately USD 62 billion) in 2003.

Fig. 5.8. Average wage loss as measured by USD PPP per capita per year due to alcohol-related labour force productivity loss across OECD countries.

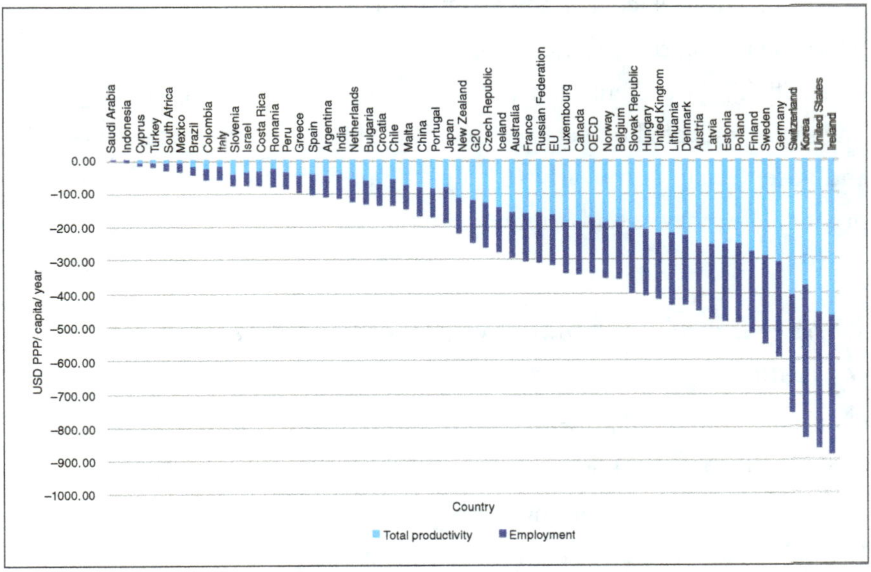

Source: Adapted from OECD Report, Preventing harmful alcohol use (2021).

[a] Purchasing power parity (PPP) is a fictitious currency that allows us to convert incomes of different countries into a common measure of living standards. That is, it is measuring the value of a currency according to how much of a 'consumption basket' of goods and services a country can buy.

Another study's analysis suggested that alcohol taxes were negatively related to employment and hours of work and positively related to wages.[32] However, the authors acknowledged imprecision and instability of their estimates and also raised concerns about the methodological reliability of the previous studies' estimates.

Nevertheless, all these findings unarguably illustrate to policymakers the benefit to public health and to an economy of either scaling-up pricing policies or introducing new ones to reduce alcohol-related productivity losses.

Finally, consumption of SSBs incurs indirect productivity costs through its contribution to obesity, premature death, diabetes and cardiovascular disease. Similar to determining costs for alcohol-related productivity loss, a comprehensive review done in 2017 on the productivity costs of obesity found the heterogeneity of the analytical approaches and data of the 50 included studies made it difficult to provide an accurate estimate of the costs incurred.[57] In Mexico, a study estimated costs of approximately USD 1.4 billion were incurred from SSB-related productivity loss due to premature mortality (57%), presenteeism (41%) and absenteeism (approximately 2%).[58] The study indicated diabetes caused over 90% of the premature mortality and absenteeism and nearly 100% of the presenteeism costs. The overall productivity cost was said to represent more than 100% of the SSB tax revenue in 2014.[58]

Working life-related productivity loss due to tobacco and alcohol consumption

Globally, tobacco and alcohol consumption has also translated into millions of working years lost. For instance, the global 13% tobacco-related mortality rate among the world's working-age population (i.e. 30–69 years) translated to 18 million labour years lost (LYL)[b] – more than double that seen in tobacco-related morbidity.[18] Interestingly, when the data were aggregated by (1) World Bank income group (Figure 5.9) and (2) WHO region (Figure 5.10), mortality and morbidity LYL were highest in the lower-middle-income group and

[b] Labour years lost (LYL) includes the future labour years (until retirement) lost.

Fig. 5.9. Productivity loss from tobacco consumption by World Bank income group.

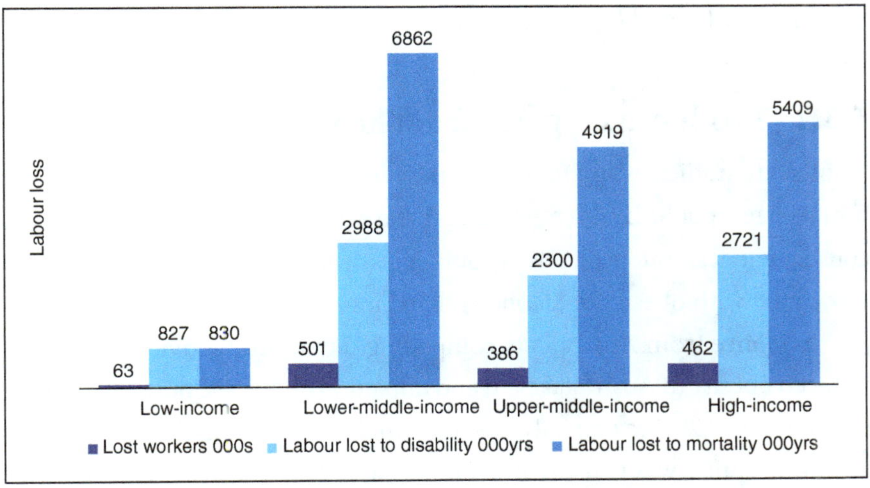

Source: Adapted from Goodchild et al. (2018).

Fig. 5.10. Productivity loss from tobacco consumption by WHO region.

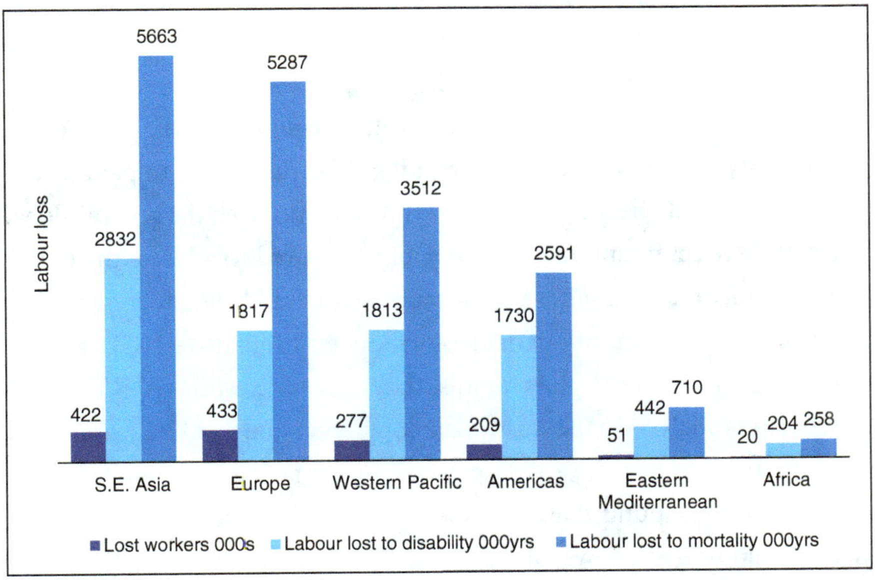

Source: Adapted from Goodchild et al. (2018).

lowest in the low-income group, and highest in South East Asia and lowest in Africa, for (1) and (2), respectively.

5.3.2. Productivity gains from health taxes

Numerous studies estimate productivity losses due to obesity and NCDs; however, few public health researchers have extended these analyses to assess consequential labour productivity outcomes of applying taxes to the products associated with obesity or alcohol-related morbidity.[7]

Evidence from Australia is compelling. First, productivity gains from reduced obesity in Australia's paid and unpaid working-age population from a hypothetical 20% tax on SSBs (i.e. unpaid defined as household, voluntary and community work) using the human capital approach were estimated.[7] The analysis found that from an approximate 2% population decrease in obesity from the tax, a total of 363,000 additional weeks of work would be gained over the model's 25-year lifetime, translating to approximately AUD 2 billion (approximately USD 1.4 billion). Interestingly, the unpaid sector's annual estimates continued to increase beyond the model's 25 years, but the paid sector's annual estimates declined after the first 5 years. These differences occurred due to the nature of the work: after retirement in the paid sector, productivity would likely decrease rapidly; however, for the unpaid sector, productivity would be sustained beyond retirement. Given the general global trend of increasing retirement age eligibility in a bid to address the global aging population, the figures for the paid sector are likely underestimated.

Second, productivity gains from reduced premature NCD-related mortality (defined as <80 years for this study) were also estimated.[19] The cost-effectiveness analysis in the Australian population due to a 10% tax on junk foods (defined as biscuits, cakes, pastries, pies, snack foods, confectionary and soft drinks) found that a total of 8,700 full-time equivalent working years would be gained over the model's 27-year lifetime, translating to an additional AUD 307 million (USD 207 million) to all future income that would have been earned if mortality were averted (or 'present value of lifetime income,' PVLI). Also, more than half of this productivity gain was from averted deaths of males aged 40–59 years. Finally, and unsurprisingly, cardiovascular disease-averted premature mortality accounted for nearly 50% of total productivity gains, followed by diabetes, stroke and colorectal cancer (19%, 14% and 9%, respectively). Figure 5.11 shows the junk food tax to be more effective and less expensive relative to a counterfactual of 'business as usual' or in other words, it was 'dominant'. The lighter points show how the cost-effectiveness improved when the productivity gains were included.

Alcohol-related taxes also show productivity gains. As discussed in the employment section above, and based on an OECD study[55] of 48 countries, 809,000 more people could be employed annually as a result of the increased tax. Additionally, 122,000 and 267,000 increased labour outputs would be attributable to reduced absenteeism and presenteeism, respectively. The study showed greatest impact in the US, Brazil, China, India and the Russian Federation. The least impact was seen in Malta and Iceland. Further, expressed in monetary terms by converting the changes in employment rate, absenteeism, presenteeism and early retirement into missed wages,

Fig. 5.11. Cost-effectiveness plan for a 10% junk food tax in Australia.

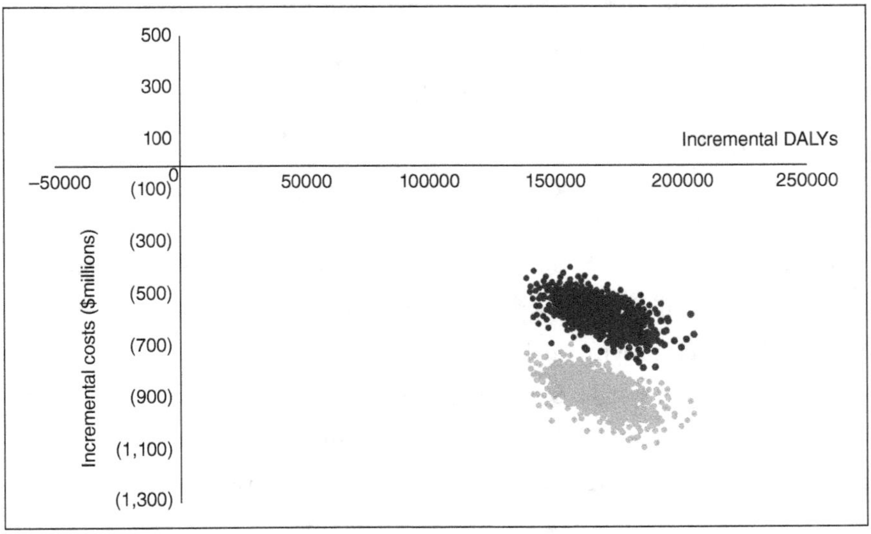

Source: Carter et al. (2019); https://doi.org/10.1371/journal.pone.0220209.g003.

the impact of cost savings was, for example, approximately USD PP 43, 37 and 27 per capita per year for the US, Korea and Switzerland, respectively.

5.3.3. Summary of productivity impacts of health taxes

The implementation of health taxes can help reverse the indirect costs to an economy from productivity losses attributable to morbidity and mortality from consumption of tobacco, alcohol and SSBs/energy-dense foods. Reversing these costs shows improved life expectancy and extra working life years are significant; however, the evidence relies on large assumptions and the extent to which different labour markets respond to the tax and actually translate it into productivity gains must be considered.

5.4. Labour impacts and achieving SDGs

In this chapter, we have highlighted how health taxes can be a key driver to support political commitment and efforts towards decreased consumption of the taxed good, significant healthcare cost savings and improved labour productivity. We have also shown these taxes are unlikely to have the negative employment impacts the taxed industries claim. But as there are both benefits and costs to the implementation of these taxes, how, as a policy tool to reduce the NCD burden, do they support the achievement of the SDGs? Indeed, literature debates that achieving SDG health goals, and particularly for utilising health taxes to reduce the global NCD burden (SDG 3.4 – to reduce NCD premature mortality by one-third by 2030), may create a complex political economy, or tension, in efforts to achieving the SDG economic goals (SDG 1.1 – eradicate extreme poverty, SDG 8.1 – sustainable economic growth, SDG 8.3 – promoting policies to support job creating or SDG 8.5 – full employment.[59]

For instance, perhaps it is the magnitude of the costs incurred in implementing the taxes that ultimately determine if the health and economic goals will conflict.[59] Hangoma and Surgey argue that job losses from SSB taxes in country contexts where sugar industries and their value chain contribute significantly to the overall economy may actually go against eradicating poverty (SDG 1.1) in the event of limited alternative industries or livelihoods (this may be extended to tobacco and alcohol industries). Furthermore, they indicate that in order for health taxes to align with *all* SDGs, the contextual factors of whether costs outweigh the benefits must be carefully assessed. These factors include: (1) the industry size and available alternative industries to provide alternative livelihoods; (2) the tax rate and how the market responds (or the price elasticity of demand and substitution; and (3) use of generated revenue. The paper concluded designing an appropriate tax as well as making available alternative industries for absorbing lost employment is critical to prevent conflicting policy agendas and thwarting the achievement of SDGs 8.1, 8.3 and 8.5. This aligns with evidence from the literature around designing effective tax policies[11] and our employment section that highlights little or neutral impact to job loss from taxes when workers are absorbed into other industries and sectors.[16,35,43]

In contrast, although the *Lancet Taskforce on NCDs and economics* recognises the political will and multisectoral commitment required for effectively achieving the SDG goals, it strongly contends that pricing policies are indispensable in contributing to controlling NCD burden which in turn, affects productivity.[60] For example, the Taskforce highlights that reduced NCD-related mortality alone, from health taxes, and the subsequent productivity gains accrued, will directly contribute to achieving not only SDG 8, but contribute towards achieving SDG 10.4 – (fiscal and social policies that promote equality), SDG 11 (sustainable cities) and SDG 12 (sustainable consumption and production); furthermore, the benefits will accrue from achieving these goals to indirectly and positively impact goals for SDG 1 (eliminating poverty), SDG 4 (education throughout the lifespan) and SDG 5 (gender equality). All aspects of health taxes and SDGs are covered in more depth in the next chapter (Chapter 6: Impacts of health taxes on the attainment of the SDGs).

5.5. Conclusion

This chapter considers a simplified conceptual framework to describe the interactions between health tax policy and labour market impacts for both employment and productivity as well as revenue generation and the drivers of structural sector change. The evidence suggests that industry's claims of negative economic consequences and net job losses are overstated based on inappropriate methodological approaches in industry-reported studies. More research is needed for country-specific data, particularly on diet-related taxes and alcohol taxes and future evaluations should include not only impacts on demand but also potential unintended consequences in order to build a robust evidence base on the impacts. It is critical for policymakers globally to understand that much of the evidence available is based on industry-funded economic reports that often provide only partial analyses. Robust, high-quality comprehensive studies on the other hand, generally show improved labour productivity, substantial indirect cost savings and government revenue and no net employment losses. Earmarking revenue generated towards the training and redirection to alternative livelihood of affected tobacco, alcohol and sugar workers is widely recommended.

Key messages

- For decades health taxes have been opposed by industry actors, with claims of negative labour impacts, particularly in lower socio-economical contexts. However, global evidence suggests instead, of neutral or even positive gains to labour markets as well as improved productivity across the supply chain due to improved health.
- The introduction or increase of health taxes, with at least some pass-through to consumers, will, depending on the size of the tax and the price elasticity of demand, lead to reduced consumption of the taxed goods.

- The taxed industry *will* see decreased *gross* revenue and *direct* job loss. *Indirect* employment will also decrease. However, individuals will substitute their spending to other products and hence generate increased demand and a new revenue stream for those products.
- Government will also generate tax revenue, introducing new spending in other sectors which will add to the increased consumer spending on other products and services.
- Together, this new spending creates demand and new employment in other sectors. In summary, instead of employment losses and economic decline as industry suggests, the balance of spending and employment ultimately – albeit with transient restructuring costs – will shift across sectors.
- In addition, and separately to the employment impacts, health taxes improve productivity across sectors, largely through improved health and more years of working life.
- With sufficiently high tax levels that induce behaviour change, these indirect benefits can offset the negative income losses caused by the taxes, particularly for low-income households, and have a largely progressive impact.
- It is critical for policymakers globally to understand that much of the evidence available is based on industry-funded economic reports that often provide only partial analyses.
- Earmarking revenue generated towards the training and redirection to alternative livelihood of affected tobacco, alcohol and sugar workers is widely recommended.
- More research is needed for country-specific data, particularly on diet-related taxes and alcohol taxes and future evaluations should include not only impacts on demand but also potential unintended consequences such as labour market impacts in order to build a robust evidence base on the impacts.

References

1. *WHO Report on the Global Tobacco Epidemic, 2017: Monitoring Tobacco Use and Prevention Policies* Geneva; Switzerland: World Health Organization; 2017. Report No.: 9241512822.
2. *WHO Report on the Global Tobacco Epidemic, 2019: Offer Help to Quit Tobacco Use.* Geneva, Switzerland: World Health Organization; 2019.
3. *Global Status Report on Alcohol and Health*, 2018. Geneva, Switzerland: World Health Organization; 2018.
4. The World Bank Group. *Obesity: Health and Economic Consequences of an Impending Global Challenge.* Washington, DC: World Bank Group; 2020.
5. World Bank Group. Taxes on Sugar-Sweetened Beverages: Summary of International Evidence and Experiences. Washington, DC: World Bank; 2020.
6. Breda J, Calvert J, Galea G, Jewell J, Mantingh M. Using Pricing Policies to Promote Healthier Diets. Geneva, Switzerland: World Health Organization Regional Office for Europe; 2015.
7. Nomaguchi T, Cunich M, Zapata-Diomedi B, Veerman JL. The impact on productivity of a hypothetical tax on sugar-sweetened beverages. *Health Policy.* 2017; 121(6): 715–725.
8. Schofield D, Cunich MM, Shrestha RN, Passey ME, Veerman L, Callander EJ, et al. The economic impact of diabetes through lost labour force participation on individuals and government: Evidence from a microsimulation model. *BMC Public Health.* 2014; 14: 220.
9. US National Cancer Institute and World Health Organization. The economics of tobacco and tobacco control. National Cancer Institute Tobacco Control Monograph 21. Geneva: World Health Organization, US Department of Health and Human Services, National Institutes of Health NCI; 2016.
10. Nolte K, Ostermeier M. Labour market effects of large-scale agricultural investment: conceptual considerations and estimated employment effects. *World Development.* 2017; 98: 430–446.
11. Chaloupka F, Powell LM, Warner KE. The use of excise taxes to reduce tobacco, alcohol and sugary beverage consumption. *Annual Review of Public Health.* 2019; (40): 187–201.
12. Fuchs A, Gonzalez Icaza F, Paz D. *Distributional Effects of Tobacco Taxation: A Comparative Analysis.* Washington, DC: World Bank Group; 2019.
13. Chavez JJ, Drope J, Li Q, Aloria MJ. *The Economics of Tobacco Farming in the Philippines.* Quezon City: American Cancer Society; 2016.
14. Gretton P. *On Input-Output Tables: Uses and Abuses.* Productivity Commission Staff Research Note. Canberra, Australia: Australian Government Productivity Commission; 2013.
15. Bonn MA, Harrington J. A comparison of three economic impact models for applied hospitality and tourism research. *Tourism Economics.* 2008; 14(4): 769–789.

16. Guerrero-Lopez CM, Molina M, Colchero MA. Employment changes associated with the introduction of taxes on sugar-sweetened beverages and nonessential energy-dense food in Mexico. *Preventive Medicine.* 2017; 105S: S43–S49.
17. Barendregt JJ, Van Oortmarssen GJ, Van Hout BA, Van Den Bosch JM, Bonneux L. Coping with multiple morbidity in a life table. *Mathematical Population Studies.* 1998; 7(1): 29–49, 109.
18. Goodchild M, Nargis N, Tursan d'Espaignet E. Global economic cost of smoking-attributable diseases. *Tobacco Control.* 2018; 27(1): 58–64.
19. Carter HE, Schofield DJ, Shrestha R, Veerman L. The productivity gains associated with a junk food tax and their impact on cost-effectiveness. *PLoS One.* 2019; 14(7): e0220209.
20. Robinson R. Cost-effective analysis. *BMJ.* 1993; 307(6907): 793–795.
21. World Bank Group. *Curbing the Epidemic: Governments and the Economics of Tobacco Control.* Development in Practice. Washington, DC: World Bank Group; 1999.
22. Warner KE, Fulton GA, Nicolas P, Grimes DR. Employment implications of declining tobacco product sales for the regional economies of the US. *JAMA.* 1996; 275(16): 1241–1245.
23. van der Merwe, Abedian I. A reduction in consumer expenditure on cigarettes and its effects on employment: A case study of South Africa. *Contemporary Economic Policy.* 1999; 17(3): 412–422.
24. International Labour Office (ILO). *Tobacco Sector Employment Statistical Update.* Geneva: International Labour Office; 2014.
25. Hu T-W, Mao Z, Shi J, Chen W. *Tobacco Taxation and its Potential Impact in China.* Paris: International Union Against Tuberculosis and Lung Disease; 2008.
26. Quimbo SLA, Miguel-Baquilod M, Xu X, Casoria AA, Medalla FM, Chaloupka FJ. *The Economics of Tobacco and Tobacco Taxation in the Philippines.* Paris: International Union Against Tuberculosis and Lung Disease; 2012.
27. Burki SJ, Pasha HA, Jha P, Kamboh GN, Pasha AG, John R, et al. *The Economics of Tobacco and Tobacco Taxation in Pakistan.* Paris: International Union Against Tuberculosis and Lung Disease; 2013.
28. Wada R, Chaloupka FJ, Powell LM, Jernigan DH. Employment impacts of alcohol taxes. *Preventive Medicine.* 2017; 105S: S50–S55.
29. Jernigan DH, Waters H, Ross C, Stewart A. The potential economic effects of alcohol excise tax increases in Maryland. Virtual Media Resources and Boston University School of Public Health: Johns Hopkins Bloomberg School of Public Health; 2011.
30. Connolly K, Bhattacharya A, Lisenkova K, McGregor PG. Can a policy-induced reduction in alcohol consumption improve health outcomes and stimulate the UK economy?: A potential 'double dividend'. *Drug and Alcohol Review.* 2019; 38: 554–560.
31. Organisation for Economic Co-operation and Development (OECD). *Preventing Harmful Alcohol Use, OECD Health Policy Studies.* Paris: OECD Publishing; 2021.

32. Dave D, Kaestner RK. Alcohol taxes and labor market outcomes. *Journal of Health Economics.* 2002; 21: 357–371.
33. World Health Organization (WHO). *Fiscal Policies for Diet and Prevention of Noncommunicable Diseases,* Technical Meeting Report, 5–6 May 2015. Geneva, Switzerland: World Health Organization; 2015.
34. Mounsey S, Veerman L, Jan S, Thow AM. The macroeconomic impacts of diet-related fiscal policy for NCD prevention: A systematic review. *Economics and Human Biology.* 2020; 37: 100854.
35. Powell LM, Wada R, Persky JJ, Chaloupka FJ. Employment impact of sugar-sweetened beverage taxes. *American Journal of Public Health.* 2014; 104: 672–677.
36. Oxford Economics. "For the Beverage Association of South Africa." Oxford Economics is based in Oxford, so for all of the Oxford Economics reports, place of publish can be assumed to be Oxford, UK; 2016.
37. Cantu JC, Curiel DF, Valero LZ. The Non-Alcoholic Beverage Industry in Mexico. Economics Research Centre (CIE), Mexico: Autonomous University of Nuevo León; 2015.
38. Oxford Economics. *The Economic Impact of Philadelphia's Beverage Tax.* Oxford, UK: Oxford Economics (for American Beverage Association); 2017.
39. Balbinotto G, Cardoso L. Measuring the economic impact of SSB Taxes in Brazil: An input-output analysis. *Value in Health.* 2016; 19(3): A101.
40. Fairhead H. An estimate of the effect of the soft drinks industry levy on employment. UK: For The Taxpayers' Alliance; 2016.
41. Oxford Economics. *The Economic Impact of the Soft Drinks Levy – Final Report.* Oxford Economics (for British Soft Drinks Association); Oxford, UK: 2016.
42. Theron N, Rossouw R, Fourie H. Economy-wide implications of the proposed tax on sugar sweetened beverages (SSBs) – Research Note 42. *ECONEX;* 2016.
43. Lawman HG, Bleich SN, Yan J, LeVasseur MT, Mitra N, Roberto CA. Unemployment claims in Philadelphia one year after implementation of the sweetened beverage tax. *PLoS One.* 2019; 14(3): e0213218.
44. Marinello S, Leider J, Pugach O, Powell L. The impact of the Philadelphia beverage tax on employment: A synthetic control analysis. *Economics & Human Biology.* 2021 January; 40: 100939. DOI: 10.1016/j.ehb.2020.100939. Epub 2020 Oct 29. PMID: 33232891.
45. International Labour Organization (ILO). Key Indicators of the Labour Market. 9th edn. Geneva: Document and Publications Production, Printing and Distribution Branch (PRODOC) of the ILO; 2016.
46. Sweeny K, Rasmussen B, Sheehan P. *The Impact of Health Worker Attendance and Productivity in Twelve Countries.* Melbourne, Australia: Victoria Institute of Strategic Economic Studies; 2015.
47. The Task Force on Fiscal Policy for Health. *Health Taxes to Save Lives: Employing Effective Excise Taxes on Tobacco, Alcohol and Sugary Beverages.* US: University of Illinois; 2019 April. https://www.tobacconomics.org/files/research/512/Health-Taxes-to-Save-Lives-Report.pdf.

48. International Agency for Research on Cancer (IARC). *Effectiveness of Tax and Price Policies for Tobacco Control.* Lyon, France: World Health Organization; 2011.
49. Chen S, Kuhn M, Prettner K, Bloom DE. The macroeconomic burden of noncommunicable diseases in the US: Estimates and projections. *PLoS One.* 2018; 13(11): e0206702.
50. Ekpu VU, Brown AK. The economic impact of smoking and of reducing smoking prevalence: Review of evidence. *Tobacco Use Insights.* 2015; 8: 1–35.
51. Thavorncharoensap M, Teerawattananon Y, Yothasamut J, Lertpitakpong C, Chaikledkaew U. The economic impact of alcohol consumption: a systematic review. *Substance Abuse Treatment, Prevention, and Policy.* 2009; 4(1): Article 20.
52. Baumberg B. The global economic burden of alcohol: a review and some suggestions. *Drug and Alcohol Review.* 2006; 25(6): 537–551.
53. Johansson P, Pekkarinen T, Verho J. Cross-border health and productivity effects of alcohol policies. *Journal of Health Economics.* 2014; 36: 125–136.
54. Johannson P, Palme M. Do economic incentives affect work absence? Empirical evidence using Swedish micro data. *Journal of Public Economics.* 1996; 59: 195–218.
55. Organization for Economic Co-operation and Development (OECD). *Preventing Harmful Alcohol Use.* Paris: OECD Health Policy Studies, OECD Publishing; 2021. https://DOI.org/10.1787/6e4b4ffb-en.
56. Devaux M, Sassi F. *The Labour Market Impacts of Obesity, Smoking, Alcohol Use and Related Chronic Diseases,* OECD Health Working Papers, No. 86. Paris: Organization for Economic Co-operation and Development (OECD); 2015.
57. Goettler A, Grosse A, Sonntag D. Productivity loss due to overweight and obesity: a systematic review of indirect costs. *BMJ Open.* 2017; 7(10): e014632.
58. Guerrero-López CM, Colchero MA. Productivity loss associated with the consumption of sugar-sweetened beverages in Mexico. *Preventive Medicine.* 2018; 115: 140–144.
59. Hangoma P, Surgey G. Contradictions within the SDGs: Are sin taxes for health improvement at odds with employment and economic growth in Zambia. *Global Health.* 2019; 15(1): Article 82.
60. Nugent R, Bertram MY, Jan S, Niessen LW, Sassi F, Jamison DT, et al. Investing in non-communicable disease prevention and management to advance the Sustainable Development Goals. *The Lancet.* 2018; 391(10134): 2029–2035.

https://doi.org/10.1142/9781800612396_0007

Chapter 6

Impacts of Health Taxes on the Attainment of the SDGs

Norman Maldonado-Vargas* **and Blanca Llorente**†

The reduction in consumption of harmful products triggered by increases in health taxes has effects in multiple development dimensions beyond health. We firstly review the evidence on health taxes' effects on Sustainable Development (SD), and secondly, we provide guidance for policymakers on how to make a stronger case for health taxes by emphasising their role as policy instruments for development. We show that the effects on SD go beyond income inequalities or the progressive/regressive nature of health taxes. In general, health taxes positively affect the three systems that sustain human life, namely, the global society, the earth's physical system and the world's economy. Despite the need for more research and for stronger monitoring and evaluation of health taxes, we provide enough evidence to support a strong case for health taxes from a SD perspective. Reframing health taxes with a SD perspective in all stages of the policy cycle has enormous potential to gain wider societal support for progress on global uptake and increase of health taxes.

* PROESA, Universidad Icesi, Colombia.

† Fundación Anáas, Colombia.

6.1. Introduction

Health is a human right[1] and is one of the conditions that define a good life. Other conditions play an essential role in achieving higher quality of life, such as access to food, education, shelter or security, which are also human rights.[2] Development, as the study of the achievement of a better life, is able to provide a thorough understanding of the elements that define and determine people's quality of life, as well as the complex interactions among those elements. In practice, the pursuit of development translates into a set of goals targeting improvements in humanity's quality of life, called sustainable development goals (SDGs).

From the health perspective, health taxes can improve people's quality of life by discouraging unhealthy habits, leading to substantial health gains over people's life course. From the wider perspective of development, this effect is only the tip of the iceberg, because health taxes also trigger a sequence of reactions that, eventually, improve society's welfare beyond the direct benefits on health. For that reason, health taxes are a policy instrument to achieve development goals. For instance, health taxes may divert people from harmful behaviours that lead to non-communicable diseases (NCDs) and catastrophic healthcare expenditure, and in that way they have the potential to prevent people falling into poverty. Another example is the fiscal space they could open through tax revenues to finance development.[3,4] In general, health taxes are a powerful instrument to leapfrog in progress to meet the targets of the 2030 agenda on SDGs,[5] and the threat that COVID-19 has imposed on progress on SDGs[6] make health taxes even more relevant for performing such vault.[a] Despite such potential, current uptake of health taxes worldwide is low, and

[a] In terms of risk factors, COVID-19 has made more evident the need to control NCDs because of the additional risk they represent in other diseases. At the same time, COVID-19 has created economic vulnerabilities that make additional taxation much harder. In addition, tax reforms have become urgent to recover from the increases in public expenditure caused by the pandemic. All these mechanisms, that go in opposite directions, suggest that the crisis caused by the pandemic will open opportunities to discuss uptake and increase of health taxes as part of tax reforms.

there are no cases of countries with health taxes designed and implemented to fully exploit their entire potential for progress on development.

By bringing to light the scope on development, policymakers can make a stronger case for health taxes in order to gain broader support from society, a necessary condition for uptake (approval and implementation) of health taxes. In general, the development perspective makes a stronger case for health taxes in three ways. First, development provides a holistic view of individuals' welfare,[b] giving the whole picture of the effects of health taxes on efficient allocation of resources and the heterogeneity of such effects (e.g. by income). Such understanding is crucial for getting health taxes' design closer to the efficiency and fairness principles of good taxation.[7] A consequence of the wider spectrum of effects is that the political capital costs of policies and regulations are spread among a broader set of sectors and stakeholders. This is critical when dealing with policy changes that require relatively fair amounts of political capital to be spent in order to overcome the political economy obstacles typical of tax reforms. Second, health taxes face significantly less trade-offs than other public policies because they deal with public health challenges and, at the same time, have the capacity to generate tax revenues. Extending their scope to development challenges make health taxes even less likely to face conflict in the public policy arena among stakeholders and decision-makers on technical grounds, and therefore agreements on health taxes are more likely to be reachable.[8] Third, health policies dealing with determinants of health require important coordination among multiple sectors and active roles from those sectors on design, funding and implementation. In contrast, health taxes are an intersectoral action[9] that needs no coordination among government areas other than the technical and political support to increase those taxes; such negligible coordination costs and roles make health taxes even more appealing as

[b] This contrasts with the traditional approach on health taxes where most of the analysis focuses only on the effects on health and tax revenue.

a development policy instrument because in development the number of sectors involved, and therefore coordination costs, are considerably high.

The purpose of this chapter is twofold. First, it intends to review the evidence of effects of health taxes on development, in order to take the discussion on health taxes beyond the fields of health and public finance and bring it into a deeper, wider and more urgent discussion on development. Second, the chapter aims to provide a guidance for the policymaker on how to make a stronger case on health taxes by recognising and positioning their role as development policy instruments, that is, as a cost-effective mechanism to guarantee people's rights and to improve their quality of life. To meet these goals, the chapter starts with a conceptual framework that provides a common ground of concepts, principles and rationale (Section 6.2). Afterwards, it moves to its core by discussing the role of health taxes on dimensions of development, specifically on SDGs and the three systems that sustain human life (Section 6.3), and based on that discussion, it gives general guidelines for people engaged in policymaking to make a stronger case for health taxes in their countries (Section 6.4). Finally, the chapter closes with conclusions and policy remarks (Section 6.5).

6.2. Conceptual framework

6.2.1. Concepts

In general, development 'is concerned with the achievement of a better life'.[10] From the perspective of human rights, United Nations (UN), the leading multilateral agency on promotion and protection of human rights, defined development as 'a multi-dimensional undertaking to achieve a higher quality of life for all people'.[11] As the effects of human action have gradually become a significant global threat to the natural systems that sustain human life (the global society, the earth's physical environment and the world's economy), the discussion on development has extended its scope to the concept of sustainable development (SD). SD was initially conceived as 'development that meets the needs of the present without compromising the ability of future generations to meet their own needs', with compromises referring to 'limitations imposed by the present state of technology and social organisation on environmental resources and by the ability of the biosphere to absorb the effects of human activities'.[12]

Since then, the concept has evolved into a more practical definition that holistically intends to 'make sense of the interactions of three complex systems: the world economy, the global society, and the earth's physical environment'.[13] As of today, UN defines SD as a multi-dimensional undertaking to achieve a higher quality of life for all people, recognising that such achievement is only possible under a balanced and integrated progress on its three dimensions, namely, the economic, the social and the environmental dimensions.[5] These dimensions are more precisely defined by UN in its commitment to achieve SD[14] as follows:

> We also reaffirm the need to achieve sustainable development by: promoting sustained, inclusive and equitable economic growth, creating greater opportunities for all, reducing inequalities, raising basic standards of living; fostering equitable social development and inclusion; and promoting integrated and sustainable management of natural resources and ecosystems that supports inter alia economic, social and human development while facilitating ecosystem conservation, regeneration and restoration and resilience in the face of new and emerging challenges.

In order to bring SD into practice and to guide and coordinate efforts on moving the world forward on SD, UN has set up a participatory global action plan (agenda) with specific goals in a prioritised set of areas of intervention. After Agenda 21[15] whose focus was on development and environment, the Millennium Development Goals (MDGs)[16] successfully mobilised the world around tackling extreme poverty in its many dimensions[17] between 2000 and 2015. Currently, the world's agenda on SD, grounded in human rights,[18] is defined by a set of 169 time-bound and quantified targets (SDG-T) for 17 global SDGs intended to be achieved by 2030,[5] where each target has a set of measurable indicators (SDG-I) that add up to 244 (see Annex). The 17 SDGs are shown in Table 6.1.[c]

In spite of the SDG's potential for worldwide improvement on people's quality of life, there are legitimate concerns about the achievement of the SDGs: 'despite the initial efforts, the world is not on track for achieving most of the 169 targets that comprise the Goals', and the main challenges to get back on track are inequalities, climate change, biodiversity loss and waste from human activity.[19] Part of the poor progress is explained by some weaknesses on SDGs' design and implementation,[18,20] and for the particular case of health-related SDGs it seems to be explained by low political commitment on national ownership and effective implementation, and by low financial commitment on mobilisation of domestic resources.[21] Moreover, COVID-19 has brought in 'an unprecedented health, economic and social crisis,..., has exposed and exacerbated existing inequalities and injustices',[22] and has cut in line ahead of those main challenges to jeopardise implementation of SDGs[23] and to become a threat for two-thirds of the 169 targets.[6] Despite those limitations, SDGs and in general SD 'provides the framework for addressing all these challenges in an interconnected and comprehensive manner'[18]; also 'far from undermining the case for the SDGs, the root causes and uneven impacts of COVID-19 demonstrate precisely why we need the 2030 Agenda, the Paris Agreement on climate change and the Addis Ababa Action Agenda, and underscore the urgency of their implementation'.[22]

Most importantly, appropriate taxation, including health taxes, is a fundamental principle underlying acceleration of progress towards SDGs. Specifically, appropriate taxation is part of the economy and finance lever, one of the four levers of change that can be applied to six critical entry points to overcome those challenges and accelerate progress towards the SDGs.[19] Specifically, health taxes can accelerate progress towards SDGs

[c] More information on SDGs and the list of targets (SDG-T) and indicators (SDG-I) can be found at https://sdgs.un.org/goals.

Table 6.1. Sustainable Development Goals (SDGs).

SDG	Description
1 No poverty	End poverty in all its forms everywhere
2 Zero hunger	End hunger, achieve food security and improved nutrition and promote sustainable agriculture
3 Good health and well-being	Ensure healthy lives and promote well-being for all at all ages
4 Quality education	Ensure inclusive and equitable quality education and promote lifelong learning opportunities for all
5 Gender equality	Achieve gender equality and empower all women and girls
6 Clean water and sanitation	Ensure availability and sustainable management of water and sanitation for all
7 Affordable and clean energy	Ensure access to affordable, reliable, sustainable and modern energy for all
8 Decent work and economic growth	Promote sustained, inclusive and sustainable economic growth, full and productive employment and decent work for all
9 Industry, innovation and infrastructure	Build resilient infrastructure, promote inclusive and sustainable industrialisation and foster innovation
10 Reduced inequality	Reduce inequality within and among countries
11 Sustainable cities and communities	Make cities and human settlements inclusive, safe, resilient and sustainable
12 Responsible consumption and production	Ensure sustainable consumption and production patterns
13 Climate action	Take urgent action to combat climate change and its impacts
14 Life below water	Conserve and sustainably use the oceans, seas and marine resources for sustainable development
15 Life on land	Protect, restore and promote sustainable use of terrestrial ecosystems, sustainably manage forests, combat desertification, and halt and reverse land degradation and halt biodiversity loss
16 Peace and justice strong institutions	Promote peaceful and inclusive societies for SD, provide access to justice for all and build effective, accountable and inclusive institutions at all levels
17 Partnerships to achieve the goal	Strengthen the means of implementation and revitalise the global partnership for SD

by (i) providing incentives to change people's behaviour, (ii) opening opportunities for firms' innovation and (iii) raising revenues to finance action on development. For instance, in the case of food taxes, 'a wise employment of taxation tools should align economic incentives with the health and environmental requirements of sustainable diets and discourage the consumption of ultra-processed food products that contain high amounts of sugar, salt and fat'.[19] Moreover, as COVID-19 has led to absence of additional financial support from the international community to accelerate progress on SDGs in developing countries, health taxes such as removal of fossil subsidies (negative taxes) or uptake of tropical carbon taxes are 'innovative policy mechanisms to achieve sustainability and development aims in a cost-effective manner', and 'affordable policies that can yield immediate progress towards several SDGs together, rather than sacrificing some goals to achieve others, and aligns economic incentives for longer term sustainable development'.[24] Furthermore, there is evidence showing that health taxes on tobacco or sugar-sweetened beverages (SSB) have contributed in overcoming the lack of financial commitment by ensuring mobilisation of domestic resources for investment on progress on health and health-related SDGs.[21]

6.2.2. Taking concepts into practice

Summarising last section, SDGs are a call for socially inclusive and environmentally sustainable economic growth,[13] and health taxes are a policy instrument to move forward on SDGs. This section highlights some practical aspects of these concepts that must be heeded when making a case for health taxes from a development perspective.

SDGs and SDG-Ts are integrated and indivisible[5]

SDGs' integrated and indivisible nature originates in having the 2030 Agenda grounded in human rights, and such nature allows to deal with the complexity of making the connections and finding comprehensive solutions to the challenges on SD.[18] The interdependence of SDGs has been well-documented,[25,26] and the goal on good health and well-being (SDG3) has been linked to around 50 health-related targets across the SDGs.[27] Despite SDGs having deficiencies in integration and indivisibility,[28] abandoning those characteristics by segmentation of SDGs is dangerous, as it leads to favour decision-making in thematic silos, that is, decision-making that leaves out causes and effects of SD challenges not directly related to a specific sector; such approach breaks the interdependence among the three systems that sustain human life, hinders intersectoral actions and tends to 'prioritize immediate economic benefits over social and environmental costs that would materialize over the long term.[19]

The integrated and indivisible nature of SDGs is preserved in making a case for health taxes when all effects on SD are considered, not just the ones on health; in other words, when a comprehensive case for health taxes is made instead of a partial case. The starting point to do so is a complete recognition of the interlinkages among SDGs (e.g. Ref.[29]) for the particular conditions of the country. Based on that, the next point is to identify trade-offs and multiplier effects in order to maximise co-benefits by taking advantage of positive synergies among SDGs and at the same time resolving negative trade-offs.[19] The nature and scope of trade-offs depend on the country's local conditions, and identification of those trade-offs provides valuable information for an accurate design of health taxes. A case for health taxes using such comprehensive SD perspective is the exception rather than the rule, because the expansion of the debate on health taxes towards fields other than public health or public finance is recent; some examples of work exploring some effects on SD are investment cases (cost-effectiveness analysis), extended cost-effectiveness analysis or microsimulation (e.g. Refs.[30–32, 195]).

The two points of interlinkages and trade-offs are essential for the health taxes diagnosis (Step 0 in Section 6.4). As a last point, all the other stages of the policy cycle (Steps 1–5 in Section 6.4) should motivate participation and engagement of stakeholders from all sectors identified in the health tax diagnostic, in order to materialise the integrated and indivisible nature of SDGs into an intersectoral mobilisation supporting health taxes, a necessary and pivotal condition for uptake (approval and implementation) of the policy. In that way, health taxes become an intersectoral action, which is the type of action necessary to achieve SDG3 (good health and well-being).[33] Such country-level mobilisation can be boosted by strengthening intersectoral actions at the multilateral level, specifically to work on the calls to 'Accelerate progress in countries through joint actions' and to 'Align, by harmonizing our [multilateral organisations'] operational and financial strategies and policies'.[27]

SD driven by consumption driven by prices. Consumption of goods and services is the core of the world's economy, one of the three complex systems that sustain human life, and therefore is at the heart of SD. Consumers' choices of some goods have a direct, negative effect on people's health and also cause either 'harms on others (externalities) or harms on themselves that they do not correctly internalise (internalities)'.[d,34] Those goods mainly include tobacco, alcohol, SSBs, excessive salt intake, trans and saturated fats, red meat and processed meat, plastic packaging (bottles, bags) and fossil fuels. In addition, such consumption indirectly affects SD through the externalities and internalities imposed on the three core systems of SD (the global society, the earth's physical environment and the world economy) caused along the stages of the product life cycle (preproduction, production, distribution, use and disposal).[37] Both internalities and externalities deteriorate people's quality of life: internalities induce individuals to wrong choices that diminish their welfare, while externalities cause that prevailing prices do not reflect the true societal costs of consuming such goods,[38] reducing other people's welfare. Therefore, reaching SD goals and targets substantially rely upon changing consumption of those goods, and prices are the main driver of consumers' choices.

---

[d] For a detailed explanation on externalities and distortions caused by externalities, see Ref.[7] (Chapter 4), Ref.[35] (Part II). For internalities, see Ref.[36].

Health taxes, that is, excise taxes[39] on goods whose consumption negatively affects people's health, are a health policy that directly increases the price of harmful goods, reducing their consumption and correcting the health externalities[e] and internalities it imposes on society.[40–44] Furthermore, such reduction in consumption makes health taxes an SD policy via the corrective effect they have on other externalities and internalities imposed on the three core systems of SD across all stages of the product life cycle; this point is particularly important for the potential of health taxes to be used as an international coordination mechanism to correct for global externalities (e.g. Ref.[45]). Also, since subsidies (negative taxes) on goods harmful to health represent a distortion in prices, they are an incentive for poor progress on health and SD. For that reason, health taxes also include removal of such subsidies and positive taxation on those goods. In particular, 'subsidies on commodities such as sugar, diesel, kerosene, and coal could be reduced and the savings redirected to nutritious food and clean energy sources.'[46] Also, because pollution control has been identified as an important element to advance on many of the SDGs, 'an end to subsidies and tax breaks for polluting industries need to be integral components of pollution control programmes'.[47]

Health taxes must be well-designed to significantly contribute to progress on SD. As a last point, for health taxes to be effective as an SD policy instrument, they must be well-designed. The definition and technicalities of design of health taxes are covered in Chapter 8. In general, well-designed health taxes means that (i) their design is based on a meticulous analysis of the country's constraints on alternatives to goods related to basic human needs (air, water, food, shelter, hygiene, transport) and the unexpected effects those constraints might trigger and (ii) they have been designed to work together to correct the distortions and negative effects of externalities and internalities (corrective taxes) and to minimise the unexpected effects of the country's constraints. The first point is particularly relevant for adopting an SD perspective

[e] For a detailed explanation on taxation and use of taxes to correct externalities, see Ref.[7] (Chapters 17–20) and Chapter 8 in this book.

on health taxes, because multiple potential effects on other products, services, communities, sectors and so on might emerge. For example, in the case of food, health taxes are effective 'when the design of the tax is adapted and its consequences on other food products or nutrients have been well assessed',[48] and similar arguments apply to SSBs,[34] alcohol, tobacco[49,50] and all other harmful goods. Regarding the second point, it is imperative to consider the immense differences in the nature of products targeted by the taxes; in particular, tobacco significantly differs from alcohol and food, and even categories in food differ from each other, let alone plastic and fossil fuels. Such consideration is important, because differences in the nature of the product translate into differences in the economic loss caused by the tax (a.k.a deadweight loss) and from there into differences and challenges in optimal tax design. Thus, in addition to a technically accurate design of the tax (types and mix, magnitude, set of products, deadweight loss, etc.), well-designed health taxes also recognise the country's constraints on alternatives to goods related to basic human needs, incorporate those constraints in the design of the tax and have a medium-term agenda on investments and actions to overcome those constraints. In this way, health taxes can become local best buys[51] and the investments and actions on overcoming the country's constraints (see Section 6.3.4) will open space for future increases on health taxes in a wider spectrum of products.

6.3. Dimensions of development

This section reviews the main mechanisms through which well-designed health taxes have an impact on different dimensions of SD. The section was developed by making a careful review of the connections (mechanisms) between health taxes and SDGs, and a meticulous identification of the literature with the widest scope on each topic. The last point is central for the purpose of the chapter because the evidence cited in this section is, in most cases, general, meaning that it can be used by any country to support a case for health taxes from an SD perspective; in that way, the evidence cited can reinforce areas where the country already has local evidence and fill the gaps in those areas where local evidence is missing.

Previous work has been done in looking at the connection between health and development[52,53] and health taxes and development,[54,55] especially from multilateral institutions. Regarding tobacco, the World Bank[56] presented the public health and economic case for tobacco taxes, with a focus on income equity, poverty and employment. The World Health Organization (WHO)[57] highlighted the role of health taxes to attain the SDGs, in particular on reducing the burden of non-communicable diseases (NCDs), on benefitting vulnerable populations (poverty-SDG1, gender-SDG5 and equity-SDG10) and on boosting economic growth through a healthier workforce (SDG8) and it suggests to move forward by identifying how health taxes fit into a country's SDG plan. The International Monetary Fund (IMF) pointed out the role of corrective health taxes to create fiscal space,[58] and its work mainly focuses on using health taxes to address environmental issues.[43,59]

In contrast to previous work, the review presented in the following sections does not intend to comprehensively cover all the evidence available around one specific mechanism or to cover every possible mechanism related to SD; instead, it aims to describe the main mechanisms behind the expected effects of health taxes from the broader perspective of SD, connecting them with SDGs and supporting those mechanisms on scientific evidence. In that way, the contribution is to present a basic SD case for health taxes supported in a solid set of general and rigorous evidence; this basic SD case can be used by any country as a starting point to make their own case, adding local context, evidence and specific proposals on health taxes. Recognising SDGs' integrity and indivisibility, all SDGs were analysed and the ones more directly related to health taxes were included as the main mechanisms. Also, the references included were selected to be as general as possible, in the sense that most of them are systematic reviews covering as many countries as possible. For that reason, the magnitudes of the mechanisms and the heterogeneity of those magnitudes across societies and people are discussed in the references included in the review.

A summary of the mechanisms presented in the following sections is useful to equip the reader with a map to navigate the section. For the purpose of clarity and despite of its indivisible nature, SDGs were classified into the three systems that sustain human life: the global society (Section 6.3.1), the earth's physical environment (Section 6.3.2) and the world's economy (Section 6.3.3). The analysis starts in the global society with the effect of health taxes on reducing consumption of harmful goods and the subsequent benefits on health (SDG3), and the averted catastrophic expenditure on healthcare contributes to reduction of poverty (SDG1); since those benefits are higher for vulnerable populations, there is a positive effect on income (SDG10) and gender (SDG5) equality. Then, it moves to the earth's physical environment, where the reduction in consumption has positive effects on reducing waste, especially from plastic packaging (SDG12) and pollution from fossil fuels (SDG7), with the ensuing effects of clean water and sanitation (SDG6), climate action (SDG13) and life below water (SDG14) and land (SDG15). Finally, in the world economy, health taxes increase productivity, economic growth and decent work (SDG8), create incentives for industrial transformation towards more sustainable technologies and consumption products (SDG9) and provide an important source of tax revenues for financing SD and for developing a robust public sector able to invest in public goods that accelerate progress on SD (SDG17). Those effects, especially the ones on financing SD, require strong institutions and continuous investment to overcome the country's constraints. The discussion on tax revenues, institutions and investment is carried out in Section 6.3.4. For a detailed graphic map, the causal diagram presented in Figure 6.1 shows the main mechanisms through which health taxes contribute to SD.

Fig. 6.1. Causal diagram of health taxes & SD.

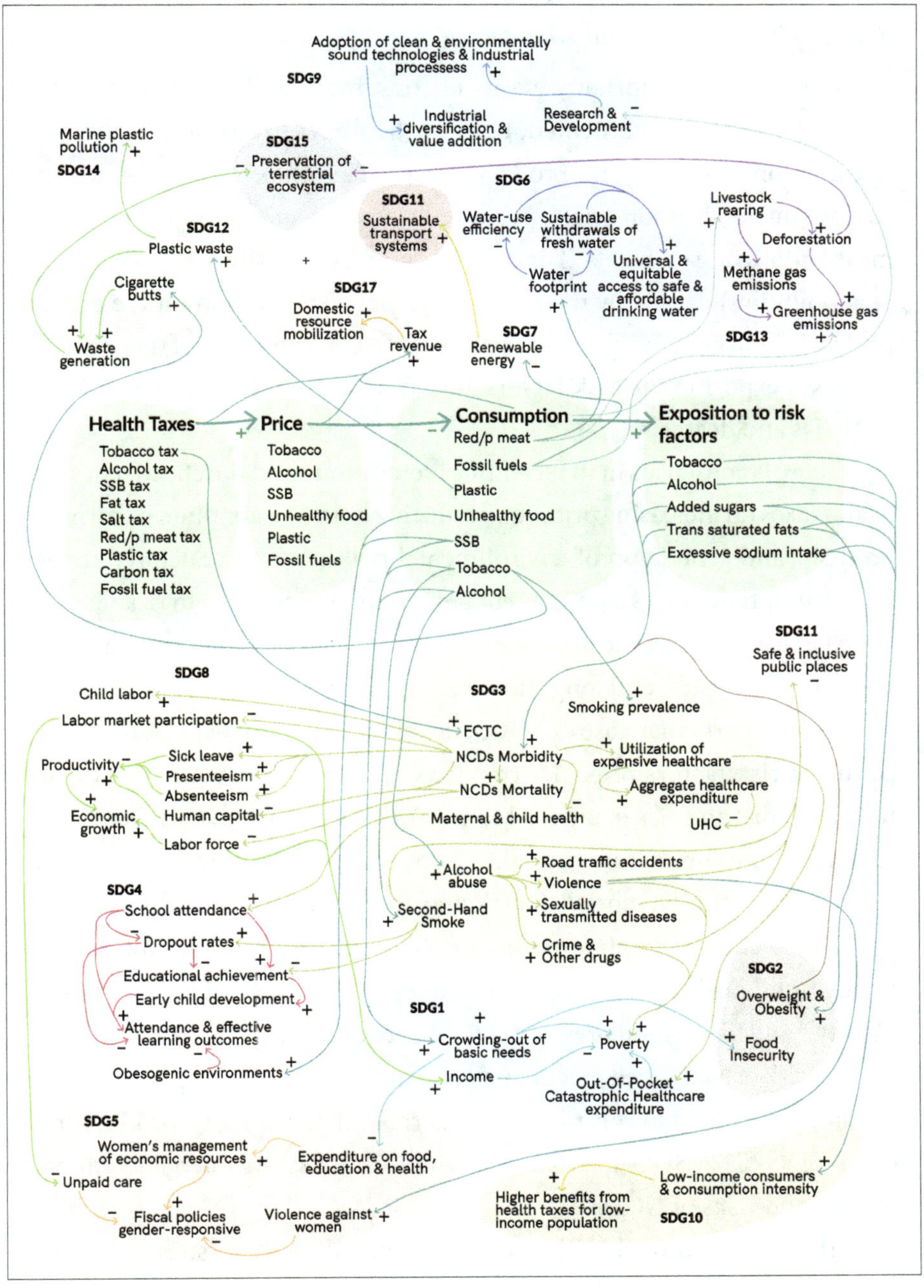

6.3.1. System 1: The global society

SDG3: Good health and well-being

The morbidity and mortality effects of consumption of harmful products have been widely documented, both in the direct exposition to the risk factor in consumption of the product (tobacco,[60] alcohol,[61] SSBs,[62,63] excessive sodium intake,[64,65] industrially produced trans fats and saturated fats,[66] red meat and processed meats[67]) and in the indirect exposition to risk factors (e.g. pollution) caused by the effects of global consumption on the earth's physical environment (plastic,[68] fossil fuels[69]). Consumption of these goods increases exposition to risk factors, and from there it increases incidence of NCDs and deaths.

There is consensus in the scientific literature around the effectiveness of health taxes on increasing prices and reducing both consumption of harmful products and generation of environmental polluters[43,70–74]. Such reduction in consumption causes a permanent reduction in exposition to risk factors, which in turn reduces the likelihood of subsequent disease and death in the medium (2–5 years) and long run (lifetime horizon).

For the particular case of SDG3, health taxes reduce exposition to the common risk factors of NCDs (tobacco use, harmful use of alcohol, an unhealthy diet and lack of physical activity)[75], contributing to the SDG Target of reduction of premature mortality from NCDs (SDG-T3.4), specifically the SDG Indicator on mortality attributed to cardiovascular disease, cancer, diabetes or chronic respiratory disease (SDG-I3.4.1). In addition it lowers populations' health risk of NCDs by reducing precursors of NCDs such as obesity[76] and high blood pressure. All these effects are magnified by the fact that the risk of NCDs and precursors starts in the womb, making health taxes a policy instrument to contribute to maternal (SDG-T3.1, SDG-I3.1.1) and child (SDG-T3.2, SDG-I3.2.1) health and to address the intergenerational burden and risks of NCDs.[77]

At the same time, health taxes contribute directly to strengthen the prevention of alcohol abuse (SDG-T3.5) and harmful use of alcohol (SDG-I3.5.2), and through this mechanism they indirectly contribute to lower deaths and injuries from road traffic accidents (SDG-T3.6, SDGI-3.6.1) from drinking and driving.[78] In addition, increases in tobacco taxes, by definition, are part of the implementation of the Framework Convention on Tobacco Control,[79] making a direct contribution to SDG-T3.A, and the reduction in consumption is progress on reducing smoking prevalence (SDG-I3.A.1). Also, health taxes on pollutants such as fossil fuels or plastic, as well as tobacco taxes through the effect on reduction of second-hand smoke, reduce deaths and illnesses from air and water pollution (SDG-T3.9, SDG-I3.9.1, SDG-I3.9.2).

Healthcare for treatment of NCDs is expensive for people and health systems[80,81] mainly because health technologies and resources for treatment of NCDs are more expensive than average costs of healthcare; at the same time, the chronic nature of NCDs requires long-term utilisation of those expensive technologies to fulfill treatment needs. Reduction of diseases and deaths from NCDs caused by health taxes is expected to lower healthcare utilisation, benefitting the country's health system through lower aggregate healthcare utilisation and expenditure; this makes health taxes an instrument for health systems financing via healthcare savings. Furthermore, conditional on the country's institutional strength on tax administration (see Section 6.3.4), the release of health systems' physical, human and financial resources opens the opportunity to advance on universal healthcare (SDG-T3.8), by expanding the population and service coverage (for instance, according to country's needs, sexual and reproductive healthcare services, making progress on SDG-T3.7).

In regard to financial protection, health taxes on food have been claimed to be a component of a health insurance system, as they contribute to correct the market failures of moral hazard, adverse selection and incomplete markets,[82] and the argument also applies to taxes on alcohol and tobacco. In addition, when there is social health insurance, health taxes create incentives to reduce the healthcare cost externality imposed over individuals who do not consume harmful goods.

Overall, health taxes have positive effects on health systems and represent an opportunity to leapfrog on achieving Universal Health Coverage (SDG-T3.8): they reduce healthcare utilisation of pricey services, avert financial risks from out-of-pocket healthcare expenditure (SDG-I3.8.2) and release resources to expand population coverage of essential health services (SDG-I3.8.1).

SDG1: No poverty

Poverty is 'the pronounced deprivation in well-being',[83] and it is usually measured as the proportion of a country's population living below the national poverty line, the last one being a minimum standard of income needed to achieve a basic living standard. The study of health taxes on development has been mostly concentrated on the link between health taxes and poverty[84], and it has identified the main mechanisms through which tobacco consumption might exacerbate poverty, known as the vicious cycle of tobacco and poverty: (i) the crowding-out effect of tobacco consumption on expenditure on basic needs, (ii) the reduction of income due to tobacco-related illnesses or lifetime disability of family members, (iii) catastrophic or impoverishing healthcare costs[85] and (iv) death (especially of the wage-earning members).

The evidence suggests that these mechanisms also work with alcohol[86,87] due, in part, to the nature of complementary behaviour between smoking and drinking.[88] As for unhealthy food (SSBs, trans and saturated fats, salt, red and processed meats), obesity and NCDs have important healthcare costs that can lead to poverty[89,90] as well as obesity-related illnesses and death.[91] Consumption of alcohol also has additional effects that might lead to or reinforce poverty, such as violence, suicide, traffic-crash, sexually transmitted diseases, use of other drugs and crime.[71] Pollution is also a causal factor of poverty through the effect that high and frequent exposition to polluters has on incidence of chronic health conditions[92]. The effect becomes a vicious circle as it is more likely that poor individuals live and work in environments with higher exposition to pollution.

Health taxes can contribute to reductions in poverty (SDG-T1.1) and extreme poverty (SDG-T1.2) by preventing catastrophic expenditure on healthcare, reduction of income due to NCDs and death of members of the family, as well as reducing violence and pollution. Despite of these positive effects, the lack of renewable sources of energy that can substitute the use of fossil fuels as well as of alternative sustainable technologies for packaging to replace plastic might have negative effects on poverty, because they can increase food prices and through that push more households below the poverty line.[93] For that reason, increases on carbon and plastic taxes must be coordinated with the country's transition to sustainable sources of energy and packaging technologies and standards.

SDG10: Reduced inequalities

Populations with lower income and education are more exposed to consumption of harmful products[94] and to dangerous environmental conditions.[95] Over time, higher exposition ultimately creates health inequalities, that is, relatively higher prevalence of disease and mortality.[96] The analysis of inequalities and health taxes has been mainly concentrated on income inequality and on tobacco.[97] The key mechanism for analysing income inequality is the fact that low-income populations have higher consumption and, at the same time, they are more sensitive to changes in prices (price-elasticity of demand), making them more likely to consume these products as long as they are cheap.

Increases on health taxes directly affect the price of taxed goods, making them less affordable and causing a reduction at both the extensive (number of consumers) and the intensive (quantity of good consumed) margins. This effect is higher in low-income populations as compared to medium- and high-income populations because low-income populations are more sensitive to changes in prices.[98] The traditional approach to study the effect of taxes on inequalities is the standard fiscal incidence analysis of short-term changes (as Ref.[99] call it). Results from standard fiscal incidence analysis suggest that health taxes are financially regressive,[72,100] as more expensive goods with small decrease in consumption at the intensive margin will increase expenditure, imposing a higher burden on low-income individuals. This analysis provides an incomplete understanding of the effects of health taxes, because it only focuses on the price paid and the expected expenditure of the ones who did not change their consumption at the extensive margin.

The analysis of inequalities based on an SD perspective overcomes those limitations, because it takes into account all the expected effects, namely, the reduction at the intensive and extensive margins, the medium- and long-term health effects from reducing or suppressing harmful consumption, and the direct and feedback effects on all three systems. Under that perspective, health taxes have proved to be a progressive policy because the health and SD benefits for low-income populations exceed by far the ones for high-income populations.[31,72,98,99,101–105] One of these progressive effects of health taxes is explicit in SDGs and occurs through the mechanism of financial protection: by protecting mostly low-income individuals from catastrophic expenditure due to NCDs, health taxes avert individuals from falling below 50% of the median income, contributing to progress on SDG-T10.2 and SDG-I-10.2.1.

SDG5: Gender equality

Gender inequality 'limits the opportunities and capabilities of half the world's population'.[19] In addition to the mechanisms highlighted in all other dimensions of SD, excessive alcohol intake can lead to intrahousehold violence against women and to sexually transmitted diseases.[71] Also, NCDs impose a lifetime homecare burden on other household's members, more likely on women.[106] Consumption of harmful products also crowds-out expenditure on other essential items such as food and education[107] and reduce intrahousehold female empowerment in managing resource allocation and expenditures.

The reduction on alcohol intake derived from increases on health taxes contributes to gender equity, specifically on reduction of violence against women (SDG-T5.2, SDG-I5.2.1, SDG-I5.2.2) and reduction of NCD burden on unpaid care (SDG-T5.4, SDG-I5.4.1). In addition, the reduction in consumption of tobacco and alcohol has positive effects on households' welfare as it releases resources to be spent on other welfare-improving goods such as food and education, and it can also give more right to women in managing economic resources in the household, especially in the cases of reductions in tobacco and alcohol consumption (SDG-5.A).

Based on these mechanisms, health taxes can be used as a tool to include gender as part of the impact analysis of fiscal systems, as well as to make fiscal policies gender-responsive[44]; these changes in fiscal systems would represent policies for the promotion of gender equality and empowerment of women (SGD-T5.C).

Other SDGs

SDG2: Zero hunger

Tobacco, alcohol and SSB taxes release resources to be spent on food and therefore they indirectly help in reducing undernourishment and food insecurity; at the same time, the expected increase in food prices derived from carbon and plastic taxes might threat undernourishment (SDG-T2.1.1) and food insecurity (SDG-T2.1.2). The net effect depends on the country's stage on transition to renewable energy sources.

In addition, by reducing consumption of unhealthy food and creating incentives for substituting for healthier food, health taxes reduce overweight and obesity (SDG-T2.2.2), and that effect is reinforced by the higher satiety and improved eating behaviour coming from lower consumption of SSBs[108] and high-energy density diets[109] (Section 6.4.8). Those effects are particularly important in children because children's obesity has long-term consequences on their health when adults.[110]

SDG 4: Quality education

Health and education are the two main components of human capital, and causality goes in both directions[111,112]: health facilitates and benefits from education. Health taxes are an instrument to prevent the effects on children's health of behaviours such as smoking,[113,114] consumption of alcohol[115] and obesity[116] and environmental conditions such as air pollution.[117] Also, NCDs related to those behaviours affect schooling attendance and dropout rates.[118] Through those mechanisms, health taxes can contribute to provide accurate conditions for early child development (SDG-T4.2) and for attendance and effective learning outcomes in primary and secondary education

(SDG-T4.1). Also, in addition to food, reduction of tobacco or alcohol changes intrahousehold allocation of resources, favouring expenditures on education.[107]

Finally, health taxes change decisions in individuals, households and organisations, including schools. The increase in price of unhealthy food changes purchase decisions of learning environments (households and schools), making them less obesogenic[119] and contributing to progress on healthier schools.[120] In this way, health taxes also contribute in having effective learning environments (SDG-T4.A). A final effect relevant for this dimension is averted deaths of teachers. NCDs cause a significant loss of human capital through disease, disability and death; teachers are also affected by NCDs and represent a special part of the stock of a country's human capital as they are providers of core education for children. Health taxes contribute to avert the loss of teachers' human capital, making an indirect contribution to SDG-T4.C.

SDG11: Sustainable cities and environments

By reducing tobacco and alcohol consumption, health taxes also contribute to reduce violence, physical and sexual harassment and second-hand smoke in public places, thus supporting progress towards safer and inclusive public spaces (SDG-T11.7, SDDG-I11.7.2) and in general towards healthier urban environments.[121–123]

6.3.2. System 2: The earth's physical environment

Health taxes have the potential to reduce the negative impact of human activities on the ecosystem, mainly by raising the price and reducing the consumption of products whose life cycle cause serious damage to the earth's physical environment, including fuels, pesticides, the use of natural capital such as timber,[44] deforestation and waste. The negative impact on the ecosystems is widely documented in the literature: tobacco,[124,125] alcohol,[126] soda drinks,[45] unhealthy foods[127]and fossil fuels for transport[128] and electricity.[129]

SDG12: Responsible consumption and production

Plastic waste is the third most important component of global waste.[130] Plastic bags, sachets and plastic bottles seem to be the most common plastic items found in waste.[131]

Taxes on SSBs can contribute in reducing plastic waste from consumption of SSBs as long as there is access to alternatives that do not use plastic packaging, namely, drinking water services. In addition, taxes on plastic bags directly reduce plastic waste. Tobacco taxes can also contribute by reducing waste of cigarette butts and plastic cigarette packaging. Through these mechanisms, health taxes can support progress on reducing waste generation through prevention (SGD-T12.5). In addition, carbon taxes and elimination of fossil-fuel subsidies can contribute to progress on SGD-T12.C.

SDG 7: Affordable and clean energy

Production of energy, in particular electricity, heat and transportation, is the most important primary source of greenhouse emissions. The world energy matrix shows that fossil fuels, namely oil, coal and gas, represent around 80% of the primary energy consumption,[132] making fossil fuels the most important source of greenhouse emissions through consumption of electricity. The externalities derived from the use of fossil fuels impose colossal costs to society not only in health (e.g. Ref.[133]) but also in global warming[f,134] and those costs ultimately translate into subsidies (negative taxes) on production of fossil fuels. The most recent estimates suggest that those subsidies represent 6.3% of global GDP and such enormous magnitude does not seem to decrease over time.[135]

Removal of fossil fuel subsidies (negative taxes) and implementation/increase of positive taxes on fossil fuels represent an incentive to transform the energy mix from fossil fuels to renewable energy (SDG-T7.2), although

[f] Of course there is an additional indirect effect on health via the effect of global warming on health (causal-loop effect). This kind of cycle effects is ubiquitous in SD mostly because of the interaction among the three systems mentioned before. To simplify the discussion, we limit the analysis to direct effects.

such transformation is expected to occur in a medium-term horizon. Because electricity, heat and transportation represent basic needs, fossil fuel taxes must be complemented with policies changing the country's energy matrix.

SDG6: Clean water and sanitation

Safe and clean drinking water and sanitation are a human right[136] and production of some harmful goods has an important water footprint. In particular, meat consumption is one of the four major determinants of a country's water footprint.[137] Also, the food and beverage industry, in particular, the soft drink beverage industry and the bottled water industry are a threat to the right to water because of the local effects of groundwater extraction.[138]

Health taxes, in particular taxes on SSBs and on red and processed meat[139] can reduce water footprint from these industries, through significant reductions in consumption. For SSBs, it is important to guarantee access to drinking water services; otherwise, consumers might substitute SSBs either for bottled water, causing no changes on water footprint, or for alcohol (beer), with the negative effects it has on health and SD. Similarly, although less restrictive given the wider variety of substitutes, having access to alternative sources of protein that can replace consumption of red and processed meat is one condition to guarantee effectiveness of the tax on that product. Through these mechanisms both taxes can contribute directly to increase water-use efficiency and to ensure sustainable withdrawals of freshwater (SDG-T6.4), and through that target, can contribute indirectly to universal and equitable access to safe and affordable drinking water (SDG-T6.1).

Other SDGs

Health taxes contribute to climate action (SDG13), life below water (SDG14), life on land (SDG15) and sustainable cities and communities (SDG11). Since livestock rearing is an important contributor to greenhouse emissions through methane gas and deforestation,[140] reduction in consumption of red and processed meat[141] through removal of agricultural subsidies[142] and subsequent positive taxation (excises) on those products can help in reducing greenhouse emissions (SDG-I13.2.1), in addition to the direct effect on greenhouse emissions from carbon taxes. For life below water, taxes on plastic bags and on SSBs reduce marine plastic pollution,[74] contributing to SDG-T14.1. Finally, the reduction of harmful products and waste derived from its consumption reduces deforestation and contributes to preservation of terrestrial ecosystems (SDG-T15.1).

The incentive for transition to renewable sources of energy and the subsequent transformation of transport systems should lead to sustainable transport systems in the medium run, contributing to SDG-T11.2. Also, the expected effect from health taxes on greenhouse emissions, particulate matter and production of waste contributes to SDG-T11.6.

6.3.3. System 3: The world economy

SDG8: Decent work and economic growth

Economic growth is mainly determined by factor accumulation, productivity and fundamentals (institutions, culture, geography, natural resources).[143] The main production factors are labour and capital, while the main components of total factor productivity are technology and efficiency. Consumption of harmful products can undermine economic growth through several mechanisms. First, the health effects on morbidity, mortality and disability explained in Section 6.3.1 directly translate in reduction of labour productivity due to reduction of labour market participation, sick leave, presenteeism, absenteeism and loss of labour force due to premature mortality.[83,144–146] Second, effects on the environment such as air pollution also reduce labour productivity.[147]

Third, impacts on labour productivity are exacerbated by the fact that an important part of the labour force has accumulated some level of human capital (education); thus, the reduction of productivity also leads to subutilisation of human capital and, in the case of premature mortality, the complete loss of that capital. Also, in young population, impacts extend to reductions in educational achievement.[117,148,149] An additional effect on growth comes from the threat to the national and global environment, which is one of the fundamentals or necessary conditions for economic growth. At the macroeconomic level, the aggregate costs represent a significant barrier to increase economic growth.[150–152]

Given those effects of consumption of harmful products, health taxes contribute to SD on decent work and economic growth with increases in labour productivity by averting disease, disability and death of the labour force in general, as well as efficient use of education human capital embedded in the labour force. Also, health taxes reduce the possibilities of unemployment, school non-attendance and dropouts through the medium-term effect on reducing smoking, alcoholism, obesity and NCDs, as well as through the reduction on pollution (SDG-T8.6, SDG-I8.6.1). Furthermore, health taxes have an indirect effect on reducing child labour (SDG-T8.7, SDG-I8.7.1), as some of the industries whose products are targeted by health taxes are also the ones that rely the most on child labour, specifically tobacco farming.[153] In addition, health taxes indirectly contribute to preserving the earth's physical environment (see Section 6.3.2), thus supporting the fundamentals of economic growth (SDG 8.1, SDG-T8.1.1).

SDG9: Industry, innovation and infrastructure

In terms of innovation and technological progress, by making harmful products less affordable, health taxes create incentives to shift the demand toward other products and services that work as substitutes, from food with lower content of sugar to alternative sources of energy. This creates an opportunity for product reformulation and diversification (SDG-T8.2), creativity and innovation (SDG-T8.3) and global resource efficiency in production to decouple economic growth from environmental degradation (SDGT-T8.4). This aspect is essential to SD for several reasons. First, because the main contribution the private sector can do to SD is the transformation of their products' life cycle in such a way that the current harm to the three systems that sustain human life is significantly reduced. In particular, transformations induced by health taxes that increase resource-use efficiency and achieve greater adoption of clean and environmentally sound technologies and industrial processes (SDG-T9.4, SDG-I9.4.1), through public and private research and development (SDG-T9.5, SDG-I9.5.1), for technology development and innovation to increase the capacity to generate added value (SDG-T9.B, SDG-T9.B.1). Second, because some industries have traditionally opposed SD through public policy and regulation interference,[154–156] it is necessary to complement health taxes with a strong complementary policy that deepens regulated competition to replace change-averse oligopolic incumbent companies. As the OECD's Programme for Effective Market Regulation asserts, such policy 'allows new firms to challenge incumbents, efficient firms to grow and inefficient ones to exit'.

A word of caveat is important. As opposed to the food, electricity or transportation industries, alcohol and tobacco do not represent basic needs, and therefore innovation from the tobacco and alcohol industries, by definition, is incompatible with SD. For that reason, the United Nations Global Compact, the world's largest corporate sustainability initiative, decided to exclude tobacco companies in 2017. Therefore, no innovation from these two industries, for example, Electronic Nicotine and Non-Nicotine Delivery System, can contribute to SDG9, to any of the SDGs, and in general, to any part of the global agenda on SD.

6.3.4. Tax revenues and financing for sustainable development

The general framework for financing SD is the Addis Ababa agenda,[3] a set of agreements and policy recommendations to pull funding from domestic public resources, domestic and international private business and international development cooperation. With regard to health taxes, the agenda explicitly recognises the need to (i) rationalise inefficient fossil-fuel subsidies that encourage wasteful consumption by removing market distortions, (ii) correct and prevent trade restrictions and distortions in world agricultural markets, (iii) prohibition of certain forms of subsidies that contribute to overcapacity and overfishing, (iv) enhance revenue administration through modernised, progressive tax systems, improved tax policy and more efficient tax collection, (v) ensure transparency in all financial transactions between governments and companies to relevant tax authorities (vi) address excessive tax incentives related to extractive industries. In addition, it recognises that 'price and tax measures on tobacco can be an effective and important means to reduce tobacco consumption and healthcare costs, and represent a revenue stream for financing for development in many countries'.

In general, tax revenues improve society's welfare through progressive redistribution of wealth and there is consensus on redistribution as a contributing factor to reduce inequality (e.g. Refs.[93,157]). In addition to that, pointing out the potential gains on redistribution of tax revenue helps in gaining public support for health taxes (e.g. potential source of funding for early childhood education[101]). A necessary condition for those positive effects on wealth redistribution is to have solid institutions, especially the ones in charge of tax collection and administration; such condition is necessary because tax administration and enforcement can be costly, and higher taxes in countries with weak institutions can introduce more corruption and taxes can be diverted to other uses (as it has been the case with donor funding[158]).

For the particular case of health taxes, their main goal is to change incentives on health-related behaviours, and in addition, as a side-effect, they generate tax revenues, giving the country a double win to reach health and revenue objectives,[44] and strengthening domestic resource mobilisation (SDG-T17.1, SGD-I17.1.1, SGD-I17.1.2). The SD perspective expands this view because, as shown in previous sections, they can contribute to progress on SD, and when designed as a package of taxes, their capacity to raise revenue for public purposes without eroding fiscal sustainability is significantly increased. Thus, health taxes are a tool for governments to expand fiscal space for financing SD. Additionally, the SD perspective shows that elimination of subsidies to production of harmful goods, for example, fossil-fuel subsidies (SDG-T12.C), releases resources that can be reallocated to support progress on SD and, at the same time, creates incentives for industrial transformation. Additionally, the integrated and indivisible nature of SD minimises the problem of fragmentation of public budget that can limit coordination across sectors,[159] and thus become an obstacle to progress on the intersectoral actions that constitute the fieldwork of SDGs.

The SD approach to health taxes suggests that tax revenues must be invested in developing a robust public sector, and part of that is to invest in public goods that accelerate progress on SD. One of those public goods is the strengthening of social protection systems, in order to cover the poor and vulnerable (SDG-T1.3) and to achieve greater equality (SDG-T10.4), reinforcing the protective effect health taxes have on poverty and inequality described in previous sections. Promotion of human capital is another public good and plays a key role in social protection systems as a way to provide capital embedded in the labour force for generation of revenue, and health taxes (corrective taxes) have been recognised as a source of funding for development of human capital.[58] Under such redistribution health taxes would have an effect on building and upgrading education facilities (SDG-T4.A) with access to drinking water and sanitation services, and to handwashing facilities (SDG-I4.A.1). In the same line, extending access to drinking water services not only to schools but also to households and workplaces contributes to achieve universal and equitable access to safe and affordable drinking water for all (SDG-T6.1), and it is an example of how to remove local constraints for further progress on taxes on SSBs.

Regarding health, investment of tax revenues on progress on Universal Health Coverage is another way to increase human capital (SDG-T3.8) as well as universal access to sexual and reproductive health (SDG-T5.6); the last one also contributes to gender equity, as well as the investment in public services to reduce unpaid care and domestic work.[44] Another public good to invest tax revenues is on reforestation and conservation of ecosystems, contributing to SDG-T13.A, SDG-T15.A, and SDG-T15.B.

Finally, investment of tax revenues on tax administration is necessary to guarantee the effectiveness of health taxes, especially to improve the domestic capacity for tax collection (SDG-T17.1). This has the potential to contribute on other fundamentals that can be a constraint for further progress of health taxes, for example, alternative sources of energy, accurate implementation of tracking and tracing systems to control and reduce illicit trade of products or development of sustainable technologies for product packaging.

6.4. Making a case for health taxes from a development perspective

Moving from analysis to action, this section presents some guidelines on how to make a case for health taxes from the SD perspective. The elements presented do not intend to be comprehensive of every possible strategy to make a case, because the domain of possible strategies changes according to the country's local conditions. Instead, it represents a set of basic steps that provide the minimum information and actions to place, keep and move up health taxes in the list of prioritised actions in the country's development agenda.

To get the guidelines close to the logic of policymaking, they have been grouped into the five stages of the policy cycle.[160] Although some might apply to several or even all steps, they have been placed in the step where, to our consideration, will be more useful and needed, so an open interpretation and adequation to local context is necessary. Because of the multiple and complex links between health taxes and SD (Section 6.3), most of the country's institutions (ministries) have some connection with health taxes, and might play an active role in all stages. However, most of the work on design, implementation and enforcement of health taxes concentrates around the country's fiscal sector capacity (usually Ministry of Finance and institutions on tax administration), and policymaking capacity from the health sector (usually Ministry of Health). For that reason, a crucial previous step to all stages is to early develop strong and credible alliances and common goals between the country's fiscal and health sector.

Step 0. SDGs and health taxes diagnosis

A precondition (Step 0) for making a case for health taxes is a sound grasp of the country's current state on SDGs and on health taxes; this requires to measure both (i) the country's observed status and (ii) the expected progress by 2030 both on health taxes and SDGs targets and indicators. For the observed status, measurement of SDGs' indicators is by itself a challenge for national statistic systems in some countries,[161] and overcoming those systemic limitations might take a long time. In those cases, an alternative to overcome limitations on information and fill the gaps on the diagnosis is to develop a qualitative analysis focused on the goals[162] and complement it with a conservative estimation of the current state of the most relevant targets and indicators; such estimation can be carried out by putting together atomised but reliable information available from several solid independent sources.

Regarding the expected progress by 2030, it consists on carrying out a diagnosis of the country's development plan and agenda, that might have incorporated the SDGs and, less likely, health taxes. The comparison of the current state and the expected progress provides a benchmark to motivate the discussion. Although doing such diagnostic for every goal, target and indicator might become a sluggish task due to all resources it needs, this chapter has proposed a prioritisation of goals and targets that might significantly reduce the domain and speed up the diagnostic.

Finally, it is important to identify the country's binding constraints for health taxes. Constraints come up when the taxed good is part of a class of goods that represent basic needs and the country's current capacities cannot guarantee access to alternative healthier goods for everyone. In those cases, increases on health taxes must go hand in hand with investments on removing constraints for healthier alternatives, with the tax revenue from health taxes as the first obvious candidate for financing such investments. For instance, tobacco or alcohol are not basic needs, and therefore tobacco and alcohol taxes have no binding constraints. In contrast, public transportation based on fossil fuels might be the only public option for urban commuting; in that case, the country has a constraint that calls for increases on health taxes accompanied by a transition to green public transport vehicles as well as infrastructure to support private sustainable mobility. The effects of investments on removing constraints might have not only local but also global positive effects; for example, investments on creating capacity for alternative sustainable sources of energy to replace fossil fuels contribute to reduce not only local but also global pollution.

Step 1. Agenda setting

SDGs allow to make a much stronger case for health taxes by giving them multiple entry points into the country's policy agenda, instead of the traditional single entry point of health. A stronger case is necessary for both to raise awareness of the need for health taxes and to gain broader support from key stakeholders and from society in general; such support is a necessary and pivotal condition for uptake (approval and implementation) of the policy.

In practice, in order to make a case in the agenda-setting stage of policymaking, a first step is to identify (i) entry points in the agenda, (ii) actors that can position health taxes in the agenda and (iii) accurate arguments favouring health taxes for each entry point in the agenda. For example, it might be the case that the country's discussion on the policy agenda is around an environmental issue such as pollution as opposed to a health issue such as obesity. In that case, there is a clear entry point for carbon taxes, but also a case can be made for tobacco taxes pointing out the benefits for the environment on reducing waste of cigarette butts[163,164]; in fact, a fiscal package on health taxes can be made by extending the argument to plastic waste from SSBs and pollutants from production of alcohol.[165]

A second step consists on diffusion of arguments among actors, in order to raise awareness of the importance of health taxes for progress on development. These actors include academia, civil society, government and private sector, as long as there is no direct or indirect conflict of interest. Using the SD perspective for health taxes significantly expands the range of actors potentially interested in supporting the case for health taxes. Solid evidence-based infographics and investment cases[166–169] could be good instruments to put together and socialise the case on uptake of health taxes and the expected benefits of such policy.

Step 2. Policy formulation

The core element to make a case in this step is to have a robust proposal for health taxes, and to share that proposal with decision makers. The robustness of the proposals comes mainly from three elements: (i) use of rigorous scientific evidence, (ii) incorporation of local constraints, trade-offs and positive synergies and (iii) connection to the country's policy agenda through the entry points identified in Step 1.

To begin with, the use of rigorous scientific evidence on all relevant areas of SD is the core component for having credibility on the case. A key ingredient for this component is to go from the general to specific scientific literature, that is, to start the review of evidence in the monographs and systematic reviews on health taxes,[60,71,76,84,89,144,170,171] as opposed to starting with articles with specific cases (e.g. Refs.[41,45,172,173]), because the general literature identifies the consensus and uncertainties around key policy parameters and provides a general framework to organise the review of evidence. Also, since discussions on health taxes under an SD perspective bring in many stakeholders as well as many vested interests, it is essential to exclude any evidence showing direct or indirect conflict of interest; otherwise, it is possible to end up formulating a policy on health taxes that protects commercial interests instead of society's welfare. This point is important as commercial determinants of health,[174,175] in particular some producers of harmful products, actively exert industry interference,[154,176] and are constantly trying to question the scientific evidence and to position studies sponsored by them to protect their own interests.

A second aspect to be considered in policy formulation is the use of ex-ante evaluation, also known as modelling studies. These evaluations estimate the expected effect of health taxes by putting together a sequence of expected events connecting the set of health taxes with final outcomes on health and on SD. The sequence is represented in a mathematical model whose parameters are calibrated based on previous estimates from scientific literature and on the country's local evidence, conditions and constraints, and it allows to explicitly incorporate the trade-offs and synergies in SD. The results of these evaluations are extremely useful for policy formulation because they clearly quantify the expected benefits and costs of the policy under different scenarios (e.g. Refs. [101,177,178]).

Some of the modelling methods to develop ex-ante evaluation have been incorporated in standardised tools for tax design, such as WHO's TaxSim for tobacco taxes, and are convenient to produce a simple, quick ex-ante evaluation of a tax proposal. Even though there are no standardised tools for other taxes and no tools at all for packages of health taxes with an SD perspective, cost-effectiveness analysis is a simple but powerful way to have a basic but rigorous ex-ante evaluation of health taxes.[179] The extended version of cost-effectiveness analysis is of particular interest for SD, as it has the flexibility to include dimensions other than health in the set of expected benefits of the taxes.[180,181] The use of scientific evidence can be complemented and strengthened by a review of experiences of other similar countries on health taxes. For example, the long experience on tobacco suggests that a non-gradual (go fast) leap (go big) in well-designed taxes[56] is an imperative principle for policy formulation.

The third aspect is to set up an ambitious but feasible design, in terms of the amount of the tax as well as on the spectrum of products included in the formulation of health taxes, taking into account local constraints and SD entry points in the current policy agenda. The SD perspective allows to make a stronger case for considerable increases, because it highlights externalities other than the ones directly related to health. Also, the SD perspective calls for taxing a set of harmful goods rather than making a separate tax design for each good, which is more likely to be perceived by ministries of finance as a fiscal package that needs technical discussion and eventual inclusion on tax reforms, instead of a specific need of the health sector.

The final aspect is that policy formulation from an SD perspective should provide incentives for industrial transformation, coming either from the incumbent companies or from new entrants under a policy of regulated competition. At the same time, the policy formulation should gradually remove subsidies on production of harmful goods because such subsidies magnify the negative effects of consumption of those goods on SD. Finally, it is key to be aware of introduction of loopholes, delays and bad design suggested by agents with conflict of interests; this is more likely to occur in a SD discussion as the range of participants is considerably wider. A policy brief with all the technical details of the proposal is a good instrument to support policy formulation. Validation of the technical content of the proposal with experts from the public sector, academia or multilateral institutions with no conflict of interest can make the proposal stronger.

Step 3. Decision-making

The core of this step is to gain society's support for health taxes; at the end, uptake of health taxes reflects the capacity of the country's citizens to be 'dignified agents of their own destiny'.[20] One way to do so is by raising awareness using judicious arguments based on scientific evidence. The SD perspective helps in this aspect by opening many additional entry points to raise awareness of and get support from, as compared to selling health taxes just as a public health measure.

A second aspect to consider in this step is to be prepared for negotiation, having second best proposals, always respecting the restriction of high increases to effectively affect consumption. One way to do so is to prioritise based on the local conditions and also based on the health taxes that face less trade-offs (e.g. tobacco and alcohol have no trade-offs). Another way is to pass the ones of easier approval first and then position the remaining ones in the political agenda, instead of passing all health taxes at the same time.

A third aspect is that gaining support requires an investment of political capital. For that reason, it is important to find allies willing to invest political capital to move forward the proposal on health taxes and SDGs. The SD perspective expands the spectrum of possible allies beyond the natural allies of ministries of health and finance. Along this process, it is important to be aware of conflicts of interests that can undermine public support for health taxes. The SD perspective contributes in this area by giving a comprehensive approach to potential conflicts of interest.

Finally, highlighting early potential victories is important to get quick and broad support for health taxes. This means to use in the public discussion not only the medium- and long-run effects of health taxes but also the short-run effects where evidence is more perceptible. For example, reduction in cigarette butts follows immediately the reduction in smokers or on smoking intensity and a similar short-run effect occurs to plastic bottles in consumption of SSBs. Politicians usually do not have a long-run perspective of SD, so short-run effects might be useful in gaining their support. Also, the wide range of benefits provided by the SD perspective on health taxes contributes to that purpose, and emphasis on sensitive areas in the society can be useful in raising public awareness of the need for health taxes (e.g. smoking initiation in children).

Step 4. Policy implementation

When using taxes as policy instruments, the capacity to collect the tax is the key part of implementation. For that, it is crucial to align the work of institutions involved in tax administration and tax collection, and implement mechanisms to strengthen tax administration[182,183] (for instance, tracking and tracing systems for tobacco[184] and alcohol). The perspective of SD might facilitate this task because the amount of expected tax revenue is significantly higher, and so the interest on improving tax administration (see Section 6.3.4).

Step 5. Policy evaluation

Ex-post evaluations (also known as intervention studies or impact evaluations) use data collected before and after changes in the tax in order to determine the effect of the increase in the tax on consumption, health and SD (e.g. Refs.[185–187]). Continuous monitoring and ex-post evaluation of the policy are essential to support a long-run agenda on health taxes and SD, because it identifies opportunities to improve the design of health taxes based on the observed effects of the policy, in order to reach further gains on public health and SD by continuously improving it, adapting it to the local context,[51] and overcoming country's constraints on SD. A side benefit of a continuous monitoring and evaluation is that it helps to fill the gap in scientific evidence on health taxes all over the world, especially in low- and middle-income countries where that gap in some dimensions of SD is bigger.[188]

In terms of action, the crucial ingredient for continuous monitoring and evaluation is to develop and use capacities on constantly measure the risks factors (consumption of harmful goods), determinants of risk factors, health outcomes and SD outcomes. This is a colossal action, because of (i) the multiple risk factors, determinants of risk factors,[189,175] health outcomes[190] and SD outcomes[13] and (ii) the complexity of the connections between them.[191–193] For that reason, it is a long-run task that can only be done by gradually and continuously improving the available information and expanding it to include additional dimensions and connections. The active involvement of multiple actors with no conflict of interest, especially academia, is an important element for permanent action in this area.

6.5. Conclusions and policy remarks

The traditional analysis of health taxes focuses on the positive effects they have on people's health and on generation of tax revenue. However, they can also significantly contribute to progress on SD by acting as strong incentives to change people's behaviour towards SD, and changes in incentives are a core strategy for successful development policies[194]; in addition they mobilise domestic public resources for financing SD. Further uptake of health taxes worldwide is crucial because the world is not on track for achieving the SDGs, and health taxes are an entry point to accelerate progress on the SD agenda. This chapter presented the evidence linking health taxes and SDGs, and provides a step-by-step guide on how to make a case for health taxes from the SD perspective.

Most of the literature on health taxes and SD has focused on the effect they have on income inequalities and the discussion around health taxes being either progressive or regressive. The chapter shows that the effects go beyond income inequalities; in general, health taxes positively affect the three systems that sustain human life, namely, the global society, the earth's physical system and the world's economy.

To rip the rewards on SD, health taxes must be well-designed, meaning that they have to consider the country's constraints on alternatives to goods related to basic human needs (air, water, food, shelter, hygiene, transport), and to work together to correct the distortions and negative effects of externalities and internalities to minimise the unexpected effects of the country's constraints.

Further research is needed to build stronger evidence around the links between health taxes and all three dimensions of SD, especially ex-post evaluation of the effects of health taxes on SD. For that to happen, it is necessary to expand the scope of health monitoring and evaluation systems to the three dimensions of development and the wider spectrum of variables and indicators presented in the chapter. Finally, despite of the need for more research and for stronger monitoring and evaluation of health taxes, the chapter shows that there is enough evidence to support a strong case for health taxes from the SD perspective; such perspective is crucial because of its enormous potential to gain wider societal support to further uptake and increase of health taxes.

Key messages

- Health taxes' effects on Sustainable Development (SD) go beyond health, tax revenue and income inequalities. In fact, they positively affect the three systems that sustain human life, namely, the global society, the earth's physical system and the world's economy.
- The world is not on track for achieving the SDGs, and bold actions are required to overcome this challenge. Meaningful progress on global uptake and increase of health taxes is an entry point to accelerate progress on the SD agenda.
- Reframing health taxes from the SD perspective in all stages of the policy cycle has an enormous potential to gain wider societal support for progress on global uptake and increase of health taxes.

Annex: Sustainable Development Goals, Targets and Indicators

Table A6.1. Sustainable Development Goals (SDG), Targets (SDG-T) and Indicators (SDG-I).

#SDG	#SDG-T	#SDG-I
1 No Poverty	1.1 By 2030, eradicate extreme poverty for all people everywhere, currently measured as people living on less than $1.25 a day	1.1.1 Proportion of population below the international poverty line, by sex, age, employment status and geographical location (urban/rural)
	1.2 By 2030, reduce at least by half the proportion of men, women and children of all ages living in poverty in all its dimensions according to national definitions	1.2.1 Proportion of population living below the national poverty line, by sex and age
	1.3 Implement nationally appropriate social protection systems and measures for all, including floors, and by 2030 achieve substantial coverage of the poor and the vulnerable	1.3.1 Proportion of population covered by social protection floors/systems, by sex, distinguishing children, unemployed persons, older persons, persons with disabilities, pregnant women, newborns, work-injury victims and the poor and the vulnerable
2 Zero Hunger	2.1 By 2030, end hunger and ensure access by all people, in particular the poor and people in vulnerable situations, including infants, to safe, nutritious and sufficient food all year round	2.1.1 Prevalence of undernourishment
	2.2 By 2030, end all forms of malnutrition, including achieving, by 2025, the internationally agreed targets on stunting and wasting in children under 5 years of age, and address the nutritional needs of adolescent girls, pregnant and lactating women and older persons	2.2.2 Prevalence of malnutrition (weight for height >+2 or <-2 standard deviation from the median of the WHO Child Growth Standards) among children under 5 years of age, by type (wasting and overweight)

(Continued)

Table A6.1. *(Continued)*

#SDG	#SDG-T	#SDG-I
3 Good health and well-being	3.1 By 2030, reduce the global maternal mortality ratio to less than 70 per 100,000 live births	3.1.1 Maternal mortality ratio
	3.2 By 2030, end preventable deaths of newborns and children under 5 years of age, with all countries aiming to reduce neonatal mortality to at least as low as 12 per 1,000 live births and under 5 mortality to at least as low as 25 per 1,000 live births	3.2.1 Under-five mortality rate
	3.4 By 2030, reduce by one-third premature mortality from non-communicable diseases through prevention and treatment and promote mental health and well-being	3.4.1 Mortality rate attributed to cardiovascular disease, cancer, diabetes or chronic respiratory disease
	3.5 Strengthen the prevention and treatment of substance abuse, including narcotic drug abuse and harmful use of alcohol	3.5.2 Harmful use of alcohol, defined according to the national context as alcohol per capita consumption (aged 15 years and older) within a calendar year in litres of pure alcohol
	3.6 By 2020, halve the number of global deaths and injuries from road traffic accidents	3.6.1 Death rate due to road traffic injuries
	3.7 By 2030, ensure universal access to sexual and reproductive healthcare services, including for family planning, information and education, and the integration of reproductive health into national strategies and programmes	

Table A6.1. *(Continued)*

#SDG	#SDG-T	#SDG-I
	3.8 Achieve universal health coverage, including financial risk protection, access to quality essential healthcare services and access to safe, effective, quality and affordable essential medicines and vaccines for all	3.8.1 Coverage of essential health services (defined as the average coverage of essential services based on tracer interventions that include reproductive, maternal, newborn and child health, infectious diseases, non-communicable diseases and service capacity and access, among the general and the most disadvantaged population)
		3.8.2 Proportion of population with large household expenditures on health as a share of total household expenditure or income
	3.9 By 2030, substantially reduce the number of deaths and illnesses from hazardous chemicals and air, water and soil pollution and contamination	3.9.1 Mortality rate attributed to household and ambient air pollution
	3.A Strengthen the implementation of the World Health Organization Framework Convention on Tobacco Control in all countries, as appropriate	3.A.1 Age-standardised prevalence of current tobacco use among persons aged 15 years and older
4 Ensure inclusive and equitable quality education and promote lifelong learning opportunities for all	4.1 By 2030, ensure that all girls and boys complete free, equitable and quality primary and secondary education leading to relevant and effective learning outcomes	4.1.1 Proportion of children and young people: (a) in grades 2/3; (b) at the end of primary and (c) at the end of lower secondary achieving at least a minimum proficiency level in (i) reading and (ii) mathematics, by sex
	4.2 By 2030, ensure that all girls and boys have access to quality early childhood development, care and pre- primary education so that they are ready for primary education	4.2.1 Proportion of children under 5 years of age who are developmentally on track in health, learning and psychosocial well-being, by sex

(Continued)

Table A6.1. *(Continued)*

#SDG	#SDG-T	#SDG-I
	4.A Build and upgrade education facilities that are child, disability and gender sensitive and provide safe, non- violent, inclusive and effective learning environments for all	4.A.1 Proportion of schools with access to: (a) electricity; (b) the Internet for pedagogical purposes; (c) computers for pedagogical purposes; (d) adapted infrastructure and materials for students with disabilities; (e) basic drinking water; (f) single-sex basic sanitation facilities and (g) basic handwashing facilities (as per the WASH indicator definitions)
	4.C By 2030, substantially increase the supply of qualified teachers, including through international cooperation for teacher training in developing countries, especially least developed countries and small island developing States	4.C.1 Proportion of teachers in: (a) pre-primary; (b) primary; (c) lower secondary; and (d) upper secondary education who have received at least the minimum organised teacher training (e.g. pedagogical training) pre-service or in-service required for teaching at the relevant level in a given country
5 Achieve gender equality and empower all women and girls	5.2 Eliminate all forms of violence against all women and girls in the public and private spheres, including trafficking and sexual and other types of exploitation	5.2.1 Proportion of ever-partnered women and girls aged 15 years and older subjected to physical, sexual or psychological violence by a current or former intimate partner in the previous 12 months, by form of violence and by age
		5.2.2 Proportion of women and girls aged 15 years and older subjected to sexual violence by persons other than an intimate partner in the previous 12 months, by age and place of occurrence

Table A6.1. *(Continued)*

#SDG	#SDG-T	#SDG-I
	5.4 Recognise and value unpaid care and domestic work through the provision of public services, infrastructure and social protection policies and the promotion of shared responsibility within the household and the family as nationally appropriate	5.4.1 Proportion of time spent on unpaid domestic and care work, by sex, age and location
	5.6 Ensure universal access to sexual and reproductive health and reproductive rights as agreed in accordance with the Programme of Action of the International Conference on Population and Development and the Beijing Platform for Action and the outcome documents of their review conferences	5.6.1 Proportion of women aged 15–49 years who make their own informed decisions regarding sexual relations, contraceptive use and reproductive healthcare
	5.A Undertake reforms to give women equal rights to economic resources, as well as access to ownership and control over land and other forms of property, financial services, inheritance and natural resources, in accordance with national laws	
	5.C Adopt and strengthen sound policies and enforceable legislation for the promotion of gender equality and the empowerment of all women and girls at all levels	
6 Ensure availability and sustainable management of water and sanitation for all	6.1 By 2030, achieve universal and equitable access to safe and affordable drinking water for all	6.1.1 Proportion of population using safely managed drinking water services

(Continued)

Table A6.1. *(Continued)*

#SDG	#SDG-T	#SDG-I
	6.4 By 2030, substantially increase water-use efficiency across all sectors and ensure sustainable withdrawals and supply of freshwater to address water scarcity and substantially reduce the number of people suffering from water scarcity	6.4.2 Level of water stress: freshwater withdrawal as a proportion of available freshwater resources
7 Ensure access to affordable, reliable, sustainable and modern energy for all	7.2 By 2030, increase substantially the share of renewable energy in the global energy mix	7.2.1 Renewable energy share in the total final energy consumption
8 **Promote sustained,** inclusive and sustainable economic growth, full and productive employment and decent work for all	8.1 **Sustain per capita economic growth in** accordance with national circumstances and, in particular, at least 7% gross domestic product growth per annum in the least developed countries	8.1.1 **Annual growth rate of real GDP per capita**
	8.2 Achieve higher levels of economic productivity through diversification, technological upgrading and innovation, including through a focus on high-value added and labour-intensive sectors	8.2.1 Annual growth rate of real GDP per employed person
	8.3 Promote development-oriented policies that support productive activities, decent job creation, entrepreneurship, creativity and innovation, and encourage the formalisation and growth of micro-, small- and medium-sized enterprises, including through access to financial services	8.3.1 Proportion of informal employment in non-agriculture employment, by sex

Table A6.1. *(Continued)*

#SDG	#SDG-T	#SDG-I
	8.4 Improve progressively, through 2030, global resource efficiency in consumption and production and endeavour to decouple economic growth from environmental degradation, in accordance with the 10-year framework of programmes on sustainable consumption and production, with developed countries taking the lead	8.4.1 Material footprint, material footprint per capita, and material footprint per GDP
	8.6 By 2020, substantially reduce the proportion of youth not in employment, education or training	8.6.1 Proportion of youth (aged 15–24 years) not in education, employment or training
	8.7 Take immediate and effective measures to eradicate forced labour, end modern slavery and human trafficking and secure the prohibition and elimination of the worst forms of child labour, including recruitment and use of child soldiers, and by 2025 end child labour in all its forms	8.7.1 Proportion and number of children aged 5–17 years engaged in child labour, by sex and age
9 Build resilient infrastructure, promote inclusive and sustainable industrialisation and foster innovation	9.4 By 2030, upgrade infrastructure and retrofit industries to make them sustainable, with increased resource use efficiency and greater adoption of clean and environmentally sound technologies and industrial processes, with all countries taking action in accordance with their respective capabilities	9.4.1 CO_2 emission per unit of value added
	9.5 Enhance scientific research, upgrade the technological capabilities of industrial sectors in all countries, in particular developing countries, including, by 2030, encouraging innovation and substantially increasing the number of research and development workers per 1 million people and public and private research and development spending	9.5.1 Research and development expenditure as a proportion of GDP

(Continued)

Table A6.1. *(Continued)*

#SDG	#SDG-T	#SDG-I
	9.B Support domestic technology development, research and innovation in developing countries, including by ensuring a conducive policy environment for, *inter alia*, industrial diversification and value addition to commodities	9.B.1 Proportion of medium and high-tech industry value added in total value added
10 Reduce inequality within and among countries	10.2 By 2030, empower and promote the social, economic and political inclusion of all, irrespective of age, sex, disability, race, ethnicity, origin, religion or economic or other status	10.2.1 Proportion of people living below 50 per cent of median income, by age, sex and persons with disabilities
	10.4 Adopt policies, especially fiscal, wage and social protection policies and progressively achieve greater equality	
11 Make cities and human settlements inclusive, safe, resilient and sustainable	11.2 By 2030, provide access to safe, affordable, accessible and sustainable transport systems for all, improving road safety, notably by expanding public transport, with special attention to the needs of those in vulnerable situations, women, children, persons with disabilities and older persons	11.2.1 Proportion of population that has convenient access to public transport, by sex, age and persons with disabilities
	11.6 By 2030, reduce the adverse per capita environmental impact of cities, including by paying special attention to air quality and municipal and other waste management	11.6.1 Proportion of urban solid waste regularly collected and with adequate final discharge out of total urban solid waste generated, by cities

Table A6.1. *(Continued)*

#SDG	#SDG-T		#SDG-I	
	11.7	By 2030, provide universal access to safe, inclusive and accessible, green and public spaces, in particular for women and children, older persons and persons with disabilities	11.7.2	Proportion of persons victim of physical or sexual harassment, by sex, age, disability status and place of occurrence, in the previous 12 months
12 Ensure sustainable consumption and production patterns	12.5	By 2030, substantially reduce waste generation through prevention, reduction, recycling and reuse	12.5.1	National recycling rate, tons of material re-cycled
	12.C	Rationalise inefficient fossil-fuel subsidies that encourage wasteful consumption by removing market distortions, in accordance with national circumstances, including by restructuring taxation and phasing out those harmful subsidies, where they exist, to reflect their environmental impacts, taking fully into account the specific needs and conditions of developing countries and minimising the possible adverse impacts on their development in a manner that protects the poor and the affected communities	12.C.1	Amount of fossil-fuel subsidies per unit of GDP (production and consumption) and as a proportion of total national expenditure on fossil fuels
13 Take urgent action to combat climate change and its impacts	13.2	Integrate climate change measures into national policies, strategies and planning	13.2.1	Number of countries that have communicated the establishment or operationalisation of an integrated policy/strategy/plan which increases their ability to adapt to the adverse impacts of climate change, and foster climate resilience and low greenhouse gas emissions development in a manner that does not threaten food production (including a national adaptation plan, nationally determined contribution, national communication, biennial update report or other)

(Continued)

Table A6.1. *(Continued)*

#SDG	#SDG-T		#SDG-I	
	13.A	Implement the commitment undertaken by developed country parties to the United Nations Framework Convention on Climate Change to a goal of mobilising jointly $100 billion annually by 2020 from all sources to address the needs of developing countries in the context of meaningful mitigation actions and transparency on implementation and fully operationalise the Green Climate Fund through its capitalisation as soon as possible	13.A.1	Mobilised amount of United States dollars per year starting in 2020 accountable towards the $100 billion commitment
14 Conserve and sustainably use the oceans, seas and marine resources for sustainable development	14.1	By 2025, prevent and significantly reduce marine pollution of all kinds, in particular from land-based activities, including marine debris and nutrient pollution	14.1.1	Index of coastal eutrophication and floating plastic debris density
15 Protect, restore and promote sustainable use of terrestrial ecosystems, sustainably manage forests, combat desertification and halt and reverse land degradation and halt biodiversity loss	15.1	By 2020, ensure the conservation, restoration and sustainable use of terrestrial and inland freshwater ecosystems and their services, in particular forests, wetlands, mountains and drylands, in line with obligations under international agreements	15.1.1	Forest area as a proportion of total land area

Table A6.1. *(Continued)*

#SDG	#SDG-T		#SDG-I	
	15.A	Mobilise and significantly increase financial resources from all sources to conserve and sustainably use biodiversity and ecosystems	15.A.1	Official development assistance and public expenditure on conservation and sustainable use of biodiversity and ecosystems
	15.B	Mobilise significant resources from all sources and at all levels to finance sustainable forest management and provide adequate incentives to developing countries to advance such management, including for conservation and reforestation	15.B.1	Official development assistance and public expenditure on conservation and sustainable use of biodiversity and ecosystems
17 Strengthen the means of implementation and revitalise the global partnership for sustainable development	17.1	Strengthen domestic resource mobilisation, including through international support to developing countries, to improve domestic capacity for tax and other revenue collection	17.1.1	Total government revenue as a proportion of GDP, by source
			17.1.2	Proportion of domestic budget funded by domestic taxes

References

1. UN. *International Covenant on Economic, Social and Cultural Rights. Tech. rep.* Adopted, opened for signature, ratification, and accession by General Assembly resolution 2200A (XXI) of 16 December 1966 entry into force 3 January 1976, in accordance with article 27. United Nations (UN), 1966.
2. UN. *Universal Declaration of Human Rights (Illustrated edition).* Tech. rep. United Nations (UN), 2015.
3. UN. *Addis Ababa Action Agenda of the Third International Conference on Financing for Development (Addis Ababa Action Agenda).* Tech. rep. The final text of the outcome document adopted at the Third International Conference on Financing for Development (Addis Ababa, Ethiopia, 13–16 July 2015) and endorsed by the General Assembly in its resolution 69/313 of 27 July 2015, United Nations (UN), 2015.
4. Le Minh T, et al. Assessing Domestic Revenue Mobilization: Analytical Tools and Techniques. 2016.
5. UN. *Transforming our world: the 2030 Agenda for Sustainable Development.* Tech. rep. A/70/L.1. United Nations (UN). General Assembly. Seventieth session, 2015.
6. Naidoo R, Fisher B. Reset sustainable development goals for a pandemic world. Nature 2020; 583: 198-201. DOI: 10.1038/d41586-020-01999-x.
7. Stiglitz, J, Rosengard, J. Chapter 17: Introduction to taxation, In: *Economics of the public sector.* 4th edn. W.W. Norton Company, 2015. ISBN: 978-0-393-92522-7.
8. Susskind L. "Arguing, bargaining and getting agreement." In: *The Oxford Handbook of Public Policy. Ed. by* Moran, Michael, Rein, Martin, and Goodin, Robert. New York, NY, USA: Oxford University Press, 2006. Chap. 13. DOI: 10.1093/oxfordhb/9780199548453.003.0013.
9. Watkins DA, et al. "Intersectoral Policy Priorities for Health." In: *Disease Control Priorities: Improving Health and Reducing Poverty (Volume 9). Ed. by* Jamison, Dean T, et al. 3rd edn. New York, NY, USA: World Bank, 2018. Chap. 2. ISBN: 978-1-4648-0528-8. DOI: 10.1596/978-1-4648-0527-1.
10. Sen A. "The concept of development." In: *Handbook of Development Economics. Ed. by* Chenery, Hollis and Srinivasan, T. Vol. 1. Washington, DC, USA: Elsevier, Jan. 1988. Chap. 1, pp. 9–26. ISBN: 9780444703378. DOI: 10.1016/S1573-4471(88)01004-6.
11. UN. *Agenda for Development.* Tech. rep. A/RES/51/240. United Nations (UN), fifty-first session, 1997. New York, NY, USA.
12. WCED. *Our Common Future. The World Commission on environment and Development (WCED).* Oxford University Press, 1987. ISBN: 0-19-282080-X.
13. Sachs J. *The Age of Sustainable Development.* Columbia University Press, 2015. ISBN: 978-1515910879.
14. UN. *The future we want.* Tech. rep. A/RES/66/288. United Nations (UN). General Assembly. Sixty-sixth session, 2012.
15. UN. *Agenda 21.* Tech. rep. United Nations (UN), Division for Sustainable Development. United Nations Conference on Environment & Development Rio de Janerio, Brazil, 3 to 14 June 1992, 1992.
16. UN. *United Nations Millennium Declaration. Tech.* rep. A/RES/55/2. United Nations (UN), fifty-fifth session, 2000.

17. UN. *The Millennium Development Goals Report. Tech. rep. United Nations (UN),* 2015.
18. Winkler IT, Williams C. The sustainable development goals and human rights: A critical early review. The International Journal of Human Rights. Oct. 2017; 21(8): 1023–1028. DOI: 10.1080/13642987.2017.1348695.
19. UN. *Global Sustainable Development Report 2019: The Future is Now – Science for Achieving Sustainable Development.* Tech. rep. Independent Group of Scientists appointed by the Secretary-General, United Nations (UN), 2019.
20. Easterly W "The SDGs Should Stand for Senseless, Dreamy, Garbled." In: *Foreign Policy* (2015).
21. Siddiqi S, et al. Global strategies and local implementation of health and health-related SDGs: lessons from consultation in countries across five regions. *BMJ Global Health. Sept.* 2020; 5(9): e002859. DOI: 10.1136/bmjgh-2020-002859.
22. UN. *The Sustainable Development Goals Report 2020. Tech. rep. United Nations (UN),* 2020.
23. Leal Filho W, et al. COVID-19 and the UN sustainable development goals: Threat to solidarity or an opportunity? Sustainability. July 2020; 12(13): 5343. DOI: 10.3390/su12135343.
24. Barbier EB, Burgess JC. Sustainability and development after COVID-19. World Development. 2020; 135: 105082. DOI: 10.1016/j.worlddev.2020.105082.
25. ICSU. *A Guide to SDG Interactions: From Science to Implementation. Ed. by* Griggs, DJ, et al. Paris: International Council for Science (ICSU), 2017. DOI: 10.24948/2017.01.
26. Nilsson M, Griggs D, Visbeck M. Policy: Map the interactions between Sustainable Development Goals. *Nature.* 2016; 534: 320-322. DOI: 10.1038/534320a.
27. WHO. *Stronger Collaboration, Better Health: Global Action Plan for Healthy Lives and Well-Being for All. Strengthening Collaboration Among Multilateral Organizations to Accelerate Country Progress on the Health-Related Sustainable Development Goals. Geneva, Switzerland: World Health Organization (WHO), 2019. ISBN:* 978-92-4-151643-3.
28. McGowan PJK, et al. An imperfect vision of indivisibility in the sustainable development goals. *Nature Sustainability.* 2019; 2(1): 43–45. DOI: 10.1038/s41893-018-0190-1.
29. Pradhan P et al. A systematic study of sustainable development goal (SDG) interactions. *Earth's Future.* Nov. 2017; 5(11): 1169-1179. DOI: 10.1002/2017EF000632.
30. Hutchinson B, et al. The investment case as a mechanism for addressing the NCD burden: Evaluating the NCD institutional context in Jamaica, and the return on investment of select interventions. *PLos One.* Oct. 2019; 14(10): e0223412.
31. Saxena A, et al. Modelling the impact of a tax on sweetened beverages in the Philippines: An extended cost-effectiveness analysis. *Bulletin of the World Health Organization.* 2019; 97(2): 97–107. DOI: 10.2471/BLT.18.219980.
32. Yang W, et al. Future health and economic impact of comprehensive tobacco control in DoD: A microsimulation approach. *Military Medicine. Jan.* 2018; 183(1-2): e104–112. DOI: 10.1093/milmed/usx015.

33. Pega F, et al. The need to monitor actions on the social determinants of health. *Bulletin of the World Health Organization*. Nov. 2017; 95(11): 784–787. DOI: 10.2471/BLT.16.184622. https://apps.who.int/iris/handle/10665/272162.
34. Allcott H, Lockwood BB, Taubinsky D. Should we tax sugar-sweetened beverages? An overview of theory and evidence. *The Journal of Economic Perspectives*. 2019; 33(3): 202–227. DOI: 10.1257/jep.33.3.202.
35. Cornes R, Sandler T. *The Theory of Externalities, Public Goods, and Club Goods*. 2nd edn. Cambridge University Press, 1996. ISBN: 0 521 47718 2.
36. Gruber J. Externalities in action: Environmental and health externalities. In: *Public Finance and Public Policy*. 4th edn. Worth Publishers, 2013. Chap. 6.
37. Vezzoli, C. "Chapter 8 – The "Material" Side of Design for Sustainability." In: *Materials Experience: Fundamentals of Materials and Design. Ed. by* Karana, Elvin, Pedgley, Owain, and Rognoli, Valentina B T Boston: Butterworth-Heinemann, 2014, pp. 105–121. ISBN: 978-0-08-099359-1. DOI: 10.1016/B978-0-08-099359-1.00008-4.
38. Mozaffarian D, Rogoff KS, Ludwig DS. The real cost of food: Can taxes and subsidies improve public health?" *JAMA. Sept.* 2014; 312(9): 889–890. DOI: 10.1001/jama.2014.8232.
39. Terra BJM. "Excises." In: *Tax Law Design and Drafting, Volume 1. Ed. by* Thuronyi, Victor. Washington, DC, USA: International Monetary Fund, 1996. Chap. 8.
40. Galizzi MM. Label, nudge or tax? A review of health policies for risky behaviours. *Journal of Public Health Research*. Feb. 2012; 1(1): 14–21. DOI: 10.4081/jphr.2012.e5.
41. Griffith R, O'Connell M, Smith K. Tax design in the alcohol market. *Journal of Public Economics*. April 2019; 172: 20–35. DOI: 10.1016/J.JPUBECO.2018.12.005.
42. Griffith R, O'Connell M, Smith K. Corrective taxation and internalities from food consumption. *CESifo Economic Studies*. Nov. 2017; 64(1): 1–14. DOI: 10.1093/cesifo/ifx018.
43. Parry IWH, et al. *Getting Energy Prices Right: From Principle to Practice*. International Monetary Fund, 2014. ISBN: 978-1-48438-857-0. DOI: 10.5089/9781484388570.071.
44. UN. *Financing for development: Progress and prospects. Report of the Inter-agency Task Force on Financing for Development*. New York, NY, USA. United Nations (UN), 2018. ISBN: 978-92-1-101386-3.
45. Ayalon O, Avnimelech Y, Shechter M. Application of a comparative multidimensional life cycle analysis in solid waste management policy: The case of soft drink containers. *Environmental Science & Policy*. 2000; 3(2): 135–144. DOI: 10.1016/S1462-9011(00)00078-2.
46. Laxminarayan R, Parry I. Health in a time of austerity. *Finance and Development* 2017; 54(3).
47. Landrigan PJ, et al. The Lancet commission on pollution and health. *Lancet (London, England). Feb. 2018;* 391(10119): 462–512. DOI: 10.1016/S0140-6736(17)32345-0.
48. Bonnet C. How to set up an effective food tax? Comment on "food taxes: A new holy grail? *International Journal of Health Policy and Management*. 2013; 1(3): 233–234. DOI: 10.15171/ijhpm.2013.45.

49. Pierani P, Tiezzi S. Addiction and interaction between alcohol and tobacco consumption. *Empirical Economics.* 2009; 37(1): 1–23. DOI: 10.1007/s00181-008-0220-3.
50. Decker SL, Schwartz AE. "Cigarettes and alcohol: Substitutes or Complements?" In: *National Bureau of Economic Research Working Paper Series No.* 7535 (2000) DOI: 10.3386/w7535.
51. Isaranuwatchai W, et al. Prevention of non-communicable disease: Best buys, wasted buys, and contestable buys. *BMJ. Jan.* 2020; 368: m141. DOI: 10.1136/bmj.m141.
52. Acharya S, Lin V, Dhingra N. The role of health in achieving the sustainable development goals. *Bulletin of the World Health Organization.* Sept. 2018; 96(9): 591–591A. DOI: 10.2471/BLT.18.221432.
53. GBD 2015 SDG Collaborators. Measuring the health-related Sustainable Development Goals in 188 countries: A baseline analysis from the Global Burden of Disease Study 2015. *Lancet (London, England). Oct. 2016;* 388(10053): 1813–1850. DOI: 10.1016/S0140-6736(16)31467-2.
54. STAX. Sugar, tobacco, and alcohol taxes to achieve the SDGs. *The Lancet.* June 2018; 391(10138): 2400–2401. DOI: 10.1016/S0140-6736(18)31219-4.
55. Nugent R, et al. Investing in non-communicable disease prevention and management to advance the Sustainable Development Goals. *The Lancet.* May 2018; 391(10134): 2029–2035. DOI: 10.1016/S0140-6736(18)30667-6.
56. Marquez P, Moreno-Dodson B, *Tobacco Tax Reform at the Crossroads of Health and Development: A Multisectoral Perspective.* Tech. rep. World Bank, 2017.
57. WHO. *Health taxes: A primer.* Tech. rep. World Health Organization (WHO), WHO/UHC/HGF/Policy brief 19.7, 2019.
58. Coady D. Creating fiscal space. *Finance and Development.* 2018; 55(4).
59. Parry, IWH, Norregaard J, Heine D. "Environmental tax reform: Principles from theory and practice to date." 2012.
60. HHS. *The Health Consequences of Smoking—50 years of progress. A Report of the Surgeon General.* Tech. rep. U.S. Department of Health and Human Services (HHS), 2014.
61. WHO. *Global Status Report on Alcohol and Health. World Health Organization (WHO),* 2018. ISBN: 978-92-4-156563-9.
62. Malik VS, Hu FB. Sugar-sweetened beverages and cardiometabolic health: An update of the evidence. *Nutrients.* 2019; 11(8). DOI: 10.3390/nu11081840.
63. Teng AM, et al. Impact of sugar-sweetened beverage taxes on purchases and dietary intake: Systematic review and meta-analysis. *Obesity Reviews. Sept.* 2019; 20(9): 1187–1204. DOI: 10.1111/obr.12868.
64. Brown IJ, et al. Salt intakes around the world: Implications for public health. *International Journal of Epidemiology.* April 2009; 38(3): 791–813. DOI: 10.1093/ije/dyp139.
65. He FJ, MacGregor GA. A comprehensive review on salt and health and current experience of worldwide salt reduction programmes. *Journal of Human Hypertension.* 2009; 23(6): 363–384. DOI: 10.1038/jhh.2008.144.

66. Forouhi NG, et al. Dietary fat and cardiometabolic health: Evidence, controversies, and consensus for guidance. *BMJ.* June 2018; 361: k2139. DOI: 10.1136/bmj.k2139.
67. IARC. *Red meat and processed meat. International Agency for Research on Cancer (IARC).* Monographs on the evaluation of carcinogenic risks to humans. Volume 114, 2018. ISBN: 978-92-832-0180-9.
68. Halden RU. Plastics and health risks. *Annual Review of Public Health.* March 2010; 1(1): 179–194. DOI: 10.1146/annurev.publhealth.012809.103714.
69. Kampa M, Castanas E. Human health effects of air pollution. *Environmental Pollution.* 2008; 151(2): 362–367. DOI: 10.1016/j.envpol.2007.06.012.
70. IARC. *Vol. 14: Effectiveness of Tax and Price Policies for Tobacco Control.* Tech. rep. International Agency for Research on Cancer - IARC, 2011.
71. Wagenaar AC, Tobler AL, Komro KA. Effects of alcohol tax and price policies on morbidity and mortality: A systematic review. *American Journal of Public Health* Nov. 2010; 100(11): 2270–2278. DOI: 10.2105/AJPH.2009.186007.
72. Backholer K, et al. The impact of a tax on sugar-sweetened beverages according to socio- economic position: A systematic review of the evidence. *Public Health Nutrition.* 2016; 19(17): 3070–3084. DOI: 10.1017/S136898001600104X.
73. Smed, S et al. The effects of the Danish saturated fat tax on food and nutrient intake and modelled health outcomes: An econometric and comparative risk assessment evaluation. *European Journal of Clinical Nutrition.* 2016; 70(6): 681–686. DOI: 10. 1038/ejcn.2016.6.
74. Xanthos D, Walker TR. International policies to reduce plastic marine pollution from single-use plastics (plastic bags and microbeads): A review. *Marine Pollution Bulletin.* May 2017; 118(1–2): 17–26. DOI: 10.1016/J.MARPOLBUL.2017.02.048.
75. UN. *Political Declaration of the High-level Meeting of the General Assembly on the Prevention and Control of Non-communicable Diseases.* Tech. rep. United Nations (UN), General Assembly resolution 66/2 (A/RES/66/2), 2011.
76. Thow AM, et al. The effect of fiscal policy on diet, obesity and chronic disease: A systematic review. *Bulletin of the World Health Organization.* 2010; 88: 609–614. DOI: 10.2471/BLT.09.070987.
77. Hanson M, et al. Intergenerational burden and risks of NCDs: Need to promote maternal and child health. *Lancet.* Dec. 2018; 392(10163): 2422–2423. DOI: 10.101 6/S0140-6736(18)33053-8.
78. Taylor B, et al. The more you drink, the harder you fall: A systematic review and meta-analysis of how acute alcohol consumption and injury or collision risk increase together. *Drug and Alcohol Dependence.* July 2010; 110(1–2): 108–116. DOI: 10.101 6/J.DRUGALCDEP.2010.02.011.
79. UN. "WHO Framework Convention on Tobacco Control." In: *Chapter 4. Health. United Nations Treaty Collection. United Nations (UN), 2015.*
80. Muka T, et al. The global impact of non-communicable diseases on healthcare spending and national income: A systematic review. *European Journal of Epidemiology.* 2015; 30(4): 251–277. DOI: 10.1007/s10654-014-9984-2.

81. Kankeu HT, et al. The financial burden from non-communicable diseases in low- and middle-income countries: A literature review. *Health Research Policy and Systems.* 2013; 11(1): 31. DOI: 10.1186/1478-4505-11-31.
82. Strnad J. Conceptualizing the "fat tax": The role of food taxes in developed economies. *Southern California Law Review.* 2005; 78.
83. Haughton J, Khandker SR. *Handbook on Poverty and Inequality.* Washington, DC, USA. The World Bank, 2009. ISBN: 978-0-8213-7613-3. DOI: 10.1596/978-0-821 3-7613-3.
84. NCI and WHO. *The Economics of Tobacco and Tobacco Control.* Tech. rep. NCI Tobacco Control Monograph Series 21. Department of Health and Human Services, National Institutes of Health, U.S. National Cancer Institute (NCI), World Health Organization (WHO), 2016.
85. WHO and The World Bank. *Tracking Universal Health Coverage: 2017 Global Monitoring Report.* World Health Organization (WHO), Geneva, CH: The World Bank, 2017. ISBN: 978 92 4 151355 5.
86. Pu C-Y, et al. The crowding-out effects of tobacco and alcohol where expenditure shares are low: Analyzing expenditure data for Taiwan. *Social Science & Medicine.* May 2008; 66(9): 1979–1989. DOI: 10.1016/J.SOCSCIMED.2008.01.007.
87. Thanh NX, et al. Fetal alcohol spectrum disorder - Poverty trap? *Journal of Population Therapeutics and Clinical Pharmacology.* 2013; 20(1).
88. Room R. Smoking and drinking as complementary behaviours. *Biomedicine & Pharmacotherapy.* March 2004; 58(2): 111–115. DOI: 10.1016/J.BIOPHA.2003.12.003.
89. Jaspers L, et al. The global impact of non-communicable diseases on households and impoverishment: A systematic review. *European Journal of Epidemiology.* 2015; 30(3): 163–188. DOI: 10.1007/s10654-014-9983-3.
90. Finkelstein E, Yang HK. "Obesity and Medical Costs." In: *The Oxford Handbook of the Social Science of Obesity. Ed. by* Cawley, John. New York, NY, USA: Oxford University Press, 2011. Chap. 29. ISBN: 9780199736362. DOI: 10.1093/oxfordhb/ 9780199736362.013.0029.
91. Mehta NK, Chang VW. "Obesity and Mortality." English. In: *The Oxford Hand-book of the Social Science of Obesity. Ed. by* Cawley, John. New York, NY, USA: Oxford University Press, 2012. Chap. 30. ISBN: 9780199736362. DOI: 10.1093/oxfordhb/9 780199736362.013.0030.
92. Lipfert FW. Air pollution and poverty: Does the sword cut both ways? *Journal of Epidemiology and Community Health.* Jan. 2004; 58(1): 2–3. DOI: 10.1136/jech.58.1.2.
93. Renner S. Poverty and distributional effects of a carbon tax in Mexico. *Energy Policy.* Jan. 2018; 112: 98–110. DOI: 10.1016/J.ENPOL.2017.10.011.
94. Hosseinpoor AR, et al. Socioeconomic inequalities in risk factors for non communicable diseases in low-income and middle-income countries: Results from the World Health Survey. *BMC Public Health.* 2012; 12(1): 912. DOI: 10.1186/147 1-2458-12-912.
95. Samet J. The environment and health inequalities: Problems and solutions. *Journal of Health Inequalities.* 2019; 5(1): 21–27. DOI: 10.5114/jhi.2019.87818.

96. WHO. *Equity, social determinants and public health programmes. Ed. by* Blas, Erik and Sivasankara Kurup, Anand. World Health Organization (WHO), Geneva, CH. 2010. ISBN: 9789241563970.
97. Jain V, et al. Equity as a consideration in evaluations of health taxes: A systematic review. *The Lancet. Nov.* 2019; **394**: S8. DOI: 10.1016/S0140-6736(19)32805-3.
98. Sassi F, et al. Equity impacts of price policies to promote healthy behaviours. *Lancet (London, England) May 2018*; 391(10134): 2059–2070. DOI: 10.1016/S0140-6736(18)30531-2.
99. Lavado RF, et al. Beyond the perceived regressivity of higher tobacco taxes. Turning short-term losers into long-term winners? *Tobacco tax reform. At the crossroads of health and development. A Multisectoral Perspective.* 2017. Chap. 6.
100. Vandenberg B, Sharma A. Are alcohol taxation and pricing policies regressive? Product-level effects of a specific tax and a minimum unit price for alcohol. *Alcohol and Alcoholism.* June 2016; 51(4): 493–502. DOI: 10.1093/alcalc/agv133.
101. Basu S, Madsen K. Effectiveness and equity of sugar-sweetened beverage taxation. *PLOS Medicine.* June 2017; 14(6): e1002327. DOI: 10.1371/journal.pmed.1002327.
102. Hall W. Socioeconomic status and susceptibility to alcohol-related harm. *The Lancet. Public health* June 2017; 2(6): e250–e251. DOI: 10.1016/S2468-2667(17)30089-0.
103. Nordström J, Thunström L. Can targeted food taxes and subsidies improve the diet? Distributional effects among income groups. *Food Policy*, 2011; 36(2): 259–271. DOI: 10.1016/j.foodpol.2010.11.023.
104. Verguet S, Gauvreau CL, Mishra S, MacLennan M, Murphy SM, Brouwer ED, Nugent RA, Zhao K, Jha P, Jamison DT. The consequences of tobacco tax on household health and finances in rich and poor smokers in China: An extended cost-effectiveness analysis. *Global Health.* 2015; 3: 206–216. DOI: 10.1016/S2214-109X(15)70095-1.
105. James EK, et al. Distributional health and financial benefits of increased tobacco taxes in Colombia: Results from a modelling study. *Tobacco Control.* July 2019; 28(4): 374–380. DOI: 10.1136/tobaccocontrol-2018-054378.
106. Shaji K, Reddy M. Caregiving: A public health priority. *Indian Journal of Psychological Medicine.* Oct. 2012; 34(4): 303–305. DOI: 10.4103/0253-7176.108191.
107. John RM. Crowding out effect of tobacco expenditure and its implications on household resource allocation in India. *Social Science & Medicine.* March 2008; 66(6): 1356–1367. DOI: 10.1016/J.SOCSCIMED.2007.11.020.
108. Hollis JH. Beverages, satiation, satiety, and energy balance. *Beverage Impacts on Health and Nutrition.* 2nd Edn. Switzerland: Humana Press, 2016. Chap. 12, pp. 181–192. ISBN: 978-3-319- 23672-8. DOI: 10.1007/978-3-319-23672-8.
109. Benelam B. Satiation, satiety and their effects on eating behaviour. *Nutrition Bulletin.* June 2009; 34(2): 126–173. DOI: 10.1111/j.1467-3010.2009.01753.x.
110. Biro FM, Wien M. Childhood obesity and adult morbidities. *The American Journal of Clinical Nutrition.* March 2010; 91(5): 1499S–1505S. DOI: 10.3945/ajcn.2010.28701B.
111. Grossman M. Chapter 10 education and nonmarket outcomes. *Handbook of the Economics of Education* 1 (Jan. 2006), pp. 577–633. DOI: 10.1016/S1574-0692(06)01010-5.

112. Grossman M. The relationship between health and schooling: What's new? *Nordic Journal of Health Economics* 2015; 3(1): 7–17. DOI: 10.5617/njhe.2362.
113. Faber T, et al. Effect of tobacco control policies on perinatal and child health: A systematic review and meta-analysis. *The Lancet Public Health.* Sept. 2017; 2(9): e420–e437. DOI: 10.1016/S2468-2667(17)30144-5.
114. Oken E, Levitan EB, Gillman MW. Maternal smoking during pregnancy and child overweight: Systematic review and meta-analysis. *International Journal of Obesity.* 2008; 32(2): 201–210. DOI: 10.1038/sj.ijo.0803760.
115. Mangiavacchi L, Piccoli L. Parental alcohol consumption and adult children's educational attainment. *Economics & Human Biology.* Feb. 2018; 28: 132–145. DOI: 10.1016/J.EHB.2017.12.006.
116. Pan L, et al. The association of obesity and school absenteeism attributed to illness or injury among adolescents in the United States, 2009. *The Journal of Adolescent Health: Official Publication of the Society for Adolescent Medicine.* Jan. 2013; 52(1): 64–69. DOI: 10.1016/j.jadohealth.2012.04.003.
117. Currie J, et al. Does pollution increase school absences?" *The Review of Economics and Statistics.* Oct. 2009; 91(4): 682–694. DOI: 10.1162/rest.91.4.682.
118. Fletcher JM, Richards MR. Diabetes's 'health shock' to schooling and earnings: Increased dropout rates and lower wages and employment in young adults. *Health Affairs. Jan.* 2012; 31(1): 27–34. DOI: 10.1377/hlthaff.2011.0862.
119. Rendina D, Campanozzi A, De Filippo G. Methodological approach to the assessment of the obesogenic environment in children and adolescents: A review of the literature. *Nutrition, Metabolism and Cardiovascular Diseases.* 2019; 29(6): 561–571. DOI: 10 .1016/j.numecd.2019.02.009.
120. CDC. *Healthy Schools. How CDC Helps Students Get a Healthy Start.* Tech. rep. Centers for Disease Control, Prevention (CDC). National Center for Chronic Disease Prevention, and Health Promotion Division of Population Health, 2019.
121. Lawrence RJ, Fudge C. Healthy cities in a global and regional context. *Health Promotion International.* Nov. 2009; 24(suppl_1): i11–i18. DOI: 10.1093/heapro/dap051.
122. Corburn J. *Toward the healthy city. People, Places, and the Politics of Urban Planning.* The MIT Press, 2009. ISBN: 978-0-262-01331-4.
123. de Leeuw E, Simos J. eds. *Healthy Cities. The Theory, Policy, and Practice of Value-Based Urban Planning.* Springer, 2017. ISBN: 978-1-4939-6694-3. DOI: 10.1007/978-1-4939-6694-3.
124. Lecours N, et al. Environmental health impacts of tobacco farming: A review of the literature. *Tobacco Control.* March 2012; 21(2): 191–196. DOI: 10.1136/tobaccocontrol-2011-050318.
125. Novotny TE, et al. The environmental and health impacts of tobacco agriculture, cigarette manufacture and consumption. *Bulletin of the World Health Organization.* Dec. 2015; 93(12): 877–880. DOI: 10.2471/BLT.15.152744.
126. Garnett T. The alcohol we drink and its contribution to the UK's greenhouse gas emissions: A discussion paper. 2007.

127. Clark MA, et al. Multiple health and environmental impacts of foods. *Proceedings of the National Academy of Sciences.* Nov. 2019; 116(46): 23357–23362. DOI: 10.1073/pnas.1906908116.
128. Colvile RN, et al. The transport sector as a source of air pollution. *Atmospheric Environment.* 2001; 35(9): 1537–1565. DOI: 10.1016/S1352-2310(00)00551-3.
129. Borenstein S. The private and public economics of renewable electricity generation. *Journal of Economic Perspectives.* 2012; 26(1): 67–92. DOI: 10.1257/jep.26.1.67.
130. Kaza S, et al. *What a waste 2.0. A global snapshot of solid waste management to 2050.* Urban Development Series. Washington DC, USA: The World Bank, 2018. ISBN: 978-1-4648-1347-4. DOI: 10.1596/978-1-4648-1329-0.
131. BFFP. *Branded.* Vol. *II: Identifying the World's Top Corporate Plastic Polluters.* Tech. rep. Break Free from Plastic (BFFP), Greenpeace, 2019.
132. Oliveira JFG, Trindade TCG. "World Energy Matrix." In: *Sustainability Performance Evaluation of Renewable Energy Sources: The Case of Brazil. Ed. by* Oliveira, João Fernando Gomes de and Trindade, Tatiana Costa Guimarães. Cham: Springer International Publishing, 2018, pp. 1–17. ISBN: 978-3-319-77607-1. DOI: 10.1007/978-3-319-77607-1_1.
133. Machol B, Rizk S. Economic value of U.S. fossil fuel electricity health impacts. *Environment International.* 2013; 52: 75–80. DOI: 10.1016/j.envint.2012.03.003.
134. Covert T, Greenstone M, Knittel CR. Will we ever stop using fossil fuels? *Journal of Economic Perspectives.* 2016; 30(1): 117–138. DOI: 10.1257/jep.30.1.117.
135. Coady D, et al. How large are global fossil fuel subsidies? *World Development.* 2017; 91: 11–27. DOI: 10.1016/j.worlddev.2016.10.004.
136. UN. The Human Right to Water and Sanitation. United Nations (UN), sixty-fourth session, 2010. Tech. rep. A/RES/64/292.
137. Hoekstra AY, Chapagain AK. "Water footprints of nations: Water use by people as a function of their consumption pattern." In: *Integrated Assessment of Water Resources and Global Change: A North-South Analysis. Ed. by* Craswell, Eric, et al. Dordrecht: Springer Netherlands, 2007, pp. 35–48. ISBN: 978-1-4020-5591-1. DOI: 10.1007/978-1-4020-5591-1_3.
138. Mahadevan P. "Troubled waters: impact of the private sector in implementing the right to water." In: *Charting the Water Regulatory Future.* Edward Elgar, Cheltenham, Gloucestershire, UK. 2017. Chap. 11. DOI: 10.4337/9781785366727.00021.
139. Springmann M, et al. Health-motivated taxes on red and processed meat: A modelling study on optimal tax levels and associated health impacts. *Plos One.* Nov. 2018; 13(11): e0204139.
140. Garnett T. Livestock-related greenhouse gas emissions: Impacts and options for policy makers. *Environmental Science & Policy.* June 2009; 12(4): 491–503. DOI: 10.1016/J.ENVSCI.2009.01.006.
141. Walker P, et al. Public health implications of meat production and consumption. *Public Health Nutrition.* 2005; 8(4): 348–356. DOI: 10.1079/PHN2005727.
142. Elinder LS. Obesity, hunger, and agriculture: The damaging role of subsidies. *BMJ.* Dec. 2005; 331(7528): 1333–1336. DOI: 10.1136/bmj.331.7528.1333.

143. Weil D. *Economic Growth*. Harlow, Essex, UK 3rd Ed., Routledge, 2014.
144. Chaker L, et al. The global impact of non-communicable diseases on macro-economic productivity: A systematic review. *European Journal of Epidemiology*. 2015; 30(5): 357–395. DOI: 10.1007/s10654-015-0026-5.
145. Averett SL. "Labor Market Consequences: Employment, Wages, Disability, and Absenteeism." English. In: *The Oxford Handbook of the Social Science of Obesity. Ed. by* Cawley, John. New York, NY, USA: Oxford University Press, 2011. Chap. 32. ISBN: 9780199736362. DOI: 10.1093/oxfordhb/9780199736362.013.0032.
146. Jørgensen MB, et al. Alcohol consumption and labour market participation: A prospective cohort study of transitions between work, unemployment, sickness absence, and social benefits. *European Journal of Epidemiology*. 2019; 34(4): 397–407. DOI: 10.1007/s10654-018-0476-7.
147. Graff Zivin J, Neidell M. The impact of pollution on worker productivity. *American Economic Review*. 2012; 102(7): 3652–3673. DOI: 10.1257/aer.102.7.3652.
148. Latvala A, et al. Drinking, smoking, and educational achievement: Cross-lagged associations from adolescence to adulthood. *Drug and Alcohol Dependence*. April 2014; 137: 106–113. DOI: 10.1016/J.DRUGALCDEP.2014.01.016.
149. Truong K, Sturm R. Schooling and human capital. English. In: *The Oxford Handbook of the Social Science of Obesity. Ed. by* Cawley, John. New York, NY, USA: Oxford University Press, 2011. Chap. 31. ISBN: 9780199736362. DOI: 10.1093/oxfordhb/9780199736362.013.0031.
150. WEF and HSPH. *The Global Economic Burden of Non-communicable Diseases*. Tech. rep. World Economic Forum (WEF), Harvard School of Public Health (HSPH), 2011.
151. Goodchild M, Nargis N, d'Espaignet ET. Global economic cost of smoking-attributable diseases. *Tobacco Control*. Jan. 2018; 27(1): 58–64. DOI: 10.1136/tobaccocontrol-2016-053305.
152. Tremmel M, et al. "Economic burden of obesity: A systematic literature review. *International Journal of Environmental Research and Public Health*. April 2017; 14(4): 435. DOI: 10.3390/ijerph14040435.
153. Lecours N. "The harsh realities of tobacco farming: a review of socioeconomic, health and environmental impacts." In: *Tobacco Control and Tobacco Farming: Separating myth from reality. Ed. by* Leppan, Wardie, Lecours, Natacha, and Buckles, Daniel. International Development Research Center. London, UK: Anthem Press, 2014. Chap. 4. ISBN: 9781552505823.
154. Tangcharoensathien V, et al. Addressing NCDs: Challenges from industry market promotion and interferences. *International Journal of Health Policy and Management*. May 2019; 8(5): 256–260. DOI: 10.15171/ijhpm.2019.02.
155. Gilmore AB, et al. Exposing and addressing tobacco industry conduct in low-income and middle-income countries. *Lancet (London, England), March 2015;* 385(9972): 1029–1043. DOI: 10.1016/S0140-6736(15)60312-9.
156. Marten R, Amul GGH, Casswell S. Alcohol: Global health's blind spot. *The Lancet Global Health*. March 2020; 8(3): e329–e330. DOI: 10.1016/S2214-109X(20)30008-5.

157. Davis LW, Knittel CR. Are fuel economy standards regressive? *Journal of the Association of Environmental and Resource Economists.* March 2019; 6(S1): S37–S63. DOI: 10.1086/701187.
158. Dieleman JL, Graves CM, Hanlon M. The fungibility of health aid: Reconsidering the reconsidered. *The Journal of Development Studies.* Dec. 2013; 49(12): 1755–1762. DOI: 10.1080/00220388.2013.844921.
159. Cashin C, Sparkes S, Bloom D. *Earmarking for Health: From Theory to Practice.* Health Financing Working Paper, World Health Organization, Geneva, CH. 2017.
160. Howlett M, Ramesh M. *Studying Public Policy: Policy Cycles and Policy Subsystems.* 2nd Edn. Ontario, Canada: Oxford University Press, 2003. ISBN: 0-19-541794-1.
161. Pfeiffer A, Middeke F, Tambour M. 2030 agenda for sustainable development: Implications for official statistics. *Statistical Journal of the IAOS.* 2017; 33: 911–918. DOI: 10.3233/SJI-170360.
162. Fukuda-Parr S, McNeill D. Knowledge and politics in setting and measuring the SDGs: Introduction to special issue. *Global Policy. Jan.* 2019; 10(S1): 5–15. DOI: 10 .1111/1758-5899.12604.
163. Smith EA, Novotny TE. Whose butt is it? Tobacco industry research about smokers and cigarette butt waste. *Tobacco Control. May* 2011; 20(Suppl 1): 2–9. DOI: 10.11 36/tc.2010.040105.
164. Novotny TE, Slaughter E. Tobacco product waste: An environmental approach to reduce tobacco consumption. *Current Environmental Health Reports.* 2014; 1(3): 208–216. DOI: 10.1007/s40572-014-0016-x.
165. Carrilho ENVM, Labuto G, and Kamogawa MY. Destination of Vinasse, a residue from alcohol industry: Resource recovery and prevention of pollution. *Environmental Materials and Waste. Jan.* 2016: 21–43. DOI: 10.1016/B978-0-12-803837-6.00002-0.
166. Bertram MY, et al. Investing in non-communicable diseases: An estimation of the return on investment for prevention and treatment services. *The Lancet.* 2018; 391(10134): 2071–2078. DOI: 10.1016/S0140-6736(18)30665-2.
167. Bertram M, et al. Using economic evidence to support policy decisions to fund interventions for non-communicable diseases. *BMJ. May* 2019; 365: l1648. DOI: 1 0.1136/bmj.l1648.
168. Kapur A, Hod M. Maternal health and non-communicable disease prevention: An investment case for the post COVID-19 world and need for better health economic data. *International Journal of Gynecology & Obstetrics.* Aug. 2020; 150(2): 151–158. DOI: 10.1002/ijgo.13198.
169. Nugent RA, et al. Introducing the PLOS special collection of economic cases for NCD prevention and control: A global perspective. *PLOS ONE. Feb.* 2020; 15(2): e0228564.
170. Singh GM, et al. Global, regional, and national consumption of sugar-sweetened beverages, fruit juices, and milk: A systematic assessment of beverage intake in 187 countries. *PLOS ONE.* 2015; 10(8): e0124845. DOI: 10.1371/journal.pone.0124845.
171. Aleksandrowicz L, et al. The impacts of dietary change on greenhouse gas emissions, land use, water use, and health: A systematic review. *PLOS ONE.* Nov. 2016; 11(11): e0165797.

172. Maldonado N, Llorente B, Deaza, J. Impuestos y demanda de cigarrillos en Colombia. *Rev Panam Salud Publica.* 2016; 40(4): 229–236.
173. Colchero MA, et al. Price elasticity of the demand for sugar sweetened beverages and soft drinks in Mexico. *Economics & Human Biology.* Dec. 2015; 19: 129–137. DOI: 10.1016/J.EHB.2015.08.007.
174. Knai C, et al. Systems thinking as a framework for analyzing commercial determinants of health. *The Milbank Quarterly. Sept.* 2018; 96(3): 472–498. DOI: 10.1111/1468-0009.12339.
175. Maani N, et al. Bringing the commercial determinants of health out of the shadows: A review of how the commercial determinants are represented in conceptual frameworks. *European Journal of Public Health.* Jan. 2020. DOI: 10.1093/eurpub/ckz197.
176. Casswell S. Vested interests in addiction research and policy. Why do we not see the corporate interests of the alcohol industry as clearly as we see those of the tobacco industry? *Addiction.* April 2013; 108(4): 680–685. DOI: 10.1111/add.12011.
177. Global Tobacco Economics Consortium. The health, poverty, and financial consequences of a cigarette price increase among 500 million male smokers in 13 middle income countries: Compartmental model study. *BMJ.* April 2018; 361: k1162. DOI: 10.1136/bmj.k1162.
178. Keyes KM, et al. Assessing the impact of alcohol taxation on rates of violent victimization in a large urban area: An agent-based modeling approach. *Addiction. Feb.* 2019; 114(2): 236–247. DOI: 10.1111/add.14470.
179. Horton S. "Cost-Effectiveness Analysis in Disease Control Priorities, Third Edition." In: *Disease Control Priorities: Improving Health and Reducing Poverty. Volume* 9. *3rd edition.* 2018.
180. Verguet S, Jamison D. "Health Policy Analysis: Applications of Extended Cost-Effectiveness Analysis Methodology in Disease Control priorities, Third Edition." In: *Disease Control Priorities: Improving Health and Reducing Poverty. Vol. 9.* Washington DC, USA: World Bank Group, 2018. Chap. 8, pp. 157–166.
181. Verguet S, Kim JJ, Jamison DT. Extended cost-effectiveness analysis for health policy assessment: A tutorial. *PharmacoEconomics.* 2016; 34(9): 913–923. DOI: 10.1007/s40273-016-0414-z.
182. WHO. *WHO Technical Manual on Tobacco Tax Administration.* Tech. rep. World Health Organization (WHO), 2011.
183. Yurekli, Ayda Aysun. *Economics of Tobacco Taxation Toolkit.* Tech. rep. World Bank Group, 2018.
184. WHO. *WHO Protocol to Eliminate Illicit Trade in Tobacco Products.* Tech. rep. 2013.
185. Gallego JM, et al. Tobacco taxes and illicit cigarette trade in Colombia. *Economics & Human Biology.* 2020; 39: 100902. DOI: 10.1016/j.ehb.2020.100902.
186. Koski A, et al. Alcohol tax cuts and increase in alcohol-positive sudden deaths — A time-series intervention analysis. *Addiction.* March 2007; 102(3): 362–368. DOI: 10.1111/j.1360-0443.2006.01715.x.

187. Colchero MA, et al. Beverage purchases from stores in Mexico under the excise tax on sugar sweetened beverages: Observational study. *BMJ.* 2016; 352. DOI: 10.1136 /bmj.h6704.
188. Allen LN, et al. "Are WHO "best buys" for non-communicable diseases effective in low- income and lower-middle-income countries? A systematic review. *The Lancet Global Health.* April 2017; 5: S17. DOI: 10.1016/S2214-109X(17)30124-9.
189. Solar O, Irwin A. *A Conceptual Framework for Action on the Social Determinants of Health.* Tech. rep. 2. World Health Organization (WHO), 2010.
190. Boslaugh S, ed. *Encyclopedia of Epidemiology.* London, UK: SAGE Publications Inc., 2008. ISBN: 9781412928168.
191. Sturmberg J, Martin C, eds. *Handbook of Systems and Complexity in Health.* New York, NY, USA: Springer, 2013. ISBN: 9781461449973. DOI: 10.1007/978-1-4614-4998-0.
192. El-Sayed AM, Galea S, eds. *Systems Science and Population Health.* New York, NY, USA: Oxford University Press, 2017. ISBN: 9780190492410. DOI: 10.1093/acprof:oso/9780190492397.001.0001.
193. Fu B, et al. Unravelling the complexity in achieving the 17 sustainable-development goals. *National Science Review.* March 2019; 6(3): 386–388. DOI: 10.1093/nsr/nwz038.
194. Easterly WR. *The Elusive Quest for Growth: Economists' Adventures and Misadventures in the Tropics.* London, UK: MIT Press, 2001. ISBN: 978-0262550420.
195. Maldonado, Norman et al. "Tobacco taxes as the unsung hero: impact of a tax increase on advancing Sustainable Development in Colombia". In: *International Journal of Public Health* (2022). DOI: 10.3389/ijph.2022.1604353.

https://doi.org/10.1142/9781800612396_0008

Chapter 7

Expanding Health Taxation to Other Unhealthy Behaviours and Harmful Activities

Andreia Costa Santos*, Thiago Hérick de Sá†, Michael Oliver Hinsch†, Ernesto Sanchez Triana‡, and Jeremy A Lauer§

The use of taxation to improve public health has been successful in tackling tobacco and alcohol, with positive and direct effect on health outcomes. However, the taxation of other unhealthy behaviours and activities negatively affecting health (e.g. the increased use of cars) has not yet been explored for the promotion of public health and societal well-being, in particular for reducing premature mortality from non-communicable diseases (NCDs), which account for 70% of global deaths. Taxation can be expanded to unhealthy behaviours and activities affecting individuals' health and well-being, in the pursuit of public health goals. For unhealthy behaviours and some other activities, taxation might be defined at local levels of government, as a way to tackle local health problems. Local governments should be actively collaborating with other levels of government (e.g. federal level), to identify taxation-based solutions for health problems that directly affect

* University of London, UK.

† World Health Organization, Switzerland.

‡ The World Bank, USA.

§ University of Strathclyde, UK (formerly World Health Organization, Switzerland).

their jurisdiction. We use the examples of air pollution, land use, gambling and farming practices to illustrate the challenges facing local authorities, and opportunities to deal with them through taxation and health promotion, particularly in tackling NCDs.

7.1. Introduction

Unhealthy behaviours are major factors behind the rise in non-communicable diseases (NCDs), an annual killer of 40 million people of all ages accounting for 70% of all global deaths, in 2016.[1–3] Pushed by increased industrialisation and urbanisation, the consumption of highly processed food and beverages, harmful use of tobacco and alcohol and physical inactivity have led to detrimental consequences to the health of individuals around the world, with an increasing shift of the burden of NCDs from high-income countries (HICs) to low- and middle-income countries (LMICs).[4–6]

The economic development brought by industrialisation and urbanisation has contributed to harmful living conditions and unhealthy behaviours, exacerbating the risk of diseases. Living conditions and unhealthy behaviours in urban areas are characterised by heavy traffic, physical inactivity, air pollution, housing insecurity and poverty. These conditions lead to premature death, disability and reduced productivity from NCDs, with the urban poor experiencing worse health outcomes compared to their rural counterparts.[7–9] The situation tends to deteriorate as the world's population in urban areas increases. Currently, more than 55% of the world's inhabitants live in urban centres, and by 2050 the proportion is expected to grow to 68%, with Asia and Africa seeing a rise of almost 90%.[10]

Outside urban centres, the prevalence of NCDs is rapidly increasing, driven by physical inactivity and poor diet.[9,11] Obesity, for example, is growing faster in rural areas than in cities, although important differences between countries' income levels are observed: rural populations in HICs, mainly women, are more obese than those in cities because of the indirect effect of their lower-income and education levels, and the direct effects of limited availability and higher price of healthy foods, and less leisure and sports facilities; in LMICs, the mechanisation of labour and increased use of cars reduce physical activity, in addition to an increased spending on low-quality, fat-rich food.[12]

While the use of taxation to improve public health has been successful in tackling unhealthy foods, tobacco and alcohol, with a positive and direct effect on health outcomes,[6,13] the taxation of unhealthy behaviours and activities negatively affecting health (e.g. replacing subsidies with taxation for the increased use of cars and their production and disposal) has not yet been explored for the promotion of public health and societal well-being, in particular for reducing premature mortality from NCDs, one of the United Nation's Sustainable Development Goals.[14]

Taxation of unhealthy products usually occurs at the highest level of government (e.g. federal level), where revenues from taxes have been used to lessen budget deficits, and to promote health, safety, energy and environmental programmes.[15–17] This top-down approach may not be the most effective way to tackle the growing burden of NCDs when dealing with specific unhealthy behaviours and activities negatively affecting health and that may be prone to taxation. Important differences in the drivers of NCDs in urban and rural, HICs and LMICs require a cooperative approach at all governmental levels, with an important role for local governments in defining priorities.[18] For example, heavy traffic and low levels of walking and cycling, as a means of transportation and physical activity, might be an issue more prominent in urban centres than rural localities, thus, defining taxation instruments for vehicles in urban centres might be more effective than at state or federal levels; while the increased gambling leading to alcoholism, drug addiction, mental health conditions and physical inactivity, might be more severe among rural and peri-urban residents than in urban settings. Hence, the revenue generated by taxation designed and applied at the local level could help local authorities to target their populations with awareness campaigns, to provide tailored treatments for those affected and to reach out and engage with the most disadvantaged.[19–23] This approach does not eliminate the role of other levels of government in taxation and regulations, rather, it empowers local governments to contribute to the efforts of combating NCDs.

Taxation at local levels for local problems can strengthen the role of local governments in combating NCDs, empower local authorities to make critical decisions for people in their jurisdiction, and help generate the necessary financial resources to deal with the health issues at hand.[24] Local administration may also increase the transparency, accountability and engagement of citizens when a tax is implemented.[25,26]

This chapter argues that taxation could be expanded to harmful products, activities and health-related behaviours negatively affecting individuals' health and well-being. It also argues that, for unhealthy behaviours and some activities, taxation can be defined and applied at local governmental levels as an efficient way to tackle local health problems. Local governments should also be actively collaborating at other levels of government to define health policies for health problems directly affecting their jurisdictions. We use the examples of air pollution, land use, problem gambling and farming practices to illustrate the challenges facing local authorities, and opportunities to deal with them through taxation and health promotion, in particular in combating NCDs.[a]

7.1.1. Local governments creating and promoting public goods that support health – The role of local taxes for health

Typically, the creation and provision of public goods occur at the highest governmental level (e.g. federal level), where revenues generated by taxation are allocated to different activities such as national defence, flood control systems and the control of water pollution. This direct provision of a public good by the highest level of government can help to overcome the free-rider

[a] Societal well-being, including the promotion and protection of health, can only be achieved when the negative effects of products and behaviours to the society – or *negative externalities*, in economic terms – are eliminated or reduced. Thus, from the perspective of public health, it is not unreasonable to promote ways to correct, reduce or even eliminate the consumption of products that cause harm to health, and to encourage better lifestyles to prevent diseases. Externalities occur when economic transactions carried out by corporations or individuals impose costs or benefits to a third party that is not part of the price. A solution is to impose a tax equivalent to the magnitude of these external costs.[27,28]

problem which leads to market failure.[b] Health – and the promotion of public health – however, requires a whole-system approach, where cooperation between various levels of government is key to achieve the national and international targets for the control of NCDs.

The concept of public goods considers the production of 'goods' that are in the interest of the society, such as the control of climate change and prevention of diseases, but that also demonstrate public good attributes (non-exclusion and non-rivalry). These attributes mean that there is often a lack of incentive to produce these goods. Thus, the central issue of concern within the concept of public goods becomes one of ensuring collective action at all levels of government.[c,30,31]

Collective action by all levels of government requires guaranteeing a degree of independence for a lower authority in relation to a higher body or for a local authority in relation to the central government, involving the sharing of powers between several levels of authority – *the principle of subsidiarity*.[d,32] Thus, local governments can be empowered to act in the production and provision of public health as a public good.

In addition, local governments can produce and provide public goods that are efficiently tailored to local needs and act on policies to address such needs. In particular, urban governments yield *agglomeration* gains, that is, they have advantages in terms of transport and infrastructure, in the concentration of highly qualified workers, in encouraging and facilitating knowledge spillovers for a diverse and productive market and in creating

---

[b] A public good refers to a good that can be accessed and consumed by anyone, without directly paying for it (non-excludable), and once consumed, its availability is not reduced by the use of others (non-rivalrous).[28] Free-riding is a type of market failure that occurs when people can benefit from a good or service without paying for it.[29]

[c] Dees (2017)[30] and Horne (2019)[31] suggest further examination on the concept of public goods to include public health. Horne (2019) stressed the fact that public goods are not the only goods that the market may fail to provide efficiently, providing a way to broaden the account of the public good of public health, without abandoning the public goods' distinctive characteristics.

[d] The principle of subsidiarity serves to regulate the exercise of the central government's non-exclusive powers. It rules out central government intervention when an issue can be dealt with effectively by other levels of government, e.g. regional or local level (European Union, 2021).

public goods.[e,34,35,37] Taxation is the mechanism that allows local governments to efficiently take advantage of local preferences and agglomerative effects, although the challenges of slums, overcrowding and a large presence of the informal sector in LMICs may reduce the benefits of agglomeration leading to free-rider problems and difficulties in financing adequate public services, due to local governments diminished ability to tax, monitor and regulate this sector.[38] Nonetheless, taxation can be effectively used as an instrument for accountability and responsiveness by governments in LMICs, and new systems have been explored to improve taxation in these lower-income settings.[25,39] At the same time, taxation can also be used to improve slums conditions and prevent overcrowding, for example, through land-use taxes.

Taxes on activities causing air pollution – from traffic caused by cars to industrial emissions – for example, have been sources of revenue for many local governments, generating a considerable amount of income.[40] The resulting revenues are rarely allocated to fund public health spending, though the health benefits generated by the taxes are well documented.[41–44] In London, for example, a congestion charge system was introduced in 2003 with the objective of reducing traffic, improving bus service, making journey times more predictable for drivers and increasing efficiency in the delivery of goods and services throughout the city. Traffic volumes in central London are now almost a quarter lower than a decade ago, with all London buses expected to have green technologies and zero emissions by 2037.[45] In 2017–2018 alone, about USD 297 million in net income (revenue minus costs) was generated.[46] The revenue generated by the congestion charges was mostly earmarked for re-investment in transport, principally on buses,

---

[e] The assumption of the efficiency of local governments in producing local public services, based on local preferences, is anchored on the original 1956's work of Charles Tiebout, *A Pure Theory of Local Expenditure*.[33] Although Tiebout's work provided the basis for the new economic geography and agglomeration economics,[34,35] agglomeration was not the focus of his work, even though the issue permeates all his discussions.

Agglomerative efficiency can be questioned as an efficient allocative mechanism for the production of public goods due to the presence of *sorting* (residents moving from one local authority to another in order to obtain better services) – see Ref.[36] *Postcode lottery* is another potential disadvantage of policy determination independent of local governmental level, as individuals may have access to social services in one local government but not in another leading to the presence of sorting.

in order to alleviate the pressure on the underground network, with some limited investments in promoting health through walking and cycling.[47]

Reducing traffic and increasing space for walking and cycling can generate health benefits. Improving physical activity leads to long-term health benefits and the prevention of over 20 common health conditions, including mental health conditions and diabetes. Physical inactivity is estimated to cost the United Kingdom National Health Service (NHS) more than USD 1.9 billion per year, in 2018 prices.[48]

Congestion charges by themselves are a limited mechanism for reducing air pollution and promoting health, although are effective in reducing traffic. In 2008, Transport for London introduced the low emission zone (LEZ) to encourage polluting diesel vehicles driving in London to become cleaner.[49] The LEZ was expected to have a significant impact on health outcomes, although recent studies have shown only limited effects on improving air quality and health outcomes in children, despite some evidence of a reduction in the prevalence of rhinitis.[50,51]

In 2019, an ultra-low emission zone (ULEZ) was introduced, with charges being applied to all vehicles entering central London (in addition to the congestion charges) that do not conform to the emissions standards defined by legislation.[52,53] However, more ambitious schemes with wider coverage of ULEZs and plans for a reduction in the use of vehicles are needed to yield significant reductions in levels of air pollution and positive changes in population health.[50] Though the marketing strategy for the new ULEZ is heavily focused on the health benefits for the NHS, the funds generated are essentially earmarked for making the fleet 'clean and green' rather than for policies to reduce the use of cars. That said, Transport for London states that plans are being put in place for further reductions in traffic, aiming to have four out of every five trips through the city of London made by public transport, walking or cycling by 2040.[52–54] Earmarking an expanded ULEZ as a contribution to the NHS, as well as for increasing the walking and cycling infrastructure, bike-sharing and the use of free public transport could generate the much-needed support among the general public, effectively reduce the use of cars and generate meaningful health benefits. Recent polls have shown signs of an increased willingness from the public to pay more tax when health is the main area of spending.[55]

Taxes targeting harmful health-related behaviours and unhealthy activities can be designated as health taxes, and the revenue can be earmarked for public health gains through investment in solutions for health and well-being, such as increasing spaces for walking and cycling, and green spaces. Unquestionably, intensive policy coordination and investments are needed for local governments to operate efficiently, and this is a particular challenge in LMICs where a reliable tax system can be difficult to implement.[54] Even with such challenges, local governments can be empowered to find solutions to plan, finance and manage sustainable and strategic fiscal interventions that lead to better public health outcomes. As we will see in subsequent sections, local governments can catalyse sustainable development through the use of health taxes that promote health in an efficient, cost-effective and equitable manner. We will explore a few examples, from non-traditional areas of taxation for health, but that directly or indirectly produces substantial effects on health and should be more actively looked at, as opportunities to create additional revenue to improve health.

7.2. Sectoral interventions in local governments for better health

7.2.1. Air pollution and taxes for health

Air pollution affects populations in all parts of the world. The World Health Organization (WHO) estimates that worldwide, 7 million people die every year from exposure to fine particles: 4.2 million from ambient (outdoor) air pollution and 3.8 from household air pollution.[f,55,56] Recent studies have also suggested that short- and long-term exposure to air pollution might

[f] Household air pollution also contributes to ambient air pollution, but the number of deaths due to this intersection is difficult to be assessed, thus some double counting is assumed.

increase the risk of complications related to COVID-19, including deaths, although more evidence is needed to support the causal link.[57–61]

Carbon taxes have been used to support the reduction in levels of air pollution and restrict the use of fossil fuels, such as petroleum, coal and natural gas, by targeting fossil fuels according to how much carbon dioxide is emitted when the fuel is burned.[62] However, carbon does not have a direct and well-defined scope for taxation, with the source of emissions not always clearly identified and measured, making it vulnerable to lobbying, or garnering weak public and political support.[63] Until now, carbon taxes have been implemented only in a small number of countries or regions, covering less than 20% of global emissions, although it is important to note that the number of carbon-pricing initiatives almost doubled in the past 5 years, with many initiatives coming from upper-middle-income countries.[64,65]

A gateway tax focusing on air pollution has been advocated as an initial step to tackle the issue of climate change and the low coverage of carbon taxes.[63] The carbon tax is important for decarbonisation, but it is not sufficient to address human health.[g] Taxes targeting air pollution have been defended as more effective due to a straightforward link to emissions sources and clearer regulatory scope.[64,67] A lump-sum tax encompassing carbon emissions and air pollution could gain support from the public if the benefits are concentrated in specific areas, especially one with health as the focus. Research has shown that fiscal policies are more likely to be successful if their costs are diffused but the benefits are concentrated[43]; carbon taxes on the other hand tend to have diffused benefits and concentrated costs.[h,51,52] By concentrating the benefits of fiscal policies on health, policymakers gain a broader spectrum for policies that

[g] The short-lived climate pollutants black carbon, methane, tropospheric ozone, hydrofluorocarbons, and other fine particulate matter (PM) are the most important contributors to the man-made global greenhouse effect after carbon dioxide. These short-lived climate pollutants remain in the atmosphere for a much shorter period of time than carbon dioxide, but they are much harmful to the atmosphere. Certain short-lived climate pollutants are also dangerous air pollutants that have harmful effects for people, ecosystems and agricultural productivity.[68]

[h] Studies show that, although a significant reduction in the amount of CO_2 emissions can be observed since carbon taxes have been introduced, it is difficult to assign the effect to the tax since other effects are more important or the tax is too low in order to clearly assign variations in the emissions to the tax. Transaction cost and bounded rationality of actors may play a

benefit health, including tackling climate change and air pollution, but also providing potential leverage to invest in other areas such as universal health coverage. This approach could be more acceptable to the public, especially in areas with low levels of political trust and awareness of climate change.[68,69]

Concomitantly, replacing subsidies with taxes on health-related behaviours and unhealthy activities will maximise the efforts to reduce the effects of climate change, particularly on health. Subsidies maintain consumer prices artificially low, leading to higher consumption of subsidised goods, which in turn results in higher consumption and pollution. Examples of harmful subsidies include those for fossil fuels that increase air pollution and congestion and discourage energy efficiency; and agricultural subsidies that can lead to the overuse of pesticides and fertilisers.[71–74] According to the International Monetary Fund (IMF), fossil fuel subsidies were estimated at USD 5.2 trillion or 6.5% of GDP in 2017. Efficient prices would have avoided 46% of the deaths caused by fossil fuel-related air pollution in 2015.[73] Mexico, for example, has successfully phased out subsidies to gasoline and diesel. During the period of 2008 and 2017, subsidies were reduced a few cents every month, in addition to the implementation of low-emission zones at cities levels. An economy-wide assessment found that elimination of all energy subsidies would be associated with a 1.5% higher GDP growth over the long-term because resources that were being used to pay for subsidies could be used instead to increase government expenditure, potentially including the expansion of public healthcare.[75]

Local governments have an important role to play in delivering reductions in carbon emission, and a gateway price at the local level, as well as the implementation of supporting interventions to cut or reduce subsidies (e.g. implementation of zero-emission zones in cities), could be effective ways to strategically counteract industry efforts to overturn policy action for air quality. This is because local governments are close to the exposure sources that directly affect their populations, potentially increasing public engagement

---

non-negligible role and can lead to a lower reaction than what has been anticipated by pre-tax evaluations models have predicted.[72]

and support for carbon or air pollution taxes. Local governments can also define green transport policies (e.g. forestalling or limiting increases in road capacity, supporting car-sharing, or taxing the use of cars or highly polluting vehicles), enforce energy-efficient construction, adopt low-cost circular economy waste policies, restrict the volumes of waste going to landfill or incineration, support and encourage (through subsidies or grants) renewable energy and closely enforce carbon policies for industries in their jurisdictions.

7.2.2. Air pollution from traffic emissions

Transport systems are core to the development of any city. High-speed trains, subway systems and vehicle technologies are in constant development to attend to the needs of growing urban and peri-urban populations. As transportation transforms, so too does the health of individuals. Transport choices, technologies and policies determine the exposure to certain environmental pollutants, the frequency and severity of traffic-related accidents and injuries, the level and types of physical activity and the exposure to noise, with associated disruption of sleep and hearing.[76–78]

Adverse health effects associated with exposure to traffic-related pollutants are well documented, with adverse cardiorespiratory effects including the exacerbation of asthma, the incidence of new cases of asthma, reduced lung function, myocardial infarction, the progression of atherosclerosis and cardiovascular mortality being identified as the main outcomes of exposure to traffic emissions.[79] Children living near roads with heavy-duty vehicle traffic have twice the risk of respiratory problems as those living near less congested streets.[80]

Urban transport policies should be more and more turned into strategies promoting zero-emission transportation, with walking and cycling at the core. Increased walking and cycling in urban areas and reduced use of private cars generate positive effects on many health outcomes, including the reduction of type 2 diabetes, dementia, cerebrovascular disease, breast cancer, colorectal cancer, depression and ischaemic heart disease.[81] Although congestion charges and taxes on fuels have achieved considerable success, especially in increasing revenues, these interventions have shown the limited effect on emissions and health benefits, mainly because the revenue generated by fiscal policies have not been used to promote aggressive policies to reduce the use of cars and encourage the use of public transport, walking and cycling. Marketing congestion charges and fuel taxes as health taxes and allocating these corresponding resources for activities that directly benefit health, including spending on construction and maintenance of safe and comfortable infrastructure, car-free zones, tax-reduction and subsidies for bicycles, as well as a review of taxation structure that benefit cheap transport fares could enhance the acceptability of such taxes to the general public and make them more sustainable in the long term.[55]

Implementing air pollution or traffic-related taxes might be a challenge, especially if lobbying and private-sector interests are dominant. Nevertheless, if the tax is specifically designed to promote health and in addition earmarked for health as a progressive redistributive mechanism, it might be acceptable. In Delhi, for example, pollution is perceived as a serious concern for public health by segments of the population, and a source of organised and growing complaints by physicians, echoed by the media, in spite of the constant and powerful vested interest of the automotive sector.[82–84] Annual mean levels of air pollution in Delhi often exceed 20 times WHO's guideline value of 5 $\mu g/m^3$ annual mean.[85,86] The public appeal of significant health problems could be a first step towards the introduction of health taxes targeting air pollution, a framing that is potentially more acceptable than if marketed as a congestion charge or a tax on fuel. Even for those working in the informal sector – a sector corresponding to more than 50% of the active workforce in India[87] – the health tax approach can be appealing since air-pollution-related diseases can have a direct and detrimental impact on the income generated by this segment of the workforce.

7.2.3. Air pollution from industrial activities

The pollution associated with industrial activities includes mainly emissions from oil combustion, coal burning in power plants, emissions from different types of industries (e.g. petrochemical, metallurgic, etc.) and harbour-related activities.[88] Industrial activities pollute the air, soil and water. Toxic gases released into the air and combined with those from automobiles on the road are the main contributors to ambient air pollution.[88] Pollution from industrial activities is also a major contributor to water and soil pollution worldwide through the legal or illegal dumping of contaminated water, gases, chemicals, heavy metals and radioactive materials into oceans, rivers and landfills, damaging marine life, the productivity of crops and the environment as a whole.[89]

Air pollution from industrial activities is still an important environmental issue even in cities in HICs. In Europe, for example, the release of pollutants to air, water and soil by industries has decreased significantly particularly during the last decade thanks to regulations such as the Clean Air Strategies,[90,91] However, the industrial pollution of water, soil and air is still causing USD 75–242 billion in damages to health and the environment.[92]

Industries have brought rapid economic growth to cities and countries, but some of these developments have been accompanied by the generation of toxins harmful to human health and the environment. China is the largest global consumer of coal and is still commissioning new coal-fired stations to supply power to its industries.[93] The city of Chongqing, located in the southwest of China, is an example of a highly urbanised megacity, with rapid urbanisation and industrialisation, and high levels of air pollution from urban industries. Coal combustion in the industry is the dominant primary source of $PM_{2.5}$ in Chongqing.[94,95] The costs of damages associated with industrial-air-pollution-related activities in Chongqing are considerable, with the effect on public health alone estimated at almost USD 3.6 billion.[96]

India is another country that experienced rapid growth in industrial production, but without a parallel growth in regulation and law enforcement to monitor and lessen levels of air pollution. The Central Pollution Control Board (CPCB) in India has identified 17 categories of polluting industries, with 77% of them contributing to water pollution, 15% to air pollution and 8% to both water and air pollution.[97] An important source of pollution in

India comes from the (mostly) informal production of bricks in small-scale kilns. In a 2017 research with brick producers in Delhi, the CPCB found that 74% of them are still using the traditional and highly polluting fixed-chimney Bulls trench kiln (FCBTK), in which bricks are just lined up and fired, although the Environment Pollution Prevention and Control Authority had ordered that all kilns in the Delhi National Capital Region (NCR) should shift to the cleaner zigzag kiln before 2018.[98]

Environmental regulations on air pollution in China have promoted important reductions in infant mortality.[99] Carbon taxes are not explicitly used in China. Instead, the country adopted, since 2017, an emissions trading system with a cap on the amount of emissions and trade through auctions or free exchange. The caps of greenhouse gas emissions vary from 30 to 350 metric tons of carbon dioxide equivalent per year, and the price for carbon from USD1.40 to USD13.00 per ton of carbon dioxide (implicitly, a carbon tax).[100] Together with the enforcement of regulations, China seems to be making important progress to achieve the 2016 Paris Agreement.[99] On the other hand, India and Nepal are still struggling with ill-regulated industries. Carbon taxes are in place in India but lobbying from the coal industry has put pressure on the government to waive the tax to help finance pollution-curbing equipment. The government of India has already pushed back a deadline to cut emission levels, with over half of the coal industry already missing the 2019 deadline to cut emissions of sulphur oxides, a carcinogen toxin.[101] Nepal does not apply a carbon tax, and regulations are in place to try and limit emissions, although the enforcement of laws is an issue.[102]

7.2.4. Other harmful lifestyles and activities that could form the object of health taxes

Land use

The level of walking and cycling and outdoor recreational activity are strongly affected by accessibility to local facilities, including green spaces.[103] The way land is taxed and used can facilitate or obstruct the creation of spaces for a healthy population, and is a key determinant of social inclusion, and consequently, of health equity. Community design influences household car ownership and use of cars in households, public spaces and the availability of recreational areas and accessible infrastructure for older people and persons with disabilities.[104,105]

Land use has been increasingly recognised for its value in enhancing the health of populations. Activities such as walking, climbing, biking, horse riding and golf are among the activities that provide physical and mental health benefits. They also generate substantial economic activity and income. It also supports the greenspace within towns and cities where a large proportion of outdoor recreation takes place.[106] Planning decisions influencing land use directly can affect the amount of land used for interventions that promote health.[107] For example, taxation of land, especially those used for market speculation, can generate the needed resource to encourage compact developments in cities, focused on walking and cycling and public transit improvements. Land use taxation can also be an advantage for LMICs as it does not require costly administrative structures and can be administrated by modern computer-assisted mass appraisal (CAMA) systems, at the lowest level of government.[39]

It is also fundamental to take into consideration socio-economic and demographic differences and people's needs when planning for taxation, transport systems and land use.

The poorest groups in any given country tend to be less mobile and to have poor access to both private and public transport services, with important consequences to their population health.[108,109] In LMICs, the poor rely on walking or cycling over long distances and under unsafe conditions to access basic services such as health and educational facilities or to reach their workplaces. Consequently, they are more exposed to traffic-related air pollution, road injuries and deaths – 93% of the global deaths related to road traffic occur in LMICs, especially among children and young adults (5–29 years old), even though these countries have only 60% of the world's vehicles.[110] Public transportation systems in LMICs range from non-existent to poor, unreliable and expensive. In middle-income countries such as Brazil, India and China, economic growth has boosted high rates of individual car use, not only as a response to the perceived lack of efficient public transport systems for mobility, especially amongst the poor and middle-class but also because of economic status and lack of climate legislation.[108,111–113] High levels of car use result in declining physical activity, increasing levels of air pollution, noise and traffic-related injuries and fatalities.[114,115]

In HICs, the poorest, usually those on short-term or zero-hour contracts, or even jobseekers from disadvantageous socio-economic backgrounds, cannot always predict or plan their travel patterns, diminishing access to their workplaces and employment opportunities. Transport-related uncertainty can make owning a car a necessity for many on lower incomes, even when affording a car is an issue in itself.[116,117] In population-dense urban or peri-urban areas where public transport is physically present, overcrowding, high costs and lack of accessibility for those with disabilities are common barriers cited by individuals for the use of public transport, as well as concerns over safety and security, particularly after nightfall.[118,119] Wheelchair users in Toronto, for example, have access to only 75% of the jobs that are accessible to individuals who are not in a wheelchair, whilst their counterparts in Montreal have access to only 46% of the jobs accessible to others.[118] In Scotland, those in the lowest income quintile spend around 40% of their income on commuting costs compared to about 15% and 16% of those in the fourth and fifth quintile.[120] In low-density areas, such as suburban and rural areas, housing developments and long distances between households make public transport costs prohibitive, with individuals relying on private motorised transport, with its consequent deleterious effects on physical activity and traffic emissions.[121]

Government taxation policies and plans to integrate transport and land use should be attentive to social needs when supporting mobility and population health. Policy planning should focus on compact cities that provide inclusive and safe infrastructure for all individuals, limit car parking, support the modal shift from private motor vehicles to walking, cycling and low emission public transport to workplace and work opportunities. It has been estimated that compact cities that match transportation to their population needs can result in overall health gains of 420 to 826 disabilities-adjusted life-years (DALYs) per 100,000 population.[122]

As being close to their communities and aware of their needs, local governments can be more effective than other governmental jurisdictions in regulating land use. Local governments can better define restrictions to and limit parking spaces, design effective and customised transport services, take into account the needs of their own populations, including supporting the elderly, people with disabilities and those on low incomes. They can also effectively identify and tax speculation on land and exempt areas for the construction of safe walking and cycling infrastructure. In low population-density areas, local governments can encourage households to limit car ownership to one car, can promote credible rural and inter-urban public transport networks that enable intermodal links to local walking, cycling, taxi and other transport options. Local governments should be allowed to take part in multi-jurisdictional decisions on fiscal expenditure, especially to focus resources on the building of infrastructure needed for social mobility and housing.[123] Limiting or restricting the role of local governments in defining land use is ineffective and costly and is especially costly to the poor.[124,125]

Farming practices

Globally, agriculture has rapidly grown to meet the demands of a fast-growing urban population. To yield the required high levels of production, traditional farming has evolved to large-scale single-crop production that is highly mechanised and dependent on fossil fuels, pesticides, antibiotics and synthetic fertilisers, all with significant implications for human health and the environment.[126–128] Monocrop farming is highly dependent on the use of pesticides and fertilisers, and while crop rotation and natural manure or compost revives the soil and control pests and insects, monocropping exhausts natural nutrients and disturbs ecosystems.[129] Pesticides impact the ground- and surface-water quality, affecting both urban and rural communities, while synthetic fertilisers reduce soil health and are moreover produced through intensive use of fossil fuels, making agriculture one of the main contributors to ambient air pollution.[129]

The use of pesticides and other chemicals, such as lead, mercury, chromium, arsenic and volatile organic compounds, also results in mortality, morbidity, disabilities and impairment to the cognitive development of individuals, especially children. Studies showed that children exposed to lead developed lifetime intellectual disabilities, with one in three children worldwide presenting elevated blood lead levels.[130]

The routine use of antibiotics in animals contributes to antibiotic resistance, reducing the effectiveness of the drugs for human use.[131] Besides, the growing number of farm animals and the associated reduction in genetic diversity have been linked with the emergence of diseases that pose a significant threat to both animal and human health.[131,132]

To break the vicious circle of environmental degradation and costs to human health, it is necessary to promote activities that encourage individuals to shift behaviours to healthy eating, through education and public health campaigns. From the supply side, a repurposing of public investments and subsidies for food and farming should be devised to incentivise the production of a range of healthy and sustainable foods, rather than focusing on foods such as cereals. Variation in production is an expensive undertaking but redirecting money from subsidies for sugar and other crops to promote research on and development of clean technologies, for example, concomitantly with a business model that prioritises environmental and social outcomes, can be a starting point for improved food security and sustainable farming practices. A taxation system that encourages farmers to invest in more diversified food production is also desirable.[133,134]

Tax structures that encourage a more diversified production and consumption of fruits and vegetables, reduce the creation of animals for meat consumption and are environmentally friendly can form a foundation for healthier economies. The Organisation for Economic Co-operation and Development (OECD) has studied the effectiveness of a range of taxes in agriculture – from the taxation of pesticides and fertilisers to environmental taxes, such as carbon and pollution taxes and resource taxes (water pollution) and have concluded that evidence has demonstrated the limited effectiveness of these taxes in promoting sustainable agriculture.[135] This limited effectiveness could be related to the fact that the costs of taxation are compensated by the widespread use of subsidies and incentives. The focus on public health should be the explicit aim of fiscal policy in agriculture, and robust evidence from health taxes from other sectors, such as the levy on sugary drinks, have proved that it is possible to promote sustainable changes in production and consumption behaviours.[136,137]

Innovative projects in local governments can ripple and spread, benefiting not only individuals' health and well-being but also contributing to relieve other societal pressures such as food crises and poverty. Urban and peri-urban farms are relevant examples. In Havana, about 30% of the urban land is dedicated to growing food that is consumed by the local population. In other Cuban regions, up to 80% of all food produced is consumed in the corresponding city or regional perimeter.[138] In Sao Paulo, large municipal allotments produce organic fruits and vegetables that are supplied to the schools of the region.[139] Other urban farms, such as those in Dallas, Texas, produce fruit and vegetables in abandoned areas that are donated to the community.[140] Many other examples of city farms exist, from New York to The Hague and Shanghai, including household urban agriculture projects in Paris, Lusaka, Kampala and Yaounde.[141–145] City farms, either directly or indirectly, help to secure the provision of public goods: such as clean air (by reducing the need for food transportation), to re-using and decreasing the waste of water and, in some cases, using *hydroponic* technologies, permitting the growing of plants in a watery solution of mineral nutrients instead of using soil. More importantly, such projects help cut the pressure on rural lands for deforestation, protect biodiversity and wildness and reduce greenhouse gas emissions.[146]

Gambling

Gambling is defined as betting money on an outcome of uncertain results to win money and includes activities of casinos, lotteries, as well as horse and dog races, among others. For most individuals, gambling is a form of entertainment, as many people can gamble without experiencing any harm. However, a minority of gamblers present gambling illnesses, such as drug and alcohol addiction and mental health conditions leading to crime and bankruptcy.[147] Gambling is a popular activity in both urban and rural areas, but it is in rural settings where its most harmful effects have been observed.[148] Gambling has been increasingly recognised as a public health issue, leading to substantial costs to the health system, individuals and societies. In the United States, for example, 2.6% of the population (or 10 million people) are estimated to have an addiction problem because of gambling, with the age group of 16-24 years old being the most susceptible. Gambling costs USD 6 billion annually in public services to the US economy, including costs of health, welfare, employment, housing and criminal justice services.[149]

The gradual liberalisation of gambling and the advent of the internet have helped the widespread expansion of the gambling industry, with exponential growth in the number of electronic gaming machines, large casinos, lotteries and online gambling sites in the last 15 years. Advertising plays a key role. In the United Kingdom, the number of gambling advertisements aired on TV has risen substantially: in 2006, approximately 152,000 advertisements were placed against 1.39 million in 2012; only in 2017, the gambling industry spent almost USD 2 billion on advertising and marketing in the country.[150] Laptops and desktop computers are the most commonly used devices for online gambling, being employed by 50% of online gamblers in the United Kingdom and 55% in the United States, although mobile phones are growing in use, with 39% and 29% of gamblers using them in the United Kingdom and United States, respectively.[149,151]

Gambling is an influential industry worldwide, with an estimated USD 565 billion global market, expected to increase at an annual rate of 5.9% through 2022.[152] The United States, Japan and Italy are the top three revenue generators in the legalised gambling industry, corresponding to about 32% of the global gambling revenues generated worldwide.[153] Even in countries where gambling is legally restricted, such as in Brazil, the industry is estimated to generate USD 13 billion, with about 60% coming from illegal gambling, mainly from the so-called 'animal game' (*jogo do bicho*).[154] Gambling is also an important source of revenue for countries. In the United Kingdom alone, the betting and gaming tax receipts reached USD 3.8 billion in the fiscal year of 2018/2019.[155]

On the other hand, the costs attributable to gambling are also substantial. Australians are estimated to spend the most on gambling per head per year worldwide (USD 1,288 per capita), followed by residents in Singapore and Ireland, who spend, on average, USD 1,174 and USD 588, in 2017 figures.[156] Citizens in the United States collectively spent USD 117 billion, while in China and Japan, the losses were, respectively, USD 62 billion and USD 24 billion in 2016 prices, with 1–4% of this population left with problems of debt and bankruptcy, divorce, lost productivity, crime (such as theft and fraud) and depression or suicide.[147,157]

Political, religious and community groups have been advocating for tighter regulation of the gambling sector, pressuring for policies to protect the most vulnerable, including the restriction of advertisements in different media, restrictions on the use of credit and debit cards for online games and increases in the price of health insurance for gamblers.[158] There is also a movement to try and shift the focus on individual responsibility only and to look at the responsibility of the industry in shaping addiction by influencing policies, research and framing of public debate.[159,160] Stronger legislations and policies, including tax increases, are being advocated in many countries, as studies have demonstrated that costs of gambling are likely to considerably outweigh the benefits in terms of tax revenues and that the harms of gambling to society should be more systematically addressed.[161–163]

The gaming industry is one of the sectors that cause the most harm to individuals, and yet public sector spending to help individuals and their families affected by the direct consequences of addiction, including a growing number of children, has been minimal.[164] The current revenue generated by the sector, even if entirely spent on health promotion and healthcare, would not match the costs of gambling-related to addiction. In the United States, for example, the societal costs of gambling are estimated to be about USD 129 billion,[i] namely 1.6 times more than the revenue of USD 79 billion generated by gambling in 2018, with the public sector paying the bulk of costs related to this harmful activity.[156,157,165]

A gambling-levy for health, in addition to the existing levels of taxation, and clearly earmarked for healthcare, research and education appears not only desirable but potentially necessary to tackle the health issues of gambling from a societal perspective. However, this approach alone is not enough to promote the public health interest. Existing taxation on gambling is highly regressive, and gambling tax reform should also be taken into consideration within the framework of a comprehensive response that considers all forms of gambling products in the context of relevant cultural differences.[166–168]

7.3. Challenges and opportunities with the implementation of health taxes

Revenue generated from the taxation of sources of air pollution, land use, farming practices and gambling and influenced by unhealthy behaviours and activities have provided substantial financial resources for many governments. However, the revenues generated from these activities are not earmarked for improving health as a primary outcome, even though the health benefits of pricing and taxing these harmful practices are well documented.[127] On the other hand, when taking into account the economic burden associated with healthcare and the loss of productivity, welfare and lives from NCDs associated with unhealthy behaviours and environmental risk factors, the unbalanced accounting of benefits and costs has left citizens

[i] It includes the annual USD 6 billion to the US economy, including costs of health, welfare, employment, housing and criminal justice services,[151] and the USD 117 billion to US citizens with losses related to gambling,[158,159] in 2018 prices.

to pick up the negative public health and economic costs of industrial and commercial activities. Increasing taxation and re-calibrating fiscal policies to embed health as the main objective of the production and promotion of public goods can result in healthier urban (and rural) populations, gain public support and make taxes more sustainable in the long term.

The non-exclusion and non-rival nature of public health as a public good provides a strong case for collective action at all levels of government, with the particular and growing importance of local governments in providing public goods at the point of use, paid for out of taxation that can be generated and administered at this level, as discussed in Section 7.2. The local government's provision of public goods may help to prevent the under-provision and under-consumption of public goods. Local government provision of public goods can also be more efficient due to agglomeration effects.

Good governance is also highly correlated to the success of the introduction of new taxes, with countries exhibiting high levels of trust in politicians, perceived low levels of corruption, extensive public dialogue and mechanisms for social deliberation having stronger fiscal policies and better health outcomes.[169] In contrast, where levels of corruption are perceived to be high or there are problems with lack of political credibility or poor quality of public debate and engagement, taxes tend to be both unpopular and unsuccessful.[169] Moreover, in countries, and in particular, cities with large informal sectors and weak tax systems, as is the case in many urban centres in LMICs, the implementation of health taxes may be difficult.[170]

7.3.1. Scope of a tax and cities' taxing authority

In the environmental taxation literature, it is frequently stated that the appropriate authority for levying a tax depends on the scope of the damage being addressed, with the implication being that the level of political jurisdiction defines the scope of the tax (e.g. city, state or national).[171] For example, for some issues like waste disposal linked to soil contamination, as the impacts are generally realised at the level of the municipality, a local tax might be more efficiently managed. On the other hand, greenhouse emissions might involve sub-national and national jurisdictions as well as other countries, and thus this issue should normally be dealt with through a national or even international instrument.[171,172] In line with this assessment, we argue that in the context of health taxes, taxation at the local level could be introduced or expanded when considering the issues addressed in this chapter. In addition, local governments might have a greater role in multi-jurisdictional decisions on fiscal expenditure, as a way to maximise public health benefits and governmental collaboration at all levels.

Local governments provide many of our most basic public goods and services and also deal with externalities caused by harmful lifestyles and activities, such as air pollution, land use, gambling and farming practices. Traditionally, though, local governments have limited power to tax or borrow funds to support their activities as laws for taxation are typically defined at the level of state and federal governments.[173] Concerns about fiscal mismanagement and the multiplication of the administrative costs of taxation are justifications for this highly verticalised system in most countries. In many countries, however, a vertical system promotes imbalances at the subnational level in terms of the lack of subsidiarity in legal and regulatory responsibilities and the uneven availability of the fiscal resources required, making it difficult for local governments to act on some of their most challenging public health issues.[170]

Allowing local governments to participate in the definition of the scope of health taxes, regulatory policies for health and public health interventions, and even the creation and application of taxes at local levels, can create the opportunity for matching local needs with local institutional frameworks and revenue generation. The suggestion here is not to make local governments independent of state or federal laws and policies, but for them to be given *presumptive taxing authority* subject to state/federal government pre-emption. Such an approach would open the door to more local revenue innovation, improve the efficiency of revenue collection and spending, capitalise on local and regional economies of scale while ensuring that the state and the federal government can maintain their policies and interests.[173]

Presumptive taxing authority is particularly important for cities in LMICs that frequently suffer from the lack of infrastructure and technical capacity, with predominantly informal-sector economies. Local governments should be able to generate tax and non-tax revenues in the form of user charges and fees that promote urban health.

Thus, once the source of health harms has been identified and it has been established that altering market prices through taxation can change consumption behaviours and generate beneficial health outcomes, the scope of the health tax, using a mix of direct taxes (e.g. congestion charges) and indirect taxes (e.g. excise taxes), can be defined. In this sense, local governments have the opportunity to broaden the scope of areas traditionally considered for taxation by policymakers, but not understood as health-enhancing, as for example 'taxation for better cities'.[127] However, it is important to ensure that such health taxes are progressive, redistributive and benefit health and equity.

7.3.2. Promoting political acceptability and community trust

Political and public acceptability are important dimensions for the adoption and implementation of a health tax. We have previously discussed that greater public distrust of politicians and perceived corruption would undermine government performance across a variety of policy domains, including taxation. However, the sensitivity of revenue policies to levels of corruption and distrust vary according to whether the mooted policy is based on market-based or non-market-based instruments. Non-market-based instruments involve non-monetary incentives to change behaviour. Market-based instruments are indirect regulatory instruments, which influence individuals' behaviour by changing their economic incentives.[174] While non-market-based climate policies, for example, are weakened by perceptions of institutional corruption; market-based policies are notably more sensitive than non-market ones to the influence of sizeable domestic energy-intensive and trade-exposed industries.[169]

The distribution of costs and benefits of a fiscal policy is also likely to influence public and political support to a tax. Other things being equal, a tax policy is expected to be more successful if its costs are diffused but its benefits are concentrated. For instance, the reduction of air pollution is costly to industry because it must pay for the installation of equipment to combat pollution and these costs are difficult to pass on to consumers. However, the benefits are diffused in both space and time, giving the industry strong incentives to lobby in opposition to such a tax. On the other hand, if the public has a strong perception of the positive impacts of environmental improvements, then the industry may bear these costs in order to gain public support.[169,171]

Policy-framing strategies can have important implications for the public acceptability of a health tax. A systematic literature review on the political and public acceptability of a sugar-sweetened beverages (SSBs) tax showed that the degree of public acceptability of an SSB tax in the United States, Australia, the United Kingdom and France tended to depend on the wording of the question. Public support for an SSBs tax was highest (66%) if the revenue was labelled as intended for health initiatives.[175] In Switzerland and in Alberta, Canada, re-labelling a carbon tax as a 'CO_2 levy' helped to overcome public distrust.[69,176]

7.4. Conclusion

Local governments play a key role in tackling issues of climate change, NCDs, poverty and even epidemics. Local governments provide the conditions to leverage local solutions for local problems. Building cities that are inclusive, healthy, resilient and sustainable requires intensive policy coordination at the local level. Health taxes are a cost-effective opportunity to support public health and gain public support. Local governments also offer the opportunity to derive public revenues from sources other than the traditional tobacco, alcohol and beverage taxes, by taxing harmful lifestyles and activities to promote social well-being. In this chapter we offered an overview of some of the pressing health issues that can be addressed by public-health interventions supported by health taxes, including those at the local government level, and through the re-calibration of fiscal policies that embed health as its main objective. Globally, when we think about taxes, direct or indirect, health can be a powerful means for transforming the way public health is promoted through fiscal policies.

Key messages

- Considerable health gains can be achieved when the negative health effects of products and behaviours are eliminated or reduced.
- Taxation should be expanded to harmful lifestyles and activities affecting individuals' health and well-being as a matter of public health policy.
- Local governments can be better placed in identifying and dealing with the health of the people in their jurisdictions, and in producing efficient local public services, based on local preferences, if the necessary human and financial resources are in place.

References

1. Afshin A, et al. Health effects of dietary risks in 195 countries, 1990–2017: a systematic analysis for the Global Burden of Disease Study 2017. *The Lancet*. 2019; 393(10184): 1958–1972.
2. Bollyky TJ, Templin T, Andridge C, Dieleman JL. Understanding the relationships between noncommunicable diseases, unhealthy lifestyles, and country wealth. *Health Affairs*. 2015; 34(9): 1464–1471.
3. Naghavi M, et al. Global, regional, and national age-sex specific mortality for 264 causes of death, 1980–2016: a systematic analysis for the Global Burden of Disease Study 2016. *The Lancet*. 2017; 390(10100): 1151–1210.
4. Bloom DE, et al. The Global Economic Burden of Noncommunicable Diseases. Working Paper Number 87, Program on the Global Demography of Aging. World Economic Forum and Harvard School of Public Health; 2012. Available at: https://cdn1.sph.harvard.edu/wp-content/uploads/sites/1288/2013/10/PGDA_WP_87.pdf (accessed 23 December 2021).

5. World Health Organization. Global status report on noncommunicable diseases 2014. Geneva, Switzerland: WHO; 2014. Available from: https://apps.who.int/iris/bitstream/handle/10665/148114/9789241564854_eng.pdf.
6. Chaloupka FJ, Powell LM, Warner KE. The use of excise taxes to reduce tobacco, alcohol, and sugary beverage consumption. *Annual Review of Public Health*. 2019; 40(1): 187–201.
7. Public Health England. Health and wellbeing in rural areas. Public Health England. Available: http://www.local.gov.uk/sites/default/files/documents/1.39_Health%20in%20rural%20areas_WEB.pdf (accessed 1 December 2020).
8. The Lancet Diabetes & Endocrinology. Urbanisation, inequality, and non-communicable disease risk. *The Lancet Diabetes & Endocrinology*. 2017; 5(5): 313.
9. Oyebode O, Pape UJ, Laverty AA, Lee JT, Bhan N, Millett C. Rural, urban and migrant differences in non-communicable disease risk-factors in middle income countries: a cross-sectional study of WHO-SAGE data. PLoS One. 2015; 10(4): e0122747.
10. United Nations. 68% of the world population projected to live in urban areas by 2050, says UN. *United Nations: Department of Economics and Social Affairs, New York*, May 2018. Available at: https://www.un.org/development/desa/en/news/population/2018-revision-of-world-urbanization-prospects.html (accessed 17 July 2020).
11. Frumkin H, Haines A. Global environmental change and noncommunicable disease risks. *Annual Review of Public Health*. 2019; 40(1): 261–282.
12. Bixby H, et al. Rising rural body-mass index is the main driver of the global obesity epidemic in adults. *Nature*. 2019; 569(7755): 260–264.
13. Wright A, Smith KE, Hellowell M. Policy lessons from health taxes: a systematic review of empirical studies. *BMC Public Health*. 2017; 17(1): 583.
14. United Nations. Transforming our World: The 2030 Agenda for Sustainable Development. United Nations, 2015. Available at: https://sustainabledevelopment.un.org/content/documents/21252030%20Agenda%20for%20Sustainable%20Development%20web.pdf (accessed 23 December 2020).
15. Hagenaars LL, Jeurissen PPT, Klazinga NS. The taxation of unhealthy energy-dense foods (EDFs) and sugar-sweetened beverages (SSBs): an overview of patterns observed in the policy content and policy context of 13 case studies. *Health Policy*. 2017; 121(8): 887–894.
16. Beech J, Cooper E, Holmes J, McKenna H. What role do taxes and regulation play in promoting better health? The Kings Fund, Mar. 2020. Available at: https://www.kingsfund.org.uk/publications/taxes-regulation-better-health (accessed 30 November 2020).
17. Cheng KJG, Estrada MAG. Price elasticity of cigarette smoking demand in the Philippines after the 2012 Sin Tax Reform Act. *Preventive Medicine*. 2020; 134: 106042.
18. Lencucha R, Drope J, Chavez JJ. Whole-of-government approaches to NCDs: the case of the Philippines Interagency Committee—tobacco: Table 1. *Health Policy Plan*. 2015; 30(7): 844–852.
19. Wen L, Kenworthy J, Guo X, Marinova D. Solving traffic congestion through Street Renaissance: a perspective from dense Asian cities. *Urban Science*. 2019; 3(1): 18.

20. Millard-Ball A, Schipper L. Are we reaching peak travel? Trends in passenger transport in eight industrialized countries. *Transport Reviews*. 2011; 31(3): 357–378.
21. Metz D. Demographic determinants of daily travel demand. *Transport Policy*. 2012; 21: 20–25.
22. Skaal L, Sinclair H, Stein DJ, Myers B. Problem gambling among urban and rural gamblers in Limpopo Province, South Africa: associations with hazardous and harmful alcohol use and psychological distress. *Journal of Gambling Studies*. 2016; 32(1): 217–230.
23. Rural Services Network. [Not] everyone is a winner: gambling participation and problem gambling in rural communities. United Kingdom, Jan. 18, 2021. Available at: https://www.rsnonline.org.uk/not-everyone-is-a-winner-gambling-participation-and-problem-gambling-in-rural-communities (accessed 23 January 2021).
24. Whaples R. Do economists agree on anything? Yes! *The Economists' Voice*. 2006; 3(9): 1–6.
25. Quack E. Taxation and Accountability: How to Improve the State-Citizen Social Contract Through Taxation. K4D Helpdesk Report No 663. Brighton, UK: Institute of Development Studies; 2019. Available at: https://opendocs.ids.ac.uk/opendocs/handle/20.500.12413/14752 (accessed 28 December 2020).
26. Waddington H, Sonnenfeld A, Finetti J, Gaarder M, John D, Stevenson J. Citizen engagement in public services in low- and middle-income countries: a mixed-methods systematic review of participation, inclusion, transparency and accountability (PITA) initiatives. *Campbell Systematic Reviews*. 2019; 15(1–2): 1–90.
27. Mankiw NG. Smart taxes: an open invitation to join the Pigou club. *Eastern Economical Journal*. 2009; 35(1): 14–23.
28. Parkin M, Powell M, Matthews KGP. Chapter 5: Efficiency and Equity. *Economics. Eight edition. Essex, UK. Person Education Limited,* 2012; 114–115.
29. Parkin M, Powell M, Matthews KGP. *Economics. Chapter 15: Public Choices and Public Goods.* 2014; 344–359.
30. Dees RH. Public health and normative public goods. *Public Health Ethics*. 2018; 11(1): 20–26.
31. Horne LC. Public health, public goods, and market failure. *Public Health Ethics*. 2019; 12(3): 287–292.
32. European Union. The principle of subsidiarity – fact sheets on the European Union. *European Union*. 2021. Available at: https://www.europarl.europa.eu/factsheets/en/sheet/7/the-principle-of-subsidiarity (accessed 1 October 2021).
33. Tiebout CM. A pure theory of local expenditures. *Journal of Political Economy*. 1956; 64(5): 416–424.
34. Krugman PR. *Development, Geography, and Economic Theory*. Cambridge, MA: MIT Press; 1995.
35. Glaeser EL. Are cities dying? *Journal of Economic Perspectives*. 1998; 12(2): 139–160.
36. Schleicher D. The city as a law and economic subject. George Mason Law & Economics Research Paper No. 09-47, *University of Illinois Law Review*. 2009; 2010(5): 1507–1564. Available at: https://papers.ssrn.com/sol3/papers.cfm?abstract_id=1471555 (accessed 14 January 2020).

37. Johnson P, et al. Securing the future: funding health and social care to the 2030s – summary. May 2018. Available at: https://www.ifs.org.uk/uploads/publications/comms/R143%20executive%20summary.pdf (accessed 20 April 2020).
38. Moretti E. Cities and growth. The International Growth Centre (IGC) directed by the London School of Economics and The University of Oxford, 11 April 2014. Available at: https://assets.publishing.service.gov.uk/media/57a089d140f0b649740002a0/IGCEvidencePaperCities.pdf (accessed 14 July 2020).
39. Kalkuhl M, Fernandez Milan B, Schwerhoff G, Jakob M, Hahnen M, Creutzig F. Can land taxes foster sustainable development? An assessment of fiscal, distributional and implementation issues. *Land Use Policy.* 2018; 78: 338–352.
40. European Automobile Manufacturers Association (ACEA). €428 billion in taxes generated by motor vehicles in EU-15, new figures show. Press Release. 24 April 2019. Available at: https://www.acea.be/press-releases/article/428-billion-in-taxes-generated-by-motor-vehicles-in-eu-15-new-figures-show (accessed 19 December 2020).
41. Wang L, et al. Air quality strategies on public health and health equity in Europe — a systematic review. *IJERPH.* 2016; 13(12): 1196.
42. Shaw C, Hales S, Edwards R, Howden-Chapman P. Health co-benefits of policies to mitigate climate change in the transport sector: systematic review. *Journal of Transport & Health.* 2017; 5: S107–S108.
43. Burns J, et al. Interventions to reduce ambient air pollution and their effects on health: An abridged Cochrane systematic review. *Environment International.* 2020; 135: 105400.
44. Yang T, Liu W. Health effects of energy intensive sectors and the potential health co-benefits of a low carbon industrial transition in China. *IJERPH.* 2019; 16(17): 3022.
45. Transport for London. Mayor's Transport Strategy. Mayor of London, March 2018. Available at: https://www.london.gov.uk/sites/default/files/mayors-transport-strategy-2018.pdf (accessed 17 April 2020).
46. Transport for London. Annual Report and Statement of Accounts. Mayor of London, 25 July 2018. Available at: http://content.tfl.gov.uk/tfl-annual-report-and-statement-of-accounts-2017-18.pdf (accessed 17 April 2020).
47. BBC London. Congestion charge – where has the money gone? 1 July 2008. Available at: http://www.bbc.co.uk/london/content/articles/2006/11/21/congestion_update_feature.shtml (accessed 16 April 2020).
48. Scarborough H. Intergenerational equity and the social discount rate: intergenerational equity and social discount rate. *Australian Journal of Agricultural and Resource Economics.* 2011; 55(2): 145–158.
49. Transport for London. Changes to the LEZ. Transport for London, Mayor of London, 2019. Available at: https://tfl.gov.uk/modes/driving/low-emission-zone/changes-to-the-lez?intcmp=52426 (accessed 14 December 2020).
50. Mudway IS, et al. Impact of London's low emission zone on air quality and children's respiratory health: a sequential annual cross-sectional study. *The Lancet Public Health.* 2019; 4(1): e28–e40.
51. Gehrsitz M. The effect of low emission zones on air pollution and infant health. *Journal of Environmental Economics and Management.* 2017; 83: 121–144.

52. Transport For London. Ultra low emission zone. Transport for London, Mayor of London; 2020. Available at: https://tfl.gov.uk/modes/driving/ultra-low-emission-zone (accessed 13 November 2020).
53. Mayor of London. World's first ultra low emission zone to save NHS billions by 2050. Mayor of London, 26 February 2020. Available at: https://www.london.gov.uk/press-releases/mayoral/ulez-to-save-billions-for- nhs#:~:text=The%20ULEZ%20has%20already%20led,per%20cent%20in%20the%20zone.&text=almost%20300%2C000%20Londoners%20saved%20from,disease%2C%20lung%20cancer%20and%20dementia (accessed 13 November 2020).
54. Tanzi V, Zee HH. *Tax Policy for Developing Countries.* Washington, DC: IMF; 2001.
55. World Health Organization (WHO). Ambient (outdoor) air pollution. *WHO: Website,* Geneva, Switzerland, 2 May 2018. Available at: https://www.who.int/news-room/fact-sheets/detail/ambient-(outdoor)-air-quality-and-health (accessed 3 June 2019).
56. World Health Organization (WHO). Household air pollution and health. *Newsroom, Fact sheets,* 8 May 2018. Available at: https://www.who.int/news-room/fact-sheets/detail/household-air-pollution-and-health (accessed 30 May 2020).
57. Comunian S, Dongo D, Milani C, Palestini P. Air pollution and COVID-19: the role of particulate matter in the spread and increase of COVID-19's morbidity and mortality. *IJERPH.* 2020; 17(12): 4487.
58. Copat C, et al. The role of air pollution (PM and NO2) in COVID-19 spread and lethality: a systematic review. *Environmental Research.* 2020; 191: 110129.
59. Wu X, Nethery RC, Sabath BM, Braun D, Dominici F. Exposure to air pollution and COVID-19 mortality in the United States: a nationwide cross-sectional study, preprint, April 2020. Available at: http://medrxiv.org/lookup/doi/10.1101/2020.04.05.20054502 (accessed 26 August 2020).
60. Hutter H-P, et al. Air pollution is associated with COVID-19 incidence and mortality in Vienna, Austria. *IJERPH.* 2020; 17(24): 9275.
61. Pope CA, Cropper M, Coggins J, Cohen A. Health benefits of air pollution abatement policy: role of the shape of the concentration–response function. *Journal of the Air & Waste Management Association.* 2015; 65(5): 516–522.
62. Zimmer A, Koch N. Fuel consumption dynamics in Europe: tax reform implications for air pollution and carbon emissions. *Transportation Research Part A: Policy and Practice.* 2017; 106: 22–50.
63. Harman O, Berland O. The gateway to carbon pricing? Air pollution policy. *World Economic Forum, Environment and Natural Resource Security,* Davos 2020, 14 January 2020. Available at: https://www.weforum.org/agenda/2020/01/a-gateway-tax-for-helping-mitigate-climate-change/ (accessed 3 July 2020).
64. Funke F, Mattauch L. Why is carbon pricing in some countries more successful than in others? *Our World in Data, University of Oxford,* 10 August 2018. Available at: https://ourworldindata.org/carbon-pricing-popular (accessed 3 July 2020).
65. The World Bank. Whats is carbon pricing? Carbon Pricing Dashborad. The World Bank, Washington, DC, 2019. Available at: https://carbonpricingdashboard.worldbank.org/what-carbon-pricing (accessed 13 November 2020).

66. Climate and Clean Air Coalition. Short-Lived Climate Pollutants (SLCPs). UN Environment Programme, 2017. Available at: https://www.ccacoalition.org/en/content/short-lived-climate-pollutants-slcps (accessed 3 September 2020).
67. Rosenbloom D, Markard J, Geels FW, Fuenfschilling L. Opinion: why carbon pricing is not sufficient to mitigate climate change—and how "sustainability transition policy" can help. *Proceedings of the National Academy of Sciences of the United States America.* 2020; 117(16): 8664–8668.
68. Olson M. *The Logic of Collective Action: Public Goods and the Theory of Groups, 21. printing.* Cambridge, MA: Harvard University Press; 2003.
69. Klenert D, et al. Making carbon pricing work for citizens. *Nature Climate Change.* 2018; 8(8): 669–677.
70. Millock K, Nauges C. Ex post evaluation of an earmarked tax on air pollution. *Land Economics.* 2006; 82(1): 68–84.
71. Smith KR, Sagar A. Fossil fuel subsidies and health. *The Lancet Global Health.* 2015; 3(11): e674.
72. Coady D, Parry I, Sears L, Shang B. How large are global fossil fuel subsidies? *World Development.* 2017; 91: 11–27.
73. Coady D. *Global Fossil Fuel Subsidies Remain Large: An Update Based on Country-Level Estimates.* International Monetary Fund; 2019. Available at: https://elibrary.imf.org/view/IMF001/25712-9781484393178/25712-9781484393178/25712-9781484393178.xml (accessed 21 October 2021).
74. Inchauste G, Victor DG, (eds). *The Political Economy of Energy Subsidy Reform.* Washington, DC: World Bank Group; 2017.
75. World Bank. United Mexican States Reducing Fuel Subsidies : Public Policy Options. Washington, DC: World Bank; 2013. Available at: https://openknowledge.worldbank.org/handle/10986/21755 (accessed 19 October 2021).
76. Zuurbier M, et al. Commuters' exposure to particulate matter air pollution is affected by mode of transport, fuel type, and route. *Environmental Health Perspectives.* 2010; 118(6): 783–789.
77. Sahlqvist S, Song Y, Ogilvie D. Is active travel associated with greater physical activity? The contribution of commuting and non-commuting active travel to total physical activity in adults. *Preventive Medicine.* 2012; 55(3): 206–211.
78. Jiang B, et al. Transport and public health in China: the road to a healthy future. *The Lancet.* 2017; 390(10104): 1781–1791.
79. Health Effects Institute. *Traffic-Related Air Pollution: A Critical Review of the Literature on Emissions, Exposure, and Health Effects.* HEI Special Report 17, Boston: Health Effects Institute. Available at: https://www.healtheffects.org/publication/traffic-related-air-pollution-critical-review-literature-emissions-exposure-and-health. (accessed 14 May 2020).
80. World Health Organization (WHO). Air pollution and climate change. *Data and Statistics.* Available at: https://www.euro.who.int/en/health-topics/environment-and-health/Transport-and-health/data-and-statistics/air-pollution-and-climate-change2 (accessed 3 March 2020).

81. Jarrett J, et al. Effect of increasing active travel in urban England and Wales on costs to the National Health Service. *The Lancet*. 2012; 379(9832): 2198–2205.
82. Irfan U. How Delhi became the most polluted city on Earth. Vox. 25 November 2017. Available at: https://www.vox.com/energy-and-environment/2017/11/22/16666808/india-air-pollution-new-delhi (accessed 14 November 2020).
83. Irfan U. Why India's air pollution is so horrendous. Vox. 31 October 2018. Available at: https://www.vox.com/2018/5/8/17316978/india-pollution-levels-air-delhi-health (accessed 30 March 2020).
84. Bernard S, Kazmin A. Dirty air: how India became the most polluted country on earth. The Financial Times. 11 December 2018. Available at: https://ig.ft.com/india-pollution/ (accessed 30 March 2020).
85. World Health Organization. *WHO Global Air Quality Guidelines: Particulate Matter (PM2.5 and PM10), Ozone, Nitrogen Dioxide, Sulfur Dioxide and Carbon Monoxide*. Geneva: World Health Organization; 2021. Available at: https://apps.who.int/iris/handle/10665/345329 (accessed 21 October 2021).
86. IQAir. 2019 World's Air Quality Report, 2019. Available at: https://www.iqair.com/world-most-polluted-cities?continent=&country=&state=&page=1&perPage=50&cities= (accessed 24 August 2020).
87. India Wage Report. Wage policies for decent work, and inclusive growth, 'India Wage Report: Wage policies for decent work and inclusive growth'. 2018. Available at: https://www.ilo.org/wcmsp5/groups/public/---asia/---ro-bangkok/---sro-new_delhi/documents/publication/wcms_638305.pdf (accessed 22 June 2020).
88. Karagulian F, et al. Contributions to cities' ambient particulate matter (PM): a systematic review of local source contributions at global level. *Atmospheric Environment*. 2015; 120: 475–483.
89. Field.org.uk. How Can Factories Affect The Environment? 2018. Available at: http://www.field.org.uk/how-can-factories-affect-the-environment/ (accessed 14 June 2020).
90. Holland M. Cost-benefit Analysis of Scenarios for Cost-Effective Emission Controls after 2020 – Version 1.02 Corresponding to IIASA TSAP Report #7. EMRC, November 2012. Available at: https://ec.europa.eu/environment/air/pdf/TSAP_CBA_corresponding_to_IIASA7_v1-02%5B1%5D.pdf (accessed 22 February 2019).
91. Holland M. Cost-benefit Analysis of Final Policy Scenarios for the EU Clean Air Package – Version 2 Corresponding to IIASA TSAP Report 11, Version 2a. EMRC, October 2014. Available at: https://ec.europa.eu/environment/air/pdf/TSAP%20CBA.pdf (accessed 22 February 2019).
92. European Environmental Agency. Costs of air pollution from European industrial facilities 2008–2012 – an updated assessment. European Environmental Agency (EEA) Technical Report, No 20/2014, 2014. Available at: https://www.eea.europa.eu/publications/costs-of-air-pollution-2008-2012 (accessed 20 June 2020).
93. Chang S, Zhuo J, Meng S, Qin S, Yao Q. Clean coal technologies in China: current status and future perspectives. *Engineering*. 2016; 2(4): 447–459.

94. Chen Y, Xie S, Luo B, Zhai C. Particulate pollution in urban Chongqing of southwest China: historical trends of variation, chemical characteristics and source apportionment. *Science of The Total Environment*. 2017; 584–585: 523–534.
95. Power AL, et al. Monitoring impacts of urbanisation and industrialisation on air quality in the anthropocene using urban pond sediments. *Frontiers in Earth Science*. 2018; 6: 131.
96. Li L, Lei Y, Pan D, Yu C, Si C. Economic evaluation of the air pollution effect on public health in China's 74 cities. *SpringerPlus*. 2016; 5(1): 402.
97. Central Pollution Control Board. Polluting Industries. Central Pollution Control Board, 9 June 2012. Available at: http://cpcbenvis.nic.in/cpcb_newsletter/Polluting%20Industries.pdf (accessed 15 January 2020).
98. Shrivastava S. 74% brick kilns in Delhi-NCR have not shifted to cleaner technology. *DownToEarth*; 2018. https://www.downtoearth.org.in/news/environment/74-brick-kilns-in-delhi-ncr-have-not-shifted-to-cleaner-technology-61624. (accessed 14 November 2020).
99. Tanaka S. Environmental regulations on air pollution in China and their impact on infant mortality. *Journal of Health Economics*. 2015; 42: 90–103.
100. Parenteau P, Cao M. Carbon trading in China: progress and challenges. *Environmental Law Reporter*. 2016; 46(3): 10194–10199.
101. Varadhan S. Over half of India's coal-fired power plants set to miss emission norm deadline. Reuters, 2019. Available at: https://uk.reuters.com/article/uk-india-pollution-coal-excluisve/exclusive-over-half-of-indias-coal-fired-power-plants-set-to-miss-emission-norm-deadline-idUKKBN1XP1O2 (accessed 20 December 2019).
102. Climate Action Tracker. Climate action tracker. Country summary: Nepal, 2020. https://climateactiontracker.org/countries/nepal/ (accessed 22 February 2021).
103. Barton H. Land use planning and health and well-being. *Land Use Policy*. 2009; 26: S115–S123.
104. Ma L, Kent J, Mulley C. Transport disadvantage, social exclusion, and subjective well-being: the role of the neighborhood environment—evidence from Sydney, Australia. *The Journal of Transport and Land Use*. 2018; 11(1); 31–47.
105. Mitra SK. Land Use, Land Value, and Transportation: Essays on Accessibility, Carless Households, and Long-distance Travel. PhD dissertation. University of California, Irvine.
106. Manchester Metropolitan University. Reconomics Plus: The Economic, Health and Social Value of Outdoor Recreation. Manchester Metropolitan University, February 2017. Available at: https://sramedia.s3.amazonaws.com/media/documents/699fec08-3f90-4e00-ac4a-c074b353a38d.pdf (accessed 10 September 2021).
107. Litman T. Evaluating Transportation Land Use Impacts: Considering the Impacts, Benefits and Costs of Different Land Use Development Patterns. Victoria Transport Policy Institute, 1 September 2021. Available at: https://www.vtpi.org/landuse.pdf (accessed 10 September 2021).

108. Lucas K, Mattioli G, Verlinghieri E, Guzman A. Transport poverty and its adverse social consequences. *Proceedings of the Institution of Civil Engineers – Transport.* 2016; 169(6): 353–365.
109. Titheridge H, Christie N, Mackett R, Oviedo Hernández D, Ye R. Transport and poverty: a review of the evidence. University College London, 2014. Available at: https://discovery.ucl.ac.uk/id/eprint/1470392/1/transport-poverty%5B1%5D.pdf (accessed 30 December 2020).
110. World Health Organization. Road traffic injuries. World Health Organization, 2020. Available at: https://www.who.int/news-room/fact-sheets/detail/road-traffic-injuries (accessed 30 December 2020).
111. Ecola L, Rohr C, Zmud J, Kuhnimhof T, Phleps P. *The Future of Driving in Developing Countries.* Santa Monica, CA: RAND Corporation; 2014.
112. Wu T, Zhao H, Ou X. Vehicle ownership analysis based on GDP per capita in China: 1963–2050. *Sustainability.* 2014; 6(8): 4877–4899.
113. Kuhnimhof T, Rohr C, Ecola L, Zmud J. Automobility in Brazil, Russia, India, and China: Quo Vadis? *Transportation Research Record.* 2014; 2451(1): 10–19.
114. Gomez LF, et al. Urban environment interventions linked to the promotion of physical activity: a mixed methods study applied to the urban context of Latin America. *Social Science & Medicine.* 2015; 131: 18–30.
115. Kopits E, Cropper M. Traffic fatalities and economic growth. *Accident Analysis & Prevention.* 2005; 37(1): 169–178.
116. DEMAND. Precarity in housing and employment: a hidden dimension of car dependency. Research Insight 14. DEMAND, 2015. Available at: http://www.demand.ac.uk/wp-content/uploads/2015/11/demand-insight-14final.pdf (accessed 9 January 2021).
117. Davis A, Hirsch D, Smith N, Beckhelling J, Padley M. A minimum income standard for the UK in 2012, keeping up in hard times. Joseph Rowntree Foundation, 2012. Available at: https://www.jrf.org.uk/report/minimum-income-standard-uk-2012 (accessed 13 January 2021).
118. Grisé E, Boisjoly G, Maguire M, El-Geneidy A. Elevating access: comparing accessibility to jobs by public transport for individuals with and without a physical disability. *Transportation Research Part A: Policy and Practice.* 2019; 125: 280–293.
119. Transport For London. Understanding the travel needs of London's diverse communities – BAME. Transport for London, Mayor of London, 2012. Available at: http://content.tfl.gov.uk/BAME.pdf (accessed 13 January 2021).
120. Cain A, Jones PM. Does urban road pricing cause hardship to low-income car drivers?: an affordability-based approach. *Transportation Research Record.* 2008; 2067(1): 47–55.
121. Ellinas T. *Healthy Transport = Healthy Lives.* London, UK. British Medical Association, 2012. Available at: https://thepep.unece.org/sites/default/files/2017-06/Healthy%20transport%20healthy%20lives%20Britsh%20Medical%20Association.pdf (accessed 3 April 2019).

122. Stevenson M, et al. Land use, transport, and population health: estimating the health benefits of compact cities. *The Lancet*. 2016; 388(10062): 2925–2935.
123. Lucas K, Stokes G, Bastiaanssen J, Burkinshaw J. Inequalities in mobility and access in the UK transport system. UK Government Office for Science, 2019. Available at: https://assets.publishing.service.gov.uk/government/uploads/system/uploads/attachment_data/file/784685/future_of_mobility_access.pdf (accessed 19 February 2021).
124. Cheshire P, Hilber CAL, Koster HRA. Empty homes, longer commutes: the unintended consequences of more restrictive local planning. *Journal of Public Economics*. 2018; 158: 126–151.
125. OECD. The Governance of Land Use in OECD Countries: Policy Analysis and Recommendations, OECD Regional Development Studies, OECD Publishing, Paris. Available at: https://doi.org/10.1787/9789264268609-en (accessed 27 February 2021).
126. Alexandratos N. *World agriculture: towards 2010. An FAO study. Chichester, UK, John Wiley and Rome, FAO,* 1995.
127. Pimpin L, Sassi F, Corbould E, Friebel R, Webber L. Fiscal and pricing policies to improve public health: a review of the evidence. *Public Health England*, 2018. Available at: https://assets.publishing.service.gov.uk/government/uploads/system/uploads/attachment_data/file/743118/Fiscal_and_Pricing_Policies_report_FINAL.pdf (accessed 25 June 2020).
128. Sugar tax and farming policy. *Perspectives in Public Health*. 2018; 138(4): 194–195.
129. Health Care Without Harm. Community health risks of industrial agriculture. *Delivering Community Benefit: Healthy food playbook*, 2018. https://foodcommunitybenefit.noharm.org/resources/community-health-needs-assessment/community-health-risks-industrial-agriculture (accessed 28 June 2020).
130. Rees N, Fuller R. The Toxic Truth: Children's Exposure to Lead Pollution Undermines a Generation of Future Potential. UNICEF and Pure Earth, 2020. Available at: https://www.unicef.org/media/73246/file/The-toxic-truth-children%E2%80%99s-exposure-to-lead-pollution-2020.pdf (accessed 24 October 2021).
131. Tomley FM, Shirley MW. Livestock infectious diseases and zoonoses. *Philosophical Transactions of the Royal Society London B, Biological Sciences*. 2009; 364(1530): 2637–2642.
132. Centers for Disease Control and Prevention (CDC). Zoonotic Diseases. U.S. Department of Health & Human Services, United States, 2021. Available at: https://www.cdc.gov/onehealth/basics/zoonotic-diseases.html (accessed 3 May 2022).
133. Shepon A, Henriksson PJG, Wu T. Conceptualizing a sustainable food system in an automated world: toward a "Eudaimonian" future. *Frontiers in Nutrition*. 2018; 5: 104.
134. Turner MM, Whitehead I, Millard N, Turner MM, Whitehead I, Millard N. The effects of public funding on farmers' attitudes to farm diversification. Report. Exeter, UK. University of Exeter, 2006. doi: 10.22004/AG.ECON.31746. Available at: https://ageconsearch.umn.edu/record/31746?ln=en (accessed 27 August 2020).
135. OECD. Taxation in Agriculture. Paris, France., OECD Publishing, 2020. Available at: https://doi.org/10.1787/073bdf99-en (accessed 14 November 2020).

136. Taillie LS, Rivera JA, Popkin BM, Batis C. Do high vs. low purchasers respond differently to a nonessential energy-dense food tax? Two-year evaluation of Mexico's 8% nonessential food tax. *Preventive Medicine*. 2017; 105: S37–S42.
137. Seferidi P, et al. Implications of Brexit on the effectiveness of the UK soft drinks industry levy upon CHD in England: a modelling study. *Public Health Nutrition*. 2018; 21(18): 3431–3439.
138. de la Cal P. Urban agriculture – towards a continuous productive-space system in the city. In C. Díez Medina and J. Monclús (eds) *Urban Visions*. Cham: Springer International Publishing, 2018, pp. 329–338. doi: 10.1007/978-3-319-59047-9_32.
139. Lorencato A, Yassuda S. Regiões da capital se destacam por produção de vegetais orgânicos. Veja Sao Paulo. 2 March 2018. Available at: https://vejasp.abril.com.br/cidades/parelheiros-produtores-rurais-organicos-escolas-municipais/ (accessed 21 August 2020).
140. The State Fair of Texas. Big Tex Urban Farms. Available at: https://bigtex.com/supporting-texans/big-tex-urban-farms/ (accessed 27 April 2020).
141. Peach J. The impact of urban farming in New York City. SmartCitiesDive. Available at: https://www.smartcitiesdive.com/ex/sustainablecitiescollective/impact-urban-farming-new-york-city/81916/ (accessed 3 May 2020).
142. Rabbani A. Urban farmers – a green thumb for the city of Den Haag, Holland. Vanguard Voyager. Available at: https://www.vanguardvoyager.com/2018/05/26/urban-farmers-den-haag-holland/ (accessed 3 May 2020).
143. Global Site Plans. Urban farming growing in Shanghai, China. SmartCitiesDive. Available at: https://www.smartcitiesdive.com/ex/sustainablecitiescollective/urban-farming-growing-shanghai-china/126531/ (accessed 3 May 2020).
144. Beach M. Urban agriculture increases food security for poor people in Africa. PRB. 4 April 2013. Available at: https://www.prb.org/urban-agriculture-poor-africa/ (accessed 3 May 2020).
145. The Guardian. World's largest urban farm to open – on a Paris rooftop. The Guardian. 13 August 2019. Available at: https://www.theguardian.com/cities/2019/aug/13/worlds-largest-urban-farm-to-open-on-a-paris-rooftop (accessed 20 April 2020).
146. Agriculture and Economic Development Analysis Division, Food and Agriculture Organization. *Food Security: Some Macroeconomic Dimensions.* Rome: Food and Agriculture Organization of the United Nations; 1996.
147. Latvala T, Lintonen T, Konu A. Public health effects of gambling – debate on a conceptual model. *BMC Public Health*. 2019; 19(1): 1077.
148. Tolchard B. The impact of gambling on rural communities worldwide: a narrative literature review. *Journal of Rural Mental Health*. 2015; 39(2): 90–107.
149. North American Foundation for Gambling Addiction Help. Statistics Of Gambling Addiction 2016, 2016. Available at: https://nafgah.org/statistics-gambling-addiction-2016/ (accessed 22 August 2019).
150. The Guardian. Rise in gambling ad spend fuels fears over impact on children. The Guardian. 24 November 2018. Available at: https://www.theguardian.com/society/

2018/nov/24/rise-in-gambling-ad-spend-fuels-fears-over-impact-on-children (accessed 23 June 2020).

151. Rogers RD, Wardle H, Sharp CA, Wood S, Hughes K, Davies TJ, Dymond S, Bellis MA. Gambling as a public health issue in Wales. Bangor, Wales. Bangor University, Public Health Wales, and Swansea University, 2019. Available at: https://www.bangor.ac.uk/psychology/research/gambling/docs/Gambling-as-Public-Health-Issue-Wales.pdf (accessed 13 June 2020).

152. Research And Markets.com. Global Gambling Market to Reach $565 Billion by 2022: Opportunities & Strategies Report, 2014 to 2022. Business Wire. 6 June 2019. Available at: https://www.businesswire.com/news/home/20190606005537/en/Global-Gambling-Market-Reach-565-Billion-2022 (accessed 23 June 2020).

153. World Casino Directory. World Casino Directory Global Gaming Summary 2019. Available at: https://www.worldcasinodirectory.com/statistics (accessed 24 June 2020).

154. Medeiros G, Grant J, Tavares H. Gambling disorder due to Brazilian animal game ("Jogo do bicho"): gambling behavior and psychopathology. *Journal of Gambling Studies*. 2016; 32(1): 231–241.

155. Clark D. United Kingdom (UK) HMRC betting and gaming tax receipts from fiscal year 2000/01 to fiscal year 2018/19. Statista. 11 September 2019. Available at: https://www.statista.com/statistics/284338/betting-and-gaming-united-kingdom-hmrc-tax-receipts/ (accessed 25 June 2019).

156. Lock S. Countries with the largest gambling losses per adult worldwide in 2017. Statista. 26 March 2020. Available at: https://www.statista.com/statistics/552821/gambling-losses-per-adult-by-country-worldwide/ (accessed 24 June 2020).

157. The Economist. The world's biggest gamblers. 9 February 2017. Available at: https://www.economist.com/graphic-detail/2017/02/09/the-worlds-biggest-gamblers (accessed 25 June 2020).

158. Reith G. Scotland, and Social Research. *Research on the Social Impacts of Gambling: Final Report*. Edinburgh: Scottish Executive; 2006. Available at: http://www.scotland.gov.uk/Publications/2006/08/17134534/0 (accessed 27 August 2020).

159. Thomas SA, et al. The PROblem Gambling RESearch Study (PROGRESS) research protocol: a pragmatic randomised controlled trial of psychological interventions for problem gambling. *BMJ Open*. 2015; 5(11): e009385.

160. Cassidy R, Loussouarn C, Pisac A. Fair Game: Producing gambling research. The Goldsmiths Report, 15 January 2015. Available at: https://www.researchgate.net/publication/270887403_Fair_Game_Producing_gambling_research/link/54b7a6ac0cf2e68eb28037e9/download (accessed 25 June 2020).

161. Wardle H, Reith G, Langham E, Rogers RD. Gambling and public health: we need policy action to prevent harm. *BMJ*. 2019; 365: l1807, doi: 10.1136/bmj.l1807.

162. Browne M, Rockloff MJ. Prevalence of gambling-related harm provides evidence for the prevention paradox. *Journal of Behavioral Addictions*. 2018; 7(2): 410–422.

163. New Zealand. Ministry of Health. *Strategy to Prevent and Minimise Gambling Harm 2016/17 to 2018/19*. Wellington, New Zealand: Ministry of Health; 2016.

164. White S. NHS chief calls for gambling tax to pay for addiction treatment. *Accountancy Daily*, 24 June 2019. Available at: https://www.accountancydaily.co/nhs-chief-calls-gambling-tax-pay-addiction-treatment (accessed 24 June 2020).
165. Lock S. Total revenue of the gambling market in the United States from 2004 to 2018. Statista. 29 May 2020. Available at: https://www.statista.com/statistics/271583/casino-gaming-market-in-the-us/ (accessed 25 June 2020).
166. Gandullia L, Leporatti L. Distributional effects of gambling taxes: empirical evidence from Italy. *The Journal of Economic Inequality*. 2019; 17(4): 565–590.
167. Adams PJ, Rossen F. A tale of missed opportunities: pursuit of a public health approach to gambling in New Zealand: Gambling and public health in New Zealand. *Addiction*. 2012; 107(6): 1051–1056.
168. van Schalkwyk MCI, et al. A public health approach to gambling regulation: countering powerful influences. *The Lancet Public Health*. 2021; 6(8): e614–e619.
169. Rafaty R. Perceptions of corruption, political distrust, and the weakening of climate policy. *Global Environmental Politics*. 2018; 18(3): 106–129.
170. United Nations Human Settlements Programme (UN-HABITAT). The Challenge of Local Government Financing in Developing Countries. United Nations Human Settlements Programme (UN-HABITAT), 2015. Available at: https://sustainabledevelopment.un.org/content/documents/1732The%20Challenge%20of%20Local%20Government%20Financing%20in%20Developing%20Countries%20_3.pdf (accessed 3 May 2020).
171. Organisation for Economic Co-operation and Development (OECD). *Environmental Taxation: A Guide for Policy Makers*. OECD Publishing, 2011. Available at: https://www.oecd.org/env/tools-evaluation/48164926.pdf (accessed 12 June 2019).
172. Fullerton D, Leicester A, Smith S. *Environmental Taxation*. OECD Publishing, 2010. Available at: https://www.ifs.org.uk/uploads/mirrleesreview/dimensions/ch5.pdf (accessed 22 June 2019).
173. Scharff EA. Powerful cities? Limits on municipal taxing authority and what to do about them. *New York University Law Review*. 2016; 91(2): 292–343.
174. Görlach B. What constitutes an optimal climate policy mix? Defining the concept of optimality, including political and legal framework conditions. CECILIA2050 WP1 Deliverable 1.1. Berlin: Ecologic Institute, 2013. Available at: https://www.ecologic.eu/14178 (accessed 22 July 2019).
175. Eykelenboom M, van Stralen MM, Olthof MR, Schoonmade LJ, Steenhuis IHM, Renders CM. Political and public acceptability of a sugar-sweetened beverages tax: a mixed-method systematic review and meta-analysis. *International Journal of Behavioral Nutrition and Physical Activity*. 2019; 16(1): 78.
176. Carattini S, Carvalho M, Fankhauser S. Overcoming public resistance to carbon taxes. *WIREs Climate Change*. 2018; 9(5): e531.

https://doi.org/10.1142/9781800612396_0009

Chapter 8

The Design of Effective Health Taxes

Lisa M Powell* and Frank J Chaloupka*

To maximise the effectiveness of health taxes in reducing consumption of tobacco, alcoholic beverages, and sugar-sweetened beverages (SSBs), the tax design must be considered. We study tax aspects including determining tax type (i.e., ad valorem, specific excise, sales, and import taxes), what products are going to be taxed (i.e., the tax base), tax structure, tax rate to be applied, and implications related to tax revenue and earmarking. We find that excise taxes, often used as 'Pigouvian' taxes, are preferable to correct for externalities from harmful consumption. We note numerous advantages of specific (applied per unit of product) versus ad valorem (applied as percentage of price) excise taxes. We find that the narrower the product tax base, the greater the opportunities for consumers to substitute away from taxed to untaxed products, reducing the effectiveness of a tax in promoting health, while also generating lower revenues. Regarding the tax level, economic theory suggests that the tax should be set so that it generates revenues that are sufficient to cover the external costs associated with the harmful consumption of the taxed product. Regarding tax structure, tiered tax structures with higher rates based on higher levels of harm associated with products (i.e., ethanol or sugar) can help to reduce consumption of the most harmful products to a greater extent and help to encourage

* University of Illinois Chicago, USA.

> reformulation. Additionally, earmarking the revenues of increased taxes can be used to offset potential unintended consequences, and to augment the health impact through other initiatives that discourage use – i.e., for education campaigns or prevention programmes. Finally, the type and magnitude of tax employed, and extent of earmarking should be based on country-specific situational analyses of public health challenges and in the context of related public health goals, revenue needs and tax administration capacity of the country.

The goals of health taxes have generally been twofold: to reduce the demand for unhealthy products such as tobacco, alcohol and unhealthy foods and beverages such as sugar-sweetened beverages (SSBs) with the aim of improving health outcomes and to raise revenue. Historically, and still the case in many countries, governments may pursue multiple objectives when designing health taxes, including revenue generation, protection of domestic industries, equity concerns and others. The focus of this chapter, however, is on the use and design of these taxes to promote health. The rationale for implementing a tax to promote health is to correct individuals' harmful consumption of products such as tobacco, alcohol and sugary beverages, given that these products' prices do not account for their external costs (e.g. medical costs, productivity losses and other consumption-related harmful outcomes), nor might individuals fully consider the costs their choices impose on their own future selves. Thus, if consumption of certain products creates externalities or internalities, a tax set to the marginal cost of these external costs, known as a Pigouvian tax, can encourage people to reduce consumption (i.e. correct for any level of harmful consumption).

In this chapter, we examine a number of important tax design considerations for maximising the effectiveness of health taxes in meeting the goal of reducing consumption of targeted products. These considerations include determining the type of tax to be applied, what products are going to be taxed (i.e. the tax base), determining the structure of how they are taxed, determining the tax rate to be applied and assessing implications related to tax revenue and earmarking.

8.1. Determining the type of tax

Taxes that are applied to a defined set of products such as tobacco, alcohol and sugary beverages, may be used as a policy instrument to increase the relative prices of such products and, thereby, influence individual-level consumption. In addition to impacting behaviour by increasing prices, excise taxes may also signal that consumption of the taxed products should be reduced. Taxes that are tied to a level's harmful constituents (e.g. ethanol or sugar) may provide stronger signals than taxes tied to units sold invariant of their content. These signals may be implicit given that the products/constituents are being targeted for taxation or they may be made explicitly through marketing campaigns by the government or other stakeholders. This latter activity often occurs as part of an implementation plan or advocacy around the tax wherein a marketing/educational campaign is used to educate the population on the harms associated with consumption. Various aspects of advocating for health taxes are addressed in greater detail in Chapter 11 of this book.

Taxes on consumption are considered indirect taxes which are passed on to the consumer and include excise taxes, value-added taxes (VAT) or general sales taxes (GST) and import tariffs. Of these, excise taxes are most important when using fiscal policy to promote health, given that they are uniquely applied to specified products and, thus, will have a greater impact on the relative price of the taxed product than will taxes on a broader range of goods and services. In addition, excise tax rates can be set at much higher rates than is likely to be feasible for broader based taxes.

VAT and GST taxes generally apply broadly to all products and, therefore, are not considered as policy tools that would change relative prices of specific products and related consumption behaviour. Whereas a VAT tax is typically incorporated into the shelf price which is important for impacting behaviour decisions, a GST is often applied only at the point of purchase and, thus, is less salient and the least favourable tax instrument for impacting behaviour. Some governments do use differential VAT or GST rates on various products that, at times, reflect health objectives. For example,

India recently adopted a GST system with five different rates (0%, 5%, 12%, 18% and 28%), and applied the highest rate to tobacco products, at least in part due to the harms caused by tobacco consumption. Likewise, several states in the United States apply higher sales taxes to alcoholic beverages and many states disfavour carbonated beverages and other soft drinks by applying their sales tax to these products while generally exempting foods and beverages from these taxes.

Import tariffs are used to raise revenue and can influence consumption and the balance of trade. Tariffs on products that do not have domestically produced substitutes may be effective in reducing the overall consumption of such products. However, tariffs on imported products that are also produced domestically will raise the relative price of the imported products and induce substitution (tax avoidance) to the domestically produced products. Tariffs may also violate trade agreements. Thus, tariffs are not considered a best practice as an effective policy tool aimed at reducing the consumption of unhealthy products. That said, several governments rely on import tariffs rather than excise taxes for taxing tobacco products, alcoholic beverages and sugary drinks, with countries that do this generally having little or no domestic industry and relying on imports for these products. For example, until recently, the Gulf Cooperation Council countries relied on import duties rather than excise taxes for taxation of tobacco products.

Excise taxes are discriminatory taxes that are applied to specific products. As noted previously, excise taxes are often used as 'Pigouvian' taxes which are implemented with the intent of inducing a behaviour change to correct for harmful consumption. Examples include those already noted with respect to tobacco and alcoholic and sugary beverage products, but also include, for example, gasoline and motor vehicles, and products packaged in plastic bottles. Excise taxes are also used to tax luxury items and other goods as a discriminatory means to raise revenue. Excise taxes apply equally to domestically produced and imported products and, therefore, do not impact trade agreements.

Excise taxes can be levied as specific taxes, based on a measure of quantity (i.e. tax amount per unit of the product), or as ad valorem taxes, based on the price of a product (i.e. tax amount as a percentage of price). In the case of alcoholic and sugary beverages, some specific taxes are at times referred to as 'unitary' taxes which are taxes based on units of volume (e.g. per ounce or litre), while specific taxes may be used to describe taxes on the ingredient being taxed (e.g. ethanol for alcoholic beverages and sugar for SSBs). In this chapter discussion, specific taxes will be used to broadly include taxes based on quantity, volume or constituents.

Specific excise taxes have many advantages over ad valorem excise taxes.[1,2] They reduce the price gaps among different brands of the taxed product, reducing opportunities for consumers to trade down to cheaper brands when taxes are increased. Also, since specific excise taxes are applied on a per unit basis rather than as a function of price, quantity discounts are still taxed at the same rate. They tend to encourage production of higher priced products. They produce more stable revenues as they are not as subject to industry price manipulation. Also, specific taxes are relatively easy to administer and are not as susceptible to industry tax avoidance and evasion, such as under-invoicing in countries which use the Cost, Insurance, Freight (CIF) or ex-factory price as the base. The main disadvantage of a specific excise tax is that it needs to be increased regularly or its value will be eroded by inflation; whereas, given that ad valorem excise taxes are a function of price they keep up with inflation. Also, some view ad valorem excises as more equitable than specific excises, because the amount of the tax levied will be greater on the higher priced premium brands more likely to be chosen by more affluent consumers.

It is important to note that a given ad valorem tax rate that is levied based on prices early in the distribution chain will have a smaller impact on retail prices than it will if levied based on retail prices. For example, in Barbados, the SSB ad valorem excise tax is applied to the producer price, which is a lower value base for taxation than the retail price or the retail price excluding VAT. In Chile, however, 18% and 10% sweetened beverage ad valorem excise taxes are applied to the retail price excluding VAT. Therefore, even in the cases where statutory ad valorem excise tax rates may be the same across two countries, if they are applied at different points in the distribution chain, their effective impact on prices (and, hence demand) may be different. In addition, ad valorem excises levied earlier are more subject to abusive transfer pricing, where producers and/or distributors set artificially low prices at the point where the tax is levied and then raise the price further along the distribution chain. This can be particularly problematic when the industry is highly vertically integrated.

Additionally, in comparing specific versus ad valorem excise taxes, it is important to note that a specific excise tax will differentially change the relative price of different types of categories of products given that their per-unit baseline prices may differ. For example, a recent evaluation of the US Cook County, Illinois, Sweetened Beverage Tax reported mean prices per ounce of sweetened beverages by category ranging from a low of 2.68 cents per ounce for soda to 13.60 cents per ounce for energy drinks.[3] Based on these different mean prices by beverage category, a specific excise tax in the amount of 1 cent per ounce would equate, on average, to an increase in the price of soda of 37% but only a 7% increase in the price of energy drinks (assuming full tax pass-through). Thus, it is important to keep in mind that when a fixed-rate specific excise tax used, it will translate into different percentage (and hence relative) increases in prices across product categories based on their differential baseline prices.

Some governments apply combinations of specific and ad valorem excises or employ an ad valorem tax with a minimum specific tax floor in an effort to capitalise on the advantages of each. This type of mixed system will have less of an impact on health than a purely specific system would have and will be more difficult to administer. Overall, countries that rely more on specific cigarette taxes generally have higher taxes and prices on average than do countries that rely more on ad valorem taxes.[4] In addition, countries that rely more on specific taxes have less variability in cigarette prices than countries that rely more on ad valorem or tiered tax structures.[5,6]

The greater variability in prices resulting from ad valorem or tiered tax structures provides more opportunities for smokers to avoid tax increases by trading down to less expensive brands, reducing the impact of a tax increase on cigarette consumption.[7] One recent study provides similar findings for the effects of alcohol tax structure on alcohol price variability.[8]

Some governments employ tiered tax structures (specific, ad valorem or mixed) where the tax varies based on price and/or product characteristics. Tiered tax structures based on price can have disadvantages of widening price gaps between brands and facilitating tax avoidance by producers who may manipulate prices or their products to reduce the tax they face. However, tiered taxes based on product characteristics may encourage product reformulation if levied on an unhealthy product ingredient, such as a sugary beverage tax levied based on sugar content or an alcoholic beverage tax based on ethanol content – see more detailed discussion of tiered taxes based on level of product harmfulness in the next section of this chapter. The supply-side response of reformulation can add to the public health impact of the tax but there may also be supply-side responses of increased marketing.

8.1.1. Tobacco taxes

Overall, tax structures with respect to tobacco vary widely, from uniform specific or ad valorem taxes, to combinations of specific and ad valorem, to complicated tiered tax structures where different rates are applied based on various product characteristics (e.g. price, cigarette length, presence/absence of a filter, source of tobacco and size of production). Based on data from the WHO's *Report on the Global Tobacco Epidemic,* which provides data on cigarette taxes in 185 countries, just over one-third (65) of countries levy a specific cigarette excise tax, about one-third (63) levy a combination of specific and ad valorem taxes; the remainder levy either an ad valorem excise (42 countries), or have no excise (15 countries).[9] Many of the countries that implement a mixed system are in the European Union (EU), where the EU's tobacco tax directive mandates that countries implement a mixed system in which the specific tax must account for between 7.5% and 76.5% of the total excise tax. Almost half of the countries that implement an ad valorem or mixed cigarette excise tax set a minimum specific tax. In the EU, for example, the minimum excise is set at 90 euros per 1,000 cigarettes and must account for at least 60% of weighted average retail price. Other countries have much more complicated tax structures. Indonesia, for example, has a complex cigarette tax structure where the rates vary by type of cigarette (white cigarette versus kretek (clove cigarette)), type of production (machine made or handmade) and production volume. Fiji and Tanzania apply different taxes based on the source of the tobacco leaf used in production (domestic versus imported). Mozambique and Uganda levy different taxes based on the type of packaging (soft versus hard pack).

8.1.2. Alcohol taxes

As with tobacco taxes, governments have taken a variety of approaches to taxing alcoholic beverages. Some apply specific taxes based on volume, while others apply ad valorem taxes. Some volume-based taxes are applied based on total volume, while others are based on the volume of ethanol contained in the product. Taxes can differ based on the type of alcoholic beverage, with taxes on beer often lowest and taxes on distilled spirits often higher. Based on WHO's Global Information System on Alcohol and Health data for 192 countries in 2012 (the most recent year available), 155 countries levied an excise tax on beer, 138 on wine and 151 on distilled spirits. Some, but not all, of the countries that did not levy taxes banned the sale of alcoholic beverages. Tax structure data available for 138 countries show that about one in three implemented an ad valorem tax, just over one in five levied a specific tax with most levying taxes based on ethanol content, and almost half implemented a mixed tax structure. Some countries used different tax structures for different types of alcoholic beverages. South Africa provides an interesting case study for alcoholic beverage excise taxes.[10] Since 1974, South Africa applied a specific excise tax on distilled spirits based on ethanol content. From 1982 through 1990, wine was untaxed; from 1991 on, a specific excise tax based on volume has been applied. Beer was taxed based on volume until 1998, when the tax was changed to one based on ethanol content. Similarly, taxes on hard ciders and other ready-to-drink alcoholic beverages were changed from volume-based to ethanol-based taxes in 2016. Sorghum beer, a popular local beverage, continues to be taxed based on overall volume. South Africa's taxes have favoured wine, with the lowest average tax per litre of ethanol, with beer taxed at somewhat higher rates and spirits taxed at a much higher level.

8.1.3. SSB taxes

While most sugary beverage taxes to date have generally used a flat specific excise tax amount per unit volume or a flat ad valorem tax rate where all taxed beverage products are subject to the same tax irrespective of their beverage type (e.g. soda, and energy, sports, juice drinks, etc.) or sugar content, some have implemented continuous or discrete tiered tax approaches based on sugar content. Mexico's sugary beverage tax, for example, is a specific tax based on volume, initially set at one peso per litre and subsequently adjusted for inflation. The United Kingdom implements a tiered specific tax based on sugar content, with a tax of 18 pence per litre for drinks with more than 5 g of sugar per 100 mL and 24 pence per litre for those with eight or more grams per 100 mL. Similar to many of its alcoholic beverage taxes, South Africa taxes based on sugar content, levying a tax of ZAR 0.021 per gram of sugar on beverages containing more than 4 g of sugar per 100 mL. Others levy ad valorem taxes, such as Saudi Arabia and the United Arab Emirates special value-added taxes that in effect act as excise taxes, with rates of 50% on soft drinks and 100% on energy drinks.

8.2. Determining the tax base

In using fiscal policy as a tool to reduce consumption of products that impose health risks as a means to maximise health impacts an important consideration for policymakers is to define which categories of products (e.g. product categories within, e.g. tobacco, alcohol and sugary beverages) will be included as part of the tax base and hence taxed; and, whether certain characteristics of such products (i.e. level of nicotine, ethanol, sugar) will further define the base and the related structure of the tax.

The appropriate tax base depends on the objective of the tax. A public health objective would suggest the inclusion of categories of a given product area for which evidence demonstrates consumption-related health risks. If the tax base does not comprehensively include all product categories that are harmful then substitution to any harmful untaxed products will occur and will undermine the health impact of the tax. The narrower the product base, the greater the opportunities for consumers to substitute away from taxed to untaxed products, reducing the effectiveness of a tax in promoting health, while also generating lower revenues.

With tobacco, for example, nearly all countries levy excise taxes on manufactured cigarettes, but taxation of other tobacco products is more variable, with some taxing cigars, bidis, roll-your-own tobacco and smokeless tobacco products, albeit at different rates that are often lower than applied to manufactured cigarettes.[4] Relatively few governments tax emerging nicotine products, including electronic nicotine and non-nicotine delivery systems (ENNDS) and heated tobacco products (HTP). There is similar variability in the taxation of emerging nicotine products. With respect to ENNDS, some governments tax only the liquids used in vaping, while others also tax the device; some tax only liquids containing nicotine while others tax all liquids used in vaping; still others tax liquids based on nicotine content. From a public health perspective, taxing all tobacco and non-pharmaceutical nicotine products is most appropriate, with comparable taxes on similar products to minimise substitution across products.

Most governments tax alcoholic beverages, but some apply taxes to one or two beverage categories (e.g. beer and spirits) but not to others (e.g. wine; see Figure 8.1).[11] Using alcoholic beverage taxation to promote public health suggests that taxes should be applied to all alcoholic beverages and that taxes on the ethanol contained in different beverages should be similar across beverages.[12]

Fig. 8.1. Alcoholic beverage excise taxes by beverage type.

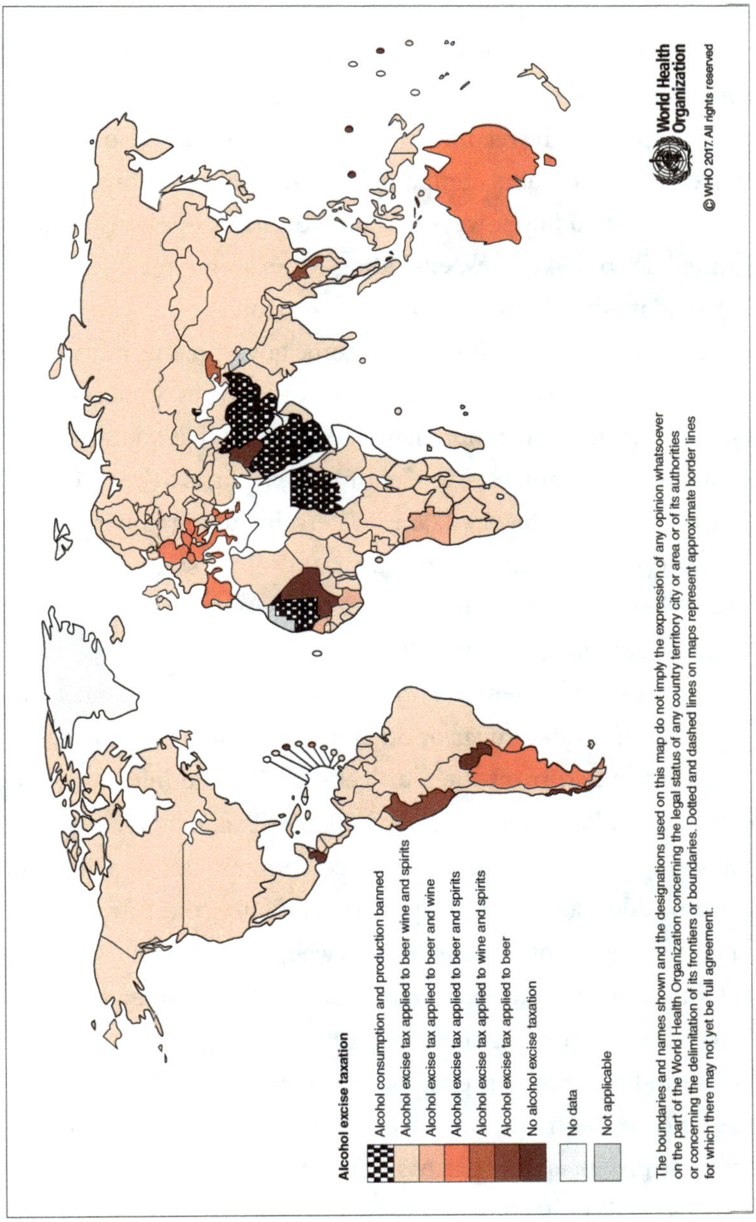

With regard to the base for sugary beverage taxation, the public health objective to reduce sugars intake suggests a tax on all SSBs including soda, fruit drinks, sports drinks, energy drinks, sweetened teas/coffees and sweetened/flavoured milk. To the extent that any 'free sugars' are considered a health risk, it would be recommended that the tax base also include 100% fruit juice, which contains comparable (and sometimes higher) amounts of free sugars as soda. However, many countries apply their SSB taxes to a limited set of beverages, excluding for example products where the first ingredient is milk, 100% fruit juices or fruit drinks with a minimum proportion of fruit juice. Additionally, some governments have focused on taxing soda (carbonated beverages) but not other types of sugary beverages.

One challenge for a comprehensive SSB tax is that countries often use the HS system (see Figure 8.2) to identify the products to be taxed, typically focusing on product category 22.02: 'Waters, including mineral waters and aerated waters, containing added sugar and other sweetening matter or flavoured'. However, SSBs can be found across a number of other HS codes. Beverages under category 20.09: 'Fruit juices (including grape must) and vegetable juices, unfermented and not containing added spirit, whether or not containing added sugar or other sweetening matter' always contain free sugars (released from the fruit cells during the mechanical juicing process), while milk products under 04.02: 'Milk and cream; concentrated or containing added sugar or other sweetening matter' may contain free sugars from added sugar, honey, syrup or fruit juice concentrates. Similarly, SSBs may be found in other categories as well, including 04.03: 'Buttermilk, curdled milk and cream, yogurt, kefir, fermented or acidified milk or cream', 04.04: 'Whey and products consisting of natural milk constituents', 18.06: 'Chocolate and other food preparations containing cocoa', 21.01: 'Extracts, essences and concentrates, of coffee, tea or maté and preparations with a basis of these products or with a basis of coffee, tea or maté; roasted chicory and other roasted coffee substitutes, and extracts, essences and concentrates thereof' and 21.06: 'Food preparations not elsewhere specified or included'.

Fig. 8.2. Categories of beverages in the HS system according to content of free sugars and non-sugar sweeteners.

Sugar-sweetened beverages	**22.02** Waters, including mineral waters and aerated waters, containing added sugar and other sweetening matter or flavored	**20.09** Fruit juices (including grape must) and vegetable juices, unfermented and not containing added spirit, whether or not containing added sugar or other sweetening matter	**04.02** Milk and cream; concentrated or containing added sugar or other sweetening matter	**04.03** Buttermilk, curdled milk and cream, yoghurt, kephir, fermented or acidified milk or cream	**18.06** Chocolate and other food preparations containing cocoa
Beverages with non-sugar sweeteners				**04.04** Whey and products consisting of natural milk constituents	**21.01** Extracts, essences, concentrates of coffee, tea or mate; preparations with a basis of these products ...; roasted chicory
Beverages that are not sweetened	**22.01** Waters, including natural or artificial mineral waters and aerated waters, not containing added sugar or other sweetening matter nor flavoured; ice and snow		**04.01** Milk and cream; not concentrated, not containing added sugar or other sweetening matter		**21.06** Food preparations not elsewhere specified or included

Source: Figure prepared by Kaia Engesveeen (WHO) based on the global training course presentation titled 'Healthy Diets and Physical Activity. Legal Issues in Policy Design and Implementation' 17–21 June 2019, Geneva, Switzerland; and based on the Harmonized Commodity Description and Coding Systems (HS). https://unstats.un.org/unsd/tradekb/Knowledgebase/50018/Harmonized-Commodity-Description-and-Coding-Systems-HS.

Under the public health objective to decrease free sugars intake, artificially sweetened beverages (ASBs) that are zero calories would not be included in the tax base. Sweetened beverage taxes have not been consistent in their application to SSB versus ASBs beverages. While most recent sweetened beverage product excise taxes have generally applied to SSBs, some taxes such as those, for example, in Chile and two jurisdictions in the United States (Cook County, IL and Philadelphia, PA) have applied their beverage taxes to both SSBs and ASBs. In relation to the HS coding system, countries that apply their taxes indiscriminately to products under HS Code 22.02 would tax a large share of sugar-sweetened beverages, but also many beverages containing non-sugar sweeteners for which there is currently no public health goal. From a public health goal of reducing intake of free sugars, one would exclude a number of products from the base including for example, in the HS coding system, 22.01: 'Waters, including natural or artificial mineral waters and aerated waters, not containing added sugar or other sweetening matter nor flavoured; ice and snow' and 04.01: 'Milk and cream; not concentrated, not containing added sugar or other sweetening matter', and some buttermilks and yogurt-based beverages (04.03), whey products (04.04), cocoa, coffee, tea, maté or chickory-based preparations (18.06 and 21.01) or other beverages (21.06) that contain neither free sugars nor non-sugar sweeteners.

8.3. Determining the tax structure

Another consideration is whether to structure the tax so that it levies different tax rates based on the level of harmfulness of the taxed products within the tax base. Applying this to tobacco could be challenging since there is considerable debate over the relative harms of different products.[13] With respect to alcohol, a tax based on ethanol would induce consumers to switch to lower taxed products containing less ethanol. At the same time, it would encourage producers to reformulate their products by reducing ethanol content in order to face a lower tax, as well as encourage them to market their lower taxed, lower ethanol products more aggressively than their higher taxed, higher ethanol products. These supply-side responses were observed in South Africa following the country's shift to a specific beer excise tax based on ethanol content rather than just volume.[12]

With respect to foods and beverages, nutrient-based tiers may be used to determine rates. As noted previously, SSB taxes to date have mostly used a uniform tax approach where all taxed beverage products are subject to the same tax irrespective of their sugar content. Although the volume-based uniform tax has the important advantage of simplicity in implementation, it does not provide incentives for consumers to switch to less calorically sweetened beverages or for the beverage industry to reformulate products to reduce sugar content per serving. An approach where beverages are taxed at different amounts depending on their sugar content (i.e. grams (g) of sugar per unit of volume or serving) has been proposed and implemented in a limited number of countries. For example, in April 2018, the United Kingdom implemented a three-tiered soft drink industry levy (SDIL) with no tax on beverages with <5 g of sugar/100 mL, and 18 pence/L and 24 pence/L on beverages with 5–8 g and >8 g of sugar/100 mL, respectively. Within two years following the SDIL announcement, there was an 11% reduction in sugar content of drinks subject to the levy, and the caloric content of such drinks fell by 6%.[14] And, recent evidence shows that between 2015 and 2018 sales volume sold of high-sugar (>8 g/100 mL) beverages fell 40% which stemmed from a combination of reformulation and reduced demand from the tax.[15] Sugar content-based SSB taxes can be designed with discrete tiers based on thresholds across which tax rates vary (i.e. Chile and the United Kingdom) or can be based on a continuum (rather than discrete tiers) of sugar content in SSBs (i.e. South African Health Promotion Levy). In the case of SSB taxes, a recent study showed that evidence on the actual distribution of the most commonly consumed SSBs by sugar content can help inform the choice of meaningful thresholds for a tiered-tax structure.[16] For example, Figure 8.3 drawn from that study revealed multiple clusters of SSB volume by sugar content and suggested threshold tiers for differential tax rates at <20 g and <5 g of sugar/8-oz (corresponding to cut points at a distance of 5 g below

Fig. 8.3. Distribution of annual sugar-sweetened beverage (SSB) sales volume by sugar content, all SSBs and by SSB category, US total, 2018.

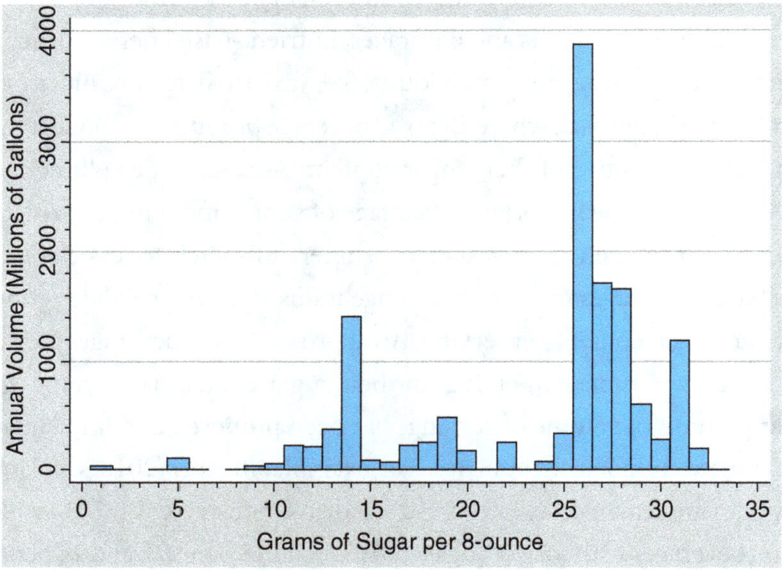

Source: Powell LM, Andreyeva T, Isgor Z. Distribution of sugar-sweetened beverage sales volume by sugar content in the United States: Implications for tiered taxation and tax revenue. *Journal of Public Health Policy.* 2020; 41(2): 125–138.

the lower bounds of the clusters; this distance should be determined based on a given jurisdiction's goals for sugar content reduction).

The Danish fat tax is an example of a tax that targets a specific nutrient found across multiple product categories as compared to the taxes based on sugar content within the single product category of SSBs. The Danish fat tax introduced in October 2011 (though subsequently repealed effective January 2013) was applied to meat, dairy, animal fat, oils, margarine and butter blends including foods containing these products at the rate of DKK 16 per kilogram of saturated fat (if the content of saturated fat exceeded 2.3 g per 100 g).[17]

It should be noted, however, that while taxes based on levels or intensity of sugar, saturated fat, nicotine or alcohol content may offer added incentives for product reformulation and greater incentives for behaviour change for the most harmful products, they may not be appropriate in jurisdictions that do not have strong tax administration.[18] Thus, when deciding on tax designs with differentially determined tax rates based on discrete or continuous levels of the harmfulness on the products' content, compared with uniform rates, it is important to do so in the context of tax administration capacity.

8.4. Determining the tax rate

It is challenging to determine an optimal recommended level of tax or magnitude of tax increases. How one defines optimal depends on the objectives of the tax. One approach could be to set the excise tax so that it generates revenues that are sufficient to cover the external costs associated with consumption of the taxed product. Another approach would be to set the tax high enough to minimise the public health harms from consumption. Yet another would be to set the tax at the level that maximises tax revenues. Still another would be to increase taxes by enough to maintain or reduce the affordability of the tax product over time.

With tobacco, the World Bank has recommended that total cigarette taxes in LMICs should be set to account for two-thirds to four-fifths of retail prices, based on tax levels in HICs that included significant tax increases as part of a comprehensive strategy for reducing tobacco use.[19] WHO has recommended that *excise* taxes should account for 70% of retail prices, a target that would require significant tax increases in nearly all countries.[20] Such targets, however, do not capture problems with tax structures or may not lead to high retail prices if industry prices are very low. The WHO's Guidelines for the Implementation of Article 6 of the Framework Convention on Tobacco Control recommend simple tax structures that emphasise uniform specific taxes or mixed systems relying on specific taxes with regular adjustments to account for inflation and income growth.

It has been recommended by WHO that sugary beverage tax rates be set high enough to raise prices by at least 20%, in order to result in net reductions in caloric intake that are potentially large enough to improve weight outcomes at the population level.[21] Lower sugary beverage tax rates such as the 1 peso per litre (approximate 10%) rate in Mexico have had a significant expected impact (in the range of 6–9% reductions) on purchases/consumption but the extent to which these changes in intake will have an impact on health outcomes such as diabetes or weight is not yet known. There are no similar recommendations for the level of taxes on alcoholic beverages.

Given that the goal of a public health-oriented tax policy is to reduce consumption of a particular good, such as tobacco, alcohol or SSBs or other foods high in nutrients recommended to limit, the tax must be passed on to consumers in the form of higher prices. The tax incidence, that is, the extent to which consumers versus producers/sellers bear the burden of the tax depends on the responsiveness (price elasticity) of demand and supply. If demand is price-insensitive (i.e. inelastic) then the entire amount of the tax is passed on to consumers but it would not impact quantity demanded and sold. Although such a setting may be ideal for raising tax revenue, it is not conducive for reducing consumption. In settings with elastic demand and supply, excise taxes generally lead to some (but not necessarily 100%) pass through (i.e. a sharing of the tax burden by consumers and producers) and lower consumption – where the level of tax pass through increases with greater consumer price sensitivity. In some settings (i.e. less than perfectly competitive markets) taxes may also lead to over-shifting. Evidence on the extent of tax pass through and various factors impacting tax pass through are discussed in detail in Chapter 4 of this book.

For a given tax pass-through rate, modest tax and price increases will have relatively small effects on consumption and health, while large increases would have a larger impact. Large tax increases may also signal to consumers that these products are dangerous and would lead to large reductions in their use. This is captured in the World Bank's recent recommendation that governments 'go big, go fast' when increasing their tobacco taxes, stating that a more gradual approach 'means condemning large numbers of people to avoidable illness and premature death'.[22]

Nearly all governments levy excise taxes on manufactured cigarettes; as noted previously, only 15 of the 185 countries who reported tax and price data for 2018 to the World Health Organization (WHO) reported that they did not levy an excise tax.[23] Tobacco taxes have increased in many countries since the entry into force of the WHO's Framework Convention on Tobacco Control in 2005, given Article 6 of the treaty's recognition of the effectiveness of tax and price increases in reducing tobacco use, particularly among young people. In 2018, cigarette excise taxes varied widely from country to country, with taxes ranging from less than $0.03 per pack in Benin and Paraguay to over $11 per pack in New Zealand, and ranging from less than 3% of price in Cabo Verde to over 77% of price in Egypt.[23]

8.4.1. Tobacco taxes

Most countries also impose a value-added tax or general sales tax on cigarettes, while several impose other special levies. On average, cigarette excise taxes account for less than one-quarter of price (22.0%) in LICs, and about two-fifths (41.3%) of price in MICs and over half of price (54.5%) in HICs (see Figure 8.4).[23] As noted previously with respect to types of taxes, about 35% of countries levy specific excise taxes only, while almost 23% levy ad valorem excises only; the remainder use a combination of specific and ad valorem taxes. The base on which the ad valorem taxes are levied varies across countries, with some levied based on producer or import prices, others on distributor prices and still others on retail prices. LMICs tend to rely more on ad valorem excises, while HICs are more likely to employ a specific or mixed tax. Of 170 countries reporting detailed tax information in 2018, 139 applied the same tax to all cigarettes, while 31 employed a tiered tax structure where the tax varied based on price and/or product characteristics (e.g. length, production type, presence/absence of a filter). LMICs are more likely to have complex tax structures. For example, Indonesia's tax structure includes 10 tiers, with taxes varying for kreteks (clove cigarettes) and white cigarettes, hand-rolled versus machine produced and so on. That said, Indonesia recognises the complications this creates and it is in the process of simplifying its tobacco tax structure. Bangladesh levies different ad valorem taxes on brands based on retail prices, with rates increasing as prices increase.

Fig. 8.4. Cigarette prices and taxes by country income, 2018.

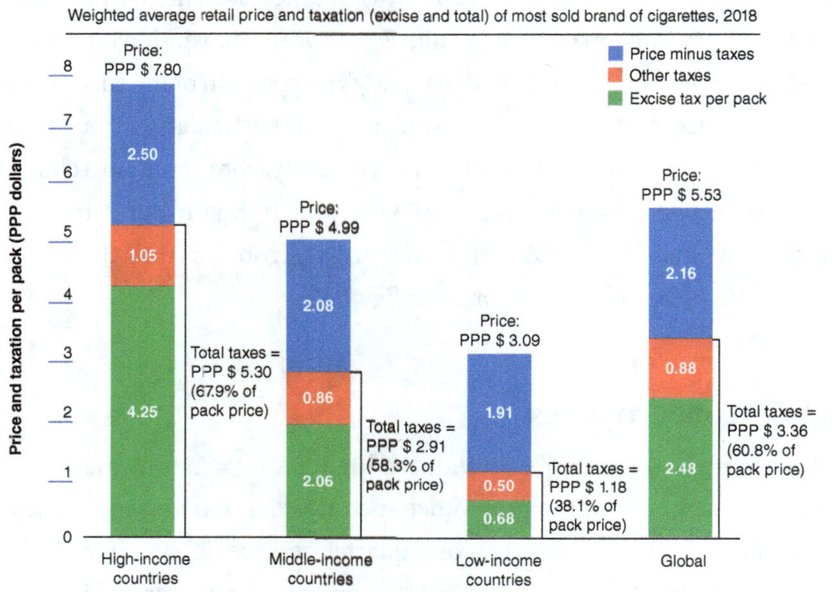

Note: Averages are weighted by WHO estimates of number of current cigarette smokers ages 15+ in each country in 2017. Prices are expressed in Purchasing Power Party (PPP) adjusted dollars or International dollars to account for differences in the purchasing power across countries. Based on 53 high-income, 97 middle-income and 28 low-income countries with data on prices of most sold brand, excise and other taxes, and PPP conversion factors. Numbers may not add exactly due to rounding.

Source: World Health Organization. *WHO Report on the Global Tobacco Epidemic, 2019: Offer Help to Quit Tobacco Use*. Geneva: World Health Organization; 2019.

Taxation of other tobacco products is more variable, with many countries taxing some or all other products, but generally at rates well below the rate imposed on manufactured cigarettes.

8.4.2. Alcohol taxes

Similarly, nearly all governments levy excise taxes and value-added or sales taxes on alcoholic beverages, although which beverages are taxed vary to some extent across countries. Also as noted previously with respect to the discussion on types of taxes, of the 192 countries that provided data for WHO's Global Information System on Alcohol and Health in 2012 (the most recent available data), 155 levied an excise tax on beer, 138 on wine and 151 on distilled spirits; alcohol sales were banned in some, but not in all of the non-taxing countries (see Figure 8.2).[24] Comprehensive data on tax rates and prices are not available, but from the limited available information, excise taxes on alcoholic beverages appear to be lower and account for a lower share of price in LMICs than in HICs, following a pattern similar to cigarette taxes. Alcoholic beverage excise taxes typical account for a lower share of price than do cigarette taxes. Among the 74 reporting countries, excise taxes as a share of retail prices ranged from a low of 0.3% in Kyrgyzstan to a high of 44.9% in Norway, with an average of 17.3%. Taxes as a percentage of price tend to be lowest on beer and highest on distilled spirits, but there was considerable variation across reporting countries. Tax structures also vary across countries; of the 138 countries reporting on tax structures, one-third levied ad valorem taxes only, just over one-fifth levied specific or unitary taxes only, and almost half used a combination of taxes. As with cigarette taxes, the base for ad valorem taxes varies across countries. The base for specific alcohol taxes also varies to some extent, with some countries levying specific taxes based on volume, and others based on alcohol content. In some countries, different tax structures are used for different beverages (e.g. a volume-based tax on beer and a tax based on ethanol content on wine and spirits).

8.4.3. SSB taxes

Based on data as of July 2021, 77 of 194 WHO Member States have adopted national level excise taxes on non-alcoholic beverages that include at least one category of SSBs. Another two Member States have sub-national level taxes and one Member State has municipality level taxes (Figure 8.5). Many of these taxes may have been implemented without a particular health objective, in order to raise tax revenue. Excise taxes targeted to SSBs as a policy tool aimed at reducing consumption and improving health have recently begun to emerge and while, in this regard, more than 30 have been implemented since 2015, they are still nowhere near the norm.[25] Of note, some countries impose targeted import duties on SSBs.[26] Finally, it should be noted that

Fig. 8.5. Sugar-sweetened beverage taxes, by location, July 2021.

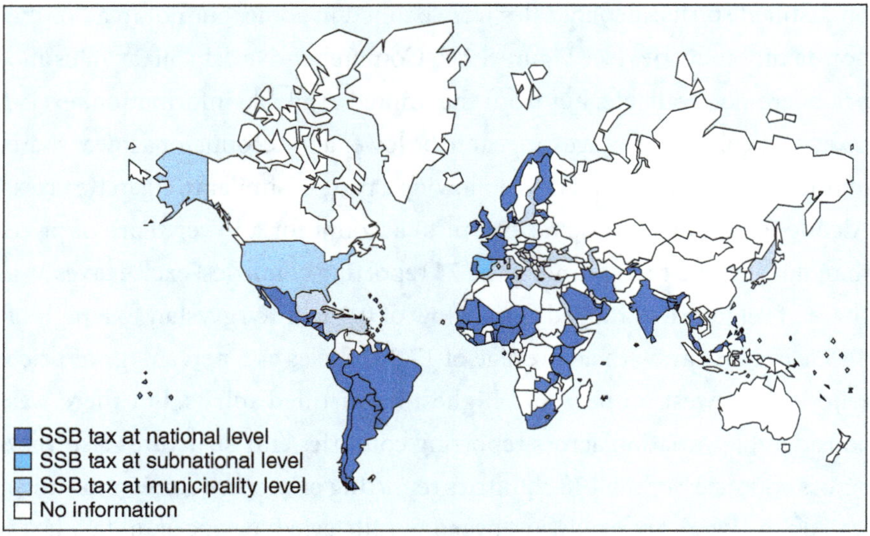

Source: WHO 2021. Country level implementation of 'WHO Best Buys and other recommended interventions for the prevention and control of NCDs' is available from progress monitoring conducted through the WHO NCD Country Capacity Survey (NCD CCS), as well as the WHO Global database on the Implementation of Nutrition Action (GINA) and the WHO Global Nutrition Policy Reviews.

in many countries and local jurisdictions soft drinks are often included in broader VAT or general sales taxes.

Within the last decade, some of the first targeted beverage taxes that emerged in countries such as Hungary were relatively small, raising prices by a few percent, although some smaller countries (e.g. Mauritius) did implement larger taxes. Mexico adopted a national tax specifically on sugary beverages of 1 peso per litre tax that was implemented in January 2014 which was equivalent to about 10% tax, on average. Several other smaller countries in the Caribbean area have followed suit with taxes in the 10% range such as Barbados and Dominica. Since then, additional countries and jurisdictions have adopted or proposed more significant excise taxes primarily aimed at reducing sugary drink consumption and promoting health, including numerous US localities where sweetened beverage taxes have ranged from 1 to 2 cents per ounce yielding increases in sweetened beverage prices, on average, for example of about 15–20% to 34%.[3,27,28] In some cases, taxes are particularly high resulting in substantial prices increases (e.g. as highlighted previously, Saudi Arabia's and the UAE's special 50% value-added tax on soft drinks and 100% value-added tax on energy drinks).

In addition to SSB taxes, countries have implemented taxes on other food products and nutrients that are considered risk factors for chronic diseases. For example, the 2011 Hungarian public health product tax included not just soft drinks with added sugar in its tax base but also a range of food products high in salt or sugars.[29] Also, at the same time as the introduction of the specific SSB excise tax in January 2014, Mexico implemented an 8% ad valorem excise tax on non-essential energy-dense (≥275 kcal per 100 g) food that included items such as chips and deep-fried salted snacks, sugar confectionery, chocolates, crème caramel and puddings, candied fruits, peanut and hazelnut spreads, caramel sauces, cereal-based products with added sugar, ice cream and popsicles.[30] And, as noted previously, the Danish fat tax introduced in 2011 and repealed in 2013 is an example of a tax that targets a specific nutrient across product types and was applied to meat, dairy, animal fat, oils, margarine and butter blends including foods containing these products.

8.5. Implications for tax revenue and earmarking

As discussed in Chapter 3 of this book, the demand for tobacco products and alcoholic beverages is generally price inelastic, implying that the relative reductions in consumption are smaller than the relative increases in price (i.e. a 10% price increase results in less than a 10% reduction in consumption). Given this and given that taxes account for only a fraction of prices, at least in the short- to medium term, increases in tobacco and alcohol taxes will generate increased revenues. For example, if half of cigarette prices are accounted for by the cigarette excise tax, doubling the tax, if fully passed on to consumers, would raise prices by 50%. With price elasticity of −0.5 in the average LMIC, the 50% price increase would reduce cigarette consumption by 25%. As a result, excise tax revenues would rise by 50%, given that the remaining 75% of consumption is taxed at twice the original rate. This will be

Fig. 8.6. Cigarette tax and tax revenues Ukraine: 2008–2015.

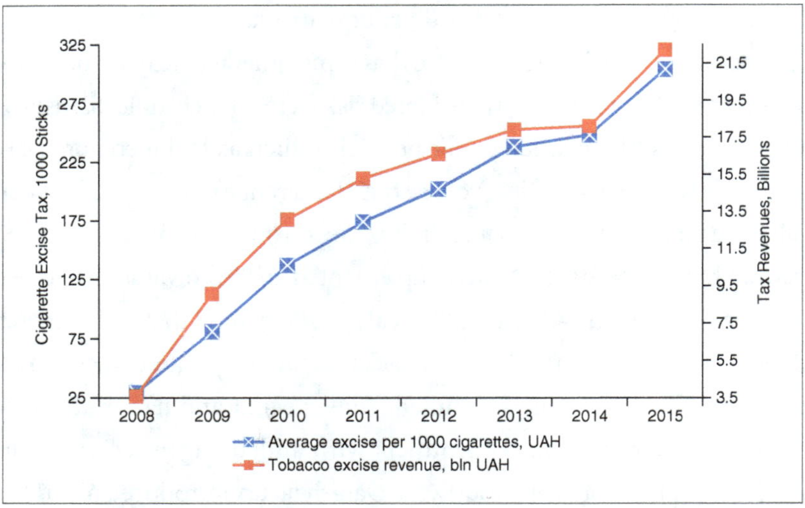

Source: Syvak O, Krasovsky K (2017). Tobacco Taxation Policy in Ukraine. Presentation at the World Bank's Tobacco Taxation Win–Win for Public Health and Domestic Resources Mobilization Conference, 18 April 2017, Washington, DC.

true even in countries with very high cigarette tax rates, as seen with recent tax increases in Australia and New Zealand. The positive impact of higher taxes on revenues is illustrated in Figure 8.6 for Ukraine, where cigarette taxes have increased sharply over the past decade, followed by increases in cigarette tax revenues (the average excise rate for cigarettes increased tenfold, while cigarette tax revenue increased sixfold).

The relative revenue impact will be even greater for alcoholic beverage tax increases given that these taxes typically account for a much smaller share of prices than do cigarette taxes. With respect to sugary drinks, the imposition of a new tax will generate significant new revenues for countries and jurisdictions that impose such taxes. A US revenue calculator for sugary drink taxes estimates potential tax revenue for each US state – for example, a 1 cent per ounce SSB tax is estimated to raise 846 million USD for the state of New York.[31] In terms of a recently implemented tax, over 2.6 billion USD was raised in the first two years post-tax implementation of Mexico's SSB tax.[32] Moreover, given the relatively low share of price accounted for by existing sugary drink taxes, increases in these taxes will still generate new revenues despite the elastic demand for these beverages. For example, the imposition of a state-wide SSB tax in the amount of 1 cent per ounce the doubling of an existing sugary drink tax that accounts for 10% of price, if fully passed on to consumers, will raise prices by 10%. Given a price elasticity of demand of −1.2 for sugary beverages, the price increase would result in a 12% drop in consumption. The remaining 88% of consumption would be taxed at twice the rate, resulting in a 76% rise in revenues. In the longer run, as taxes are increased and other policies aimed at curbing consumption are implemented, tax revenues will eventually fall, but this turning point is a long way off in nearly all countries.

Finally, the use of the increased revenues that result from increases in excise taxes on tobacco products and alcoholic beverages, and the new revenues that are generated by new sugary drink taxes can add to the health impact of these taxes. Earmarking these revenues for programmes that discourage consumption of these products, such as mass media public education campaigns, cessation and prevention programmes, enforcement of related policies and other efforts to reduce the harms caused by consumption can result in greater reductions in use and its consequences. Similarly, using these revenues for other health promotion efforts, such as programmes to support increased physical activity, healthy eating and universal health coverage, can also add to the health benefits that accrue from the tax. Moreover, public support for tax increases may be much stronger when there is a clear connection between the use of the tax revenues and the behaviours targeted by the tax. For example, data from the Global Adult Tobacco Surveys in many countries show that many smokers support increases in cigarette taxes when the revenues are used to support or improve health programmes.[33] While hard earmarking (earmarking required by law) can be difficult in some environments, soft earmarking (earmarking that is outlined/recommended but not legally binding) may be a more viable option. Indeed, there is often significant push back from governments on hard earmarking. A key argument often made against hypothecating revenue from new taxes for specific expenditures is that a marginal additional dollar of revenue should be allocated to whatever use is most effective regardless of which tax the dollar is raised from. It is argued that if the use is worthy, it makes no sense to tie expenditure on it to whatever revenue a particular tax raises. A counterargument (noted previously) is that there may be political reasons for hypothecation associated with it increasing the tax's acceptance among the public.

Earmarking a portion of tax revenue for specific government programmes is an aspect of fiscal policy that can help to maximise public health benefits and garner public support for the tax and, it can also help to alleviate opposition around potential unintended consequences. For example, to address concerns about job losses in the taxed sector, governments can dedicate some of the new revenues to programmes to facilitate worker transitions to other livelihoods, as Turkey did by earmarking some of its tobacco tax revenues to help tobacco farmers shift to other crops.[34] To address concerns about the regressivity of beverage taxes, earmarking can be targeted toward low-income populations. For example, earmarking of sugary beverage tax revenue for subsidies for fruits and vegetables for low-income families could have dual benefits of providing income assistance to offset regressive aspects of the consumption tax and improving access to healthy foods which would provide a complementary health benefit.

For a more detailed discussion related to the use of earmarking as a means of maximising resources for health and to bolster public support for health taxes, please see Chapter 10 of this book. Additionally, a discussion related to tax revenue and sustainable development and the distributional impacts of health taxes is provided in Chapter 6.

8.6. Conclusion

Several different types of health taxes are employed worldwide. Taxes on tobacco and alcohol products have a long history and taxes on unhealthy foods and beverages such as SSBs are increasingly being implemented. These taxes have included both ad valorem and specific excise taxes and have been applied at uniform or differential rates based on the level of the harmfulness on the products' content (i.e. level of sugar, saturated fat, nicotine or ethanol). Many countries use combinations of various tax types. The defined base of products to which the taxes are applied should generally be comprehensive as exclusions can lead to substitution to the excluded non-taxed products which will undermine both the health and revenue the goals of the tax. The particular type and magnitude of tax employed and extent of earmarking should be based on country-specific situational analyses of public health challenges and in the context of related public health goals, revenue needs and tax administration capacity of the country.

Key messages

- Excise taxes are often used as "Pigouvian" taxes and are implemented with the intent of inducing a behaviour change to correct for an externality of overconsumption. The amount of the tax is ideally set to equal the full cost of the externality.
- Specific excise taxes have many advantages over ad valorem excise taxes, in that they reduce price gaps among different brands of the taxed product, which can reduce opportunities for consumers to trade down to cheaper brands when taxes are increased. Specific excise taxes are also advantageous in that they tax products at the same rate regardless of quantity discounts, encourage production of higher priced products, generate more stable revenues as they are not as subject to industry price manipulation and are relatively easy to administer and are not as susceptible to industry tax avoidance and evasion.
- However, one main disadvantage of a specific excise tax is that it needs to be increased regularly or its value will be eroded by inflation.
- The base to which the tax applies should be comprehensive to include all product types, otherwise substitution to untaxed harmful products will occur reducing the effectiveness of the tax in promoting health and lowering potential tax revenue.

- Tiered tax structures with higher rates based on higher levels of harm associated with products (i.e. ethanol or sugar) can help to reduce consumption of the most harmful products to a greater extent and can also help to encourage reformulation.
- Earmarking of tax revenue can help to garner support for health taxes, augment the health impacts of health taxes and offset potential unintended consequences of health taxes.

References

1. World Health Organization. *WHO Technical Manual on Tobacco Tax Administration.* Geneva: World Health Organization; 2010.
2. Chriqui JF, Chaloupka FJ, Powell LM, Eidson SS. A typology of beverage taxation: multiple approaches for obesity prevention and obesity prevention-related revenue generation. *Journal of Public Health Policy.* 2013; 34(3): 403–423.
3. Powell LM, Leider J, Leger PT. The impact of the Cook County, IL, Sweetened Beverage Tax on beverage prices. *Economics & Human Biology.* 2020; 37: 100855.
4. World Health Organization. *WHO Report on the Global Tobacco Epidemic, 2017: Monitoring Tobacco Use and Prevention Policies*; Appendix IX. Geneva: World Health Organization; 2017. https://www.who.int/publications/i/item/9789241512824.
5. Chaloupka FJ, Kostova D, Shang C. Cigarette excise tax structure and cigarette prices: evidence from the Global Adult Tobacco Survey and the US National Adult Tobacco Survey. *Nicotine & Tobacco Research.* 2014; 16(S1): S3–S9.
6. Shang C, Chaloupka FJ, Fong GT, Thompson M. The association between tax structure and cigarette price variability: Findings from the ITC project. *Tobacco Control.* 2015; 24: iii88–iii93.
7. Shang C, Lee HM, Chaloupka FJ, Fong GT. Association between tax structure and cigarette consumption: findings from the International Tobacco Control Policy Evaluation (ITC) Project. *Tobacco Control.* 2019; 28(S1): s31–s36.
8. Shang C, Wang X, Chaloupka FJ. The association between excise tax structures and the price variability of alcoholic beverages in the United States. *PLoS One.* 2018; 13(12): e0208509.
9. World Health Organization. *Report on the Global Tobacco Epidemic: Appendix I.* Geneva: World Health Organization; 2019.
10. Chaloupka FJ, Powell LM. *Health Taxes to Save Lives – Background Materials: Case Studies.* New York: Bloomberg Philanthropies Task Force on Fiscal Policy for Health; 2019.
11. Sornpaisarn B, Shield KD, Österberg E, Rehm J. *Resource Tool on Alcohol Taxation and Pricing Policies.* Geneva. World Health Organization; 2017.

12. Blecher E. Taxes on tobacco, alcohol, and sugar sweetened beverages: Linkages and lessons learned. *Social Science & Medicine.* 2015; 136–137: 175–179.
13. Chaloupka FJ, Sweanor D, Warner KE. Differential taxes for differential risks – Toward reduced harm from nicotine yielding products. *New England Journal of Medicine.* 2015; 373(7): 594–597.
14. Public Health England. *Sugar Reduction and Wider Reformulation Programme: Report on Progress towards the First 5% Reduction and Next Steps.* London, England: Public Health England; 2018.
15. Bandy LK, Scarborough P, Harrington RA, Rayner M, Jebb SA. Reductions in sugar sales from soft drinks in the UK from 2015 to 2018. *BMC Medicine.* 2020; 18: 20.
16. Powell LM, Andreyeva T, Isgor Z. Distribution of sugar-sweetened beverage sales volume by sugar content in the United States: Implications for tiered taxation and tax revenue. *Journal of Public Health Policy.* 2020; 41(2): 125–138.
17. Jensen JD, Smed S. The Danish tax on saturated fat – short run effects on consumption, substitution patterns and consumer prices of fats. *Food Policy.* 2013; 42: 18–31.
18. World Health Organization. Fiscal policies for diet and prevention of noncommunicable diseases: Technical meeting report, 5–6 May 2015, Geneva, Switzerland; 2016.
19. Jha P, Chaloupka FJ. *Curbing the Epidemic: Governments and the Economics of Tobacco Control.* Washington DC: The World Bank; 1999.
20. World Health Organization. WHO technical manual on tobacco tax administration. Rep., WHO, Geneva; 2010. https://apps.who.int/iris/bitstream/handle/10665/44316/9789241563994_eng.pdf;sequence=1.
21. World Health Organization. *Fiscal Policies for Diet and Prevention of Noncommunicable Diseases.* Geneva, CH: World Health Organization; 2016.
22. World Bank. *Tobacco Tax Reform at the Crossroads of Health and Development – A Multisectoral Perspective.* Washington, DC: The World Bank; 2017.
23. World Health Organization. *WHO Report on the Global Tobacco Epidemic, 2019: Offer Help to Quit Tobacco Use.* Geneva: World Health Organization; 2019.
24. World Health Organization. *Global Information System on Alcohol and Health.* Geneva: World Health Organization; 2018. http://www.who.int/gho/alcohol/en/.
25. World Bank. *Taxes on Sugar-Sweetened Beverages: Summary of International Evidence and Experiences.* Washington, DC: World Bank; 2020.
26. University of North Carolina Global Food Research Programme. Sugary drink taxes around the world. 2019. Available online at: https://www.globalfoodresearchprogram.org/wp-content/uploads/2021/04/SSB_sugary_drink_taxes_maps.pdf.
27. Roberto CA, Lawman HG, LeVasseur MT, Mitra N, Peterhans A, Herring B, Bleich SN. Association of a beverage tax on sugar-sweetened and artificially sweetened beverages with changes in beverage prices and sales at chain retailers in a large urban setting. *Journal of the American Medical Association.* 2019; 321(18): 1799–1810.
28. Powell LM, Leider J. The impact of Seattle's sweetened beverage tax on beverage prices and volume sold. *Economics & Human Biology.* 2020; 37: 100856.

29. World Health Organization. Public Health Product Tax in Hungary: An example of successful intersectoral action using a fiscal tool to promote healthier food choices and raise revenues for public health. WHO Regional Office for Europe; 2015. Available at: https://www.euro.who.int/en/health-topics/Health-systems/health-systems-response-to-ncds/publications/2015/public-health-product-tax-in-hungary-an-example-of-successful-intersectoral-action-using-a-fiscal-tool-to-promote-healthier-food-choices-and-raise-revenues-for-public-health-2015.
30. Batis C, Rivera JA, Popkin BM, Taillie LS. First-year evaluation of Mexico's tax on nonessential energy-dense foods: An observational study. *PLoS Med.* 2016; 13: e1002057.
31. UCONN Rudd Center for Food Policy & Obesity. Revenue Calculator for Sugary Drink Taxes. 2020. Available at: https://uconnruddcenter.org/tax-calculator/.
32. Secretaría De Hacienda Y Créddito Públicao (SHCP). Quarterly reports on the economic situation, public finances and public debt from the 2014–2016 period. Mexico City: SHCP. Cited in: The Nutritional Health Alliance Fact Sheet Uncapping the Truth: The Mexican Sugar Sweetened Beverage Tax Works. 2016. Available at: https://apps.who.int/iris/bitstream/handle/10665/44316/9789241563994_eng.pdf;sequence=1.
33. World Health Organization. *WHO Report on the Global Tobacco Epidemic, 2015: Raising Taxes on Tobacco Products.* Geneva: World Health Organization; 2015.
34. Yürekli A, Önder Z, Elibol M, Erk N, Cabuk A, Fisunoglu M, Erk SF, Chaloupka FJ. *The Economics of Tobacco and Tobacco Taxation In Turkey.* Paris: International Union Against Tuberculosis and Lung Disease; 2010.

https://doi.org/10.1142/9781800612396_0010

Special Focus 2

Health Taxes and Illicit Trade: Evidence and Courses of Action

Norman Maldonado-Vargas*

Well-designed health taxes increase the price of the taxed good, leading to important price differentials with other countries, and potentially creating incentives to exploit arbitrage of price differences through illicit trade.[a] This section reviews the discussion on health taxes and illicit trade, in order to give technicians and policymakers guidance on the available evidence on magnitude, effects, causes and possible courses of action to deal with the problem while simultaneously moving forward on health taxes. The section does not intend to be a systematic literature review about health taxes and illicit trade; instead, it focuses on the most robust evidence on this area, and the references cited provide a rich set of additional information for the reader to deepen the discussion in much further detail. The section focuses on illicit trade of tobacco and alcohol, because there is no evidence on illicit trade on sugar-sweetened beverages (SSBs).[2] Finally, as a word of caveat,

* PROESA, Universidad Icesi, Colombia.

[a] Illicit trade is defined by The Framework Convention on Tobacco Control – FCTC as 'any practice or conduct prohibited by law and which relates to production, shipment, receipt, possession, distribution, sale or purchase, including any practice or conduct intended to facilitate such activity.'[1]

the evidence and policies on tobacco control are more robust than those on alcohol and that is also the case on illicit trade.

Independence from industry and lack of conflict of interest is the starting point of the discussion of illicit trade because industries subject to health taxes might play an important role in illicit trade itself and in the design of policies to counter illicit trade. Estimates that involve directly or indirectly the industry systematically exaggerate the magnitude of the problem; in contrast, independent evidence (i.e., with no conflict of interest) provides unbiased estimates and, in general, it is significantly more reliable because it meets standards of academic research. Clearly identifying independent and non-independent studies is crucial because each one leads to a completely different story on causes, effects, and actions, although only independent studies are able to rigorously support their claims and findings.

SF 2.1. Magnitude of illicit trade

Illicit trade is by definition an economic activity that does not comply with national laws and therefore is missing in official records. Even though this represents an important challenge for estimating its magnitude, there are several methodologies for estimation of tobacco illicit trade that, when applied under scientific standards, can provide reliable estimates of such magnitude[3,4]; these methodologies can also be adapted and extended to estimate alcohol illicit trade.

Worldwide tobacco illicit trade by independent evidence was estimated at 11.6% for 2007, with wide variations across countries,[5,38] and the estimates are even lower (3.4% for 1999) when discrepancies on trade data are taken into account,[6] and over time, illicit trade seems to be a stable share in a shrinking market.[43] To our knowledge, more recent independent estimates at the global level are not available because there is no regular monitoring. However, recent independent estimates at the country level are available, and the ones with good quality can be identified by their adherence to a set of 11 criteria for good quality (Ref.[4], Table 3). Some independent technical reports on tobacco control[7,8] have compiled much of this country-level evidence as part of their analysis, and together with the recently launched e-library on tobacco taxation and illicit trade[b] can be used as one-stop source for policymakers and researchers on independent and reliable evidence.

Estimates of illicit trade directly or indirectly developed by the tobacco industry have low or none adherence to the quality criteria, making them unreliable for use in public policy. For instance, in Colombia in 2017, the tobacco industry estimated the proportion of illicit cigarettes at 18%,[9] while independent estimation was only 6.4%.[10] Worldwide, it has been shown in the scientific literature that industry-funded studies systematically overestimate the magnitude of the problem,[11,12] and such overestimation of illicit trade is part of the narrative to undermine progress on tobacco taxes[13] and, more broadly, part of its global strategy.[14]

Compared to tobacco, regulation on the alcohol industry has been less stringent[15]; that fact, combined with the wider diversity of products and production processes in the alcohol industry, makes it more difficult to define and estimate illicit trade of alcohol. A more general concept is unrecorded alcohol, which includes five categories, one of them being illegal production and smuggling on a commercial (industrial) scale.[16] Global independent estimates of unrecorded alcohol are around 30% of the market, with more recent estimates by WHO around 25%.[17] Out of the five categories, 'relatively little is known about the smuggling of alcohol [and] available data . . . point to a sizable problem.'[18] As opposed to independent evidence, industry estimates claim illicit trade of alcohol to be higher (25.8% only for illicit trade)[19] and misleadingly present excise taxes as one of the main determinants of it.

SF 2.2. Effects of illicit trade

The main effect of illicit trade of tobacco and alcohol products is the increased access (e.g. informal distribution channels or sales to minors) and affordability (cheaper products) for consumers,[1] undermining the

[b] https://untobaccocontrol.org/taxation/e-library/.

reduction in consumption targeted by health taxes. From there, a second-level effect is the loss of tax revenues from all the products getting to final consumers without paying taxes. In a third level, getting illicit products to the marketplace requires illicit and informal parts of the supply chain to be working, and to do so they exert of specific skills and the use of power through violent and nonviolent mechanisms.[20] In addition, illicit trade funds some criminal activities and it is a way to hide the illegal origin of their income.[7,21] Thus, the gains of illicit trade mainly go to producers of those products (whether legal corporations or illegal manufacturers) and to actors involved in the supply chain of these products; meanwhile, the losses concentrate primarily in people's health and, in second place, in governments' revenue.

The story presented in studies supported by the industry[19,22–25] suggests that (i) given the high magnitude of illicit trade, there are supposedly colossal amounts of lost tax revenues for governments worldwide, and increases in health taxes will only make the problem of illicit trade and the losses of tax revenues much worse; (ii) the industry is dubiously depicted as a victim of the illicit trade problem and, (iii) given its knowledge about the market, it should be considered a key stakeholder in policy design and implementation. A corollary of this narrative is that health taxes should be low and actions to counter illicit trade should involve public–private partnerships.

In contrast, independent evidence[7,16] tells a different, more real, scientific and complex story. First, even though health taxes might have an effect on illicit trade, tax revenues rarely decrease, even in countries where illicit trade is high.[26] Second, there is a historical involvement of the tobacco industry in illicit trade as well as ongoing complicity.[14,21] Thus, scientific evidence points toward (i) the industry having vested interests in the illicit trade activity rather than being its victim and (ii) a negligible risk of permanent reduction in net tax revenues due to illicit trade.

There is no doubt of the increased access and affordability of alcohol and tobacco products caused by illicit trade and the negative effects it has on society's welfare, which make a strong case for public policy intervention.[27] For the particular case of tobacco, elimination of illicit trade worldwide is estimated to avoid millions of deaths and to recover 47.4 billion dollars of tax revenue per year.[38] Effective public policies are the ones that tackle the underlying causes of illicit trade. Those causes are summarised in the next section.

SF 2.3. Causes of illicit trade

Illicit trade of tobacco and alcohol products is a complex, multicausal phenomenon. Causes of illicit trade of these products cover a wide spectrum, with prices, governance and industry's behaviour ranking at the top of the list.

Regarding prices, excise taxation and the subsequent effect it has on increasing prices are continuously mentioned by the industry as the main driver of illicit trade.[19,23] However, there is independent and robust evidence worldwide showing that health taxes and prices play a negligible positive role on illicit trade[7,28]; in fact, independent evidence shows weak negative relationship between prices and illicit trade.[29]

With respect to governance, it includes a diverse set of causes, mainly corruption,[30] weak tax and customs enforcement agencies,[31] small penalties and insufficient capacity of judiciary systems,[16,32] the existence of informal distribution[33] and of organised crime networks,[34] and having borders with countries suffering from similar problems.[7]

The relative importance of these two causes is documented in independent studies. Cross-country data show that high-income countries with high taxes usually have a low percentage of smuggled cigarettes, and the opposite occurs in low- and middle-income countries. This stylised fact suggests 'that it is the quality of tax administration (and to some extent geographic factors) that is the prime determinant of high levels of illicit trade, not high taxes'.[31]

A third cause of illicit trade is the industry's behaviour. In general, the tobacco industry acts as a vector of the smoking epidemic,[35] and there is evidence showing that despite the differences with tobacco, the alcohol industry behaves also as a vector in terms of market and political strategy.[15] For the particular case of illicit trade, the industry plays three roles: (i) passive role by 'turning a blind eye to the fact that their cigarettes are being funneled into illicit channels, typically through small countries with no significant domestic cigarette market,'[21] (ii) an active role with 'historical involvement in cigarette smuggling [and] ongoing complicity,'[14] and (iii) a role of interference in regulation by campaigning against effective strategies and for ineffective strategies, including regulations in illicit trade.[36,37]

In fact, causes of illicit trade related to governance are also recognised in studies funded by the industry; however, one of the critical differences with independent evidence is that in industry-funded studies the industry portraits itself as an injured party and completely omits its passive and active role on illicit trade activities. Furthermore, independent evidence has also shown that the argument of high taxes and prices as the main drivers of illicit trade is actually part of the industry's strategy to keep products cheap.[14]

SF 2.4. What to do?

Control of the illicit market of harmful products such as tobacco and alcohol is needed to maximise the effect of health taxes on public health and development; effective control generates additional gains on premature deaths and tax revenues.[5,38] Based on the current state of regulation in illicit trade of tobacco and alcohol, as well as on the experiences from multiple countries and regions around the world,[7] three takeaways on illicit trade are relevant for this book.

Move forward on effective policies dealing with illicit trade

Move forward on effective policies dealing with illicit trade. A good starting point for moving forward is to gain an adequate understanding of the complexity of illicit trade, using reliable (scientific) evidence free of conflict of interest, many of them cited along this chapter.[3,4,7,17,39,40]

From there, the next step is to adopt and accurately implement the most effective policies for dealing with illicit trade on tobacco and alcohol. For illicit trade in tobacco, the Framework Convention on Tobacco Control—FCTC,[41] and specifically the Protocol to Eliminate Illicit Trade in Tobacco Products[1] contain the set of effective interventions to control illicit trade (Ref.[42] presents an overview of those interventions).[43] One of the structural elements of the protocol is that it projects a pathway toward supranational governance mechanisms that encourage a better response to transboundary crime.

Regarding alcohol, it has a weaker regulation compared to tobacco[15] and currently it does not have a framework convention. However, 'The other provisions concerning international trade in the FCTC in support of this principle, including provisions on product markings, tracking and tracing regimes, and exchange of information, are also appropriate for alcoholic beverages,'[44] and 'alcohol policymakers may look to tobacco control, and the range of policy measures implemented in this area, as a source of effective and justifiable regulatory approaches (e.g. on pricing, promotion, and availability).'[15] In fact, there is a recent discussion on the contents to be included in a framework convention on alcohol control as well as a draft convention,[45] developed to meet the need of progress in global governance of alcohol.[46]

Protect health taxes and implementation of policies to control illicit trade from industry interference

Again, a good starting point is to have a good grasp of industry's behaviour from independent evidence because, as transnational companies working in oligopolic markets, the set of strategies they have and the decisions they make go well beyond what is publicly perceived. For that, Ref.[14] has a comprehensive review of industry's strategies and Ref.[36] presents a review for the particular case of illicit trade.

After that, the next step is implementation of article 5.3 of the FCTC,[41] and adherence to articles 4.2, 8.12, and 8.13 of the Protocol.[1] Such implementation has been a challenge worldwide[47] because the industry has made multiple efforts to interfere with the development and approval of the Protocol[36] as well as with an accurate implementation.[48–50] A set of practical steps and a framework for action present in Ref.[51] can help to progress in such implementation. In general, the challenge is to take action on the commercial determinants of health[52,53] by denormalising industry interference in public policies when there is conflict of interest. One particular case is the one on autoregulation and voluntary agreements, which has proven to be 'underinterpreted, underenforced, and unstable.'[37]

Keep progress on health taxes on the policy agenda while acting effectively on illicit trade

At the end, the best solution for illicit trade is to significantly reduce consumption, and health taxes are one of the most effective policies to do so. Therefore, an accurate strategy is to gain significant progress on the implementation of effective measures to eliminate illicit trade and, at the same time, keep progress on health taxes as the focus of the health and development policy. Such focus can even allow to use part of the collected revenues from health taxes to strenghten the institutions needed for correct implementation of those measures.

References

1. WHO. *WHO Protocol to Eliminate Illicit Trade in Tobacco Products*. Tech. rep. Geneva: World Health Organization (WHO), 2013.
2. Hattersley Libby, et al. *Countering Common Arguments Against Taxes on Sugary Drinks*. Tech. rep. Knowledge Brief. Health, Nutrition and Population Global Practice. Washington, DC: World Bank Group, 2020.
3. Merriman D, Yurekli A, Beyer J de. Economics of tobacco toolkit, tool 7: understand, measure, and combat tobacco smuggling. In: *Economics of Tobacco Toolkit*. Washington, DC: The World Bank, 2013.
4. Ross H. *Understanding and Measuring Cigarette Tax Avoidance and Tax Evasion. A Methodological Guide*. Tech. rep. Prepared for the Economics of Tobacco Control Project, School of Economics, University of Cape Town, Tobacconomics, Health

Policy Center, Institute for Health Research, and Policy, University of Illinois at Chicago, Chicago, IL, 2015.

5. Joossens L, et al. The impact of eliminating the global illicit cigarette trade on health and revenue. *Addiction* 2010; 105(9): 1640–1649. DOI: 10.1111/j.1360-0443.2010.03018.x.
6. Yürekli A, Sayginsoy Ö. Worldwide organized cigarette smuggling: an empirical analysis. *Applied Economics* 2010; 42(5): 545–561. DOI: 10.1080/00036840701720721.
7. World Bank. *Confronting Illicit Tobacco Trade: A Global Review of Country Experiences.* In: Dutta S (ed). Washington, DC: The World Bank, 2019.
8. Stoklosa M, Paraje G, Blecher E. *A Toolkit on Measuring Illicit Trade in Tobacco Products. A Tobacconomics and American Cancer Society Toolkit.* Tech. rep. Tobacconomics, Health Policy Center, Institute for Health Research and Policy, University of Illinois at Chicago, Chicago, Illinois, 2020.
9. INVAMER and ANDI. *Incidencia de cigarrillos ilegales en Colombia 2017.* Tech. rep. Investigación y Asesoría de Mercado (INVAMER), Asociación Nacional de Empresarios de Colombia (ANDI), 2017.
10. Maldonado N, et al. Smoke signals: monitoring illicit cigarettes and smoking behaviour in Colombia to support tobacco taxes. *Tobacco Control* 2020 (29): s243–s248. DOI: 10.1136/tobaccocontrol-2018-054820.
11. Gallagher AWA, et al. Tobacco industry data on illicit tobacco trade: a systematic review of existing assessments. *Tobacco Control* 2019; 28(3): 334 LP–345. DOI: 10.1136/tobaccocontrol-2018-054295.
12. Blecher E, et al. Euromonitor data on the illicit trade in cigarettes. *Tobacco Control* 2015; 24(1): 100 LP–101. DOI: 10.1136/tobaccocontrol-2013-051034.
13. Smith KE, Savell E, Gilmore AB. What is known about tobacco industry efforts to influence tobacco tax? A systematic review of empirical studies. *Tobacco Control* 2013; 22.2: e1 LP–e1. DOI: 10.1136/tobaccocontrol-2011-050098.
14. Gilmore AB, et al. Exposing and addressing tobacco industry conduct in low-income and middle-income countries. *Lancet* 2015; 385(9972): 1029–1043. DOI: 10.1016/S0140-6736(15)60312-9.
15. Hawkins B, et al. Reassessing policy paradigms: a comparison of the global tobacco and alcohol industries. *Global Public Health* 2018; 13(1): 1–19. DOI: 10.1080/17441692.2016.1161815.
16. Sornpaisarn B, et al., eds. *Resource Tool on Alcohol Taxation and Pricing Policies.* Geneva: World Health Organization (WHO); 2017. ISBN: 978-92-4-151270-1.
17. WHO. *Global Status Report on Alcohol and Health 2018.* Geneva: World Health Organization (WHO); 2018. ISBN: 978-92-4-156563-9.
18. Rehm J, et al. A systematic review of the epidemiology of unrecorded alcohol consumption and the chemical composition of unrecorded alcohol. *Addiction* 2014; 109(6): 880–893. DOI: https://doi.org/10.1111/add.12498.
19. Euromonitor International. *Size and Shape of the Global Illicit Alcohol Market.* Tech. rep. 2018. https://go.euromonitor.com/white-paper-alcoholic-drinks-2018-size-and-shape-of-the-global-illicit-alcohol-market.html.

20. Beltrán I de L, Salcedo-Albarán E *El crimen como oficio: ensayos sobre economía del crimen en Colombia.* 2nd edn. Bogota: Universidad Externado de Colombia; 2014: 396. ISBN: 9789587622263.
21. Lampe K von. The illegal cigarette trade. In: Natarajan M (ed) *International Crime and Justice.* Cambridge: Cambridge University Press, 2011. Chap. 19, pp. 148–154. ISBN: 9780521196192. DOI: 10.1017/CBO9780511762116.025.
22. Melzer S, Martin C. A brief overview of illicit trade in tobacco products. In: *OECD Reviews of Risk Management Policies. Illicit Trade: Converging Criminal Networks. Organisation for Economic Co-operation and Development (OECD),* 2016. Chap. 5, pp. 123–178. DOI: 10.1787/9789264251847-en.
23. Euromonitor International. *Illicit Trade in Tobacco Products.* Tech. rep. Strategy Briefing, 2018. https://www.euromonitor.com/illicit-trade-in-tobacco-products/report.
24. Skehan P, Sanchez I, Hastings L. The size, impacts and drivers of illicit trade in alcohol. In: *OECD Reviews of Risk Management Policies. Illicit Trade: Converging Criminal Networks. OECD,* 2016. Chap. 7. ISBN: 978-92-64-25184-7. https://www.oecd-ilibrary.org/governance/charting-illicit-trade_9789264251847-en.
25. Comolli V, ed. *Organized Crime and Illicit Trade. How to Respond to This Strategic Challenge in Old and New Domains.* Cham: Palgrave Macmillan, 2018. ISBN: 978-3-319-72968-8. DOI: 10.1007/978-3-319-72968-8.
26. Iglesias RM. Increasing excise taxes in the presence of an illegal cigarette market: the 2011 Brazil tobacco tax reform. *Pan American Journal of Public Health* 2016; 40(4): 243–249.
27. Sassi F, et al. Health and economic impacts of key alcohol policy options. In: Sassi (ed) *Tackling Harmful Alcohol Use. Economics and Public Health Policy.* Franco. OECD, 2015. Chap. 5. ISBN: 978-92-64-18106-9. DOI: 10.1787/9789264181069-en.
28. Fanta E, Garcia M. Preventing and controlling illicit tobacco flows. In: Marquez P, Moreno-Dodson B (eds) *Tobacco Tax Reform at the Crossroads of Health and Development: A Multisectoral Perspective.* The World Bank, 2017. Chap. 9, pp.197–216.
29. NCI and WHO. Tobacco tax avoidance and tax evasion. In: *The Economics of Tobacco and Tobacco Control.* Bethesda; Geneva: U.S. Department of Health, Human Services, National Institutes of Health, National Cancer Institute (NCI), and World Health Organization (WHO), 2016. Chap. 14, pp. 503–542.
30. Shelley LI. Corruption & illicit trade. *Daedalus* 2018; 147(3): 127–143. DOI: 10.1162/daed_a_00506.
31. Yurekli AA. *Economics of Tobacco Taxation Toolkit.* Tech. rep. Washington, DC: World Bank Group, 2018.
32. WHO. *WHO Technical Manual on Tobacco Tax Administration. Tech. rep.* Geneva: World Health Organization (WHO), 2011.
33. Walls H, et al. Advancing alcohol research in low-income and middle-income countries: a global alcohol environment framework. *BMJ Global Health* 2020; 5(4): e001958. DOI: 10.1136/bmjgh-2019-001958.

34. OECD. *Governance Frameworks to Counter Illicit Trade.* Paris: OECD Publishing; 2018. ISBN: 978-92-64-29165-2. DOI: 10.1787/9789264291652-en.
35. Lam T-H, Ho S-Y. Tobacco. In: Detels R, et al. (eds) *Oxford Textbook of Global Public Health.* 6th edn. Oxford: Oxford University Press; 2015. Chap. 9.1. ISBN: 9780199661756. DOI: 10.1093/med/9780199661756.003.0219.
36. Bialous, Stella Aguinaga. *Impact of implementation of the WHO FCTC on the tobacco industry's behaviour.* In: Tobacco Control 28. Suppl 2 (June 2019). s94 LP–s96. DOI. 10.1136/tobaccocontrol-2018-054808.
37. Casswell S, Thamarangsi T. Reducing harm from alcohol: call to action. *The Lancet* 2009; 373(9682): 2247–2257. DOI: 10.1016/S0140-6736(09)60745-5.
38. Goodchild M, et al. Potential impact of eliminating illicit trade in cigarettes: a demand-side perspective. *Tobacco Control 2020: 2020–055980.* DOI: 10.1136/tobaccocontrol-2020-055980.
39. Babor T, et al. *Alcohol: No Ordinary Commodity. Research and Public Policy.* 2nd edn. Washington, DC: Oxford University Press, Pan American Health Organization, 2010. ISBN: 978-0-19-955114-9.
40. WHO. *WHO Report on the Global Tobacco Epidemic, 2019: Offer Help to Quit Tobacco Use.* World Health Organization (WHO); 2019. ISBN: 978-92-4-151620-4.
41. WHO. *WHO Framework Convention on Tobacco Control.* Tech. rep. Washington, DC: World Health Organization (WHO); 2004.
42. WHO FCTC. *The Protocol to Eliminate Illicit Trade in Tobacco Products: An Overview.* Tech. rep. World Health Organization Framework Convention on Tobacco Control (WHO FCTC); 2018.
43. Paraje G, Stoklosa M, Blecher E. "Illicit trade in tobacco products: Recent trends and coming challenges". In: Tobacco Control 31.2 (2022), pp. 257–262. DOI: 10.1136/tobaccocontrol-2021-056557.
44. Room R. International control of alcohol: alternative paths forward. *Drug and Alcohol Review* 2006; 25(6): 581–595. DOI: https://doi.org/10.1080/09595230600944503.
45. Room R, Cisneros Örnberg J. A framework convention on alcohol control: getting concrete about its contents. *European Journal of Risk Regulation* 2020: 12(2): 433–443. DOI: 10.1017/err.2020.73.
46. Room R, Gleeson D, Miller M. Alcoholic beverages in trade agreements: industry lobbying and the public health interest. *Drug and Alcohol Review* 2021; 40(1): 19–21. DOI: 10.1111/dar.13214.
47. Malone RE, Bialous Stella A. WHO FCTC article 5.3: promise but little progress. *Tobacco Control* 2014; 23(4): 279 LP–280. DOI: 10.1136/tobaccocontrol-2014-051817.
48. Gilmore Anna B, et al. Towards a greater understanding of the illicit tobacco trade in Europe: a review of the PMI funded 'Project Star' report. *Tobacco Control* 2014 (23): e51–e61. DOI: 10.1136/tobaccocontrol-2013-051240.
49. Gilmore AB, Gallagher AWA, Rowell A. Tobacco industry's elaborate attempts to control a global track and trace system and fundamentally undermine the Illicit

Trade Protocol. *Tobacco Control* 2019; 28(21)27 LP–140. DOI: 10.1136/tobaccoco ntrol-2017-054191.

50. Crosbie E, Bialous S, Glantz SA. Memoranda of understanding: a tobacco industry strategy to undermine illicit tobacco trade policies. *Tobacco Control* 2019; 28(e2): e110 LP–e118. DOI: 10.1136/tobaccocontrol-2018-054668.
51. WHO. *Technical Resource for Country Implementation of WHO Framework Convention on Tobacco Control Article 5.3 on the Protection of Public Health Policies with Respect to Tobacco Control from Commercial and Other Vested Interests of the Tobacco Industry.* World Health Organization (WHO); 2012. ISBN: 978 92 4 1503730.
52. Kickbusch I, Allen L, Franz C. The commercial determinants of health. *The Lancet Global Health* 2016; 4(12): e895–896. DOI: 10.1016/S2214-109X(16)30217-0.
53. Wood B, Baker P, Gary S. Conceptualising the commercial determinants of health using a power lens: a review and synthesis of existing frameworks. *International Journal of Health Policy and Management* 2021; 10. DOI: 10.34172/ijhpm.2021.05.

https://doi.org/10.1142/9781800612396_0011

Chapter 9

Public Governance and Financing, and Earmarking Health Taxes

Ceren Ozer* **and Susan P Sparkes**†

We examine the nature and impact of health taxes within the broader context of public financing systems, including considerations around earmarking of health tax revenue. As health taxes are part of larger tax systems, policies and administrations, the design and implementation of these taxes should be analysed within the context of countries' overall tax, budgeting and governance systems. Part of these public financing issues include how the revenue from health taxes is ultimately allocated and used. As of 2017, at least 80 countries earmarked a specific source of revenues for health. While many of these country examples involve earmarking payroll or income taxes to fund healthcare, they also represent at least 54 countries that earmark all or a portion of tobacco, alcohol, or sugar-sweetened beverage (SSB) taxation for the health sector. Despite their prevalence, significant care must be exercised when considering earmarks due to clear concerns around fungibility with other sources of revenue for the sector and potential rigidities and inefficiencies that can be introduced. The specificities of earmarking

* World Bank, USA.

† World Health Organization, Switzerland.

vary greatly in practice and range from a spectrum of soft to hard. From a political economy perspective, soft earmarking has been shown to help to advance the adoption of new health taxes in some settings as having a notional revenue-expenditure link can boost public support. In general, the closer the practice is to standard budget process, where revenues are matched with political priorities and population needs, the more effective it is.

9.1. Introduction

Health taxes are part of the broader fiscal framework both in terms of the revenues they generate and the expenditures they support. Therefore, this tax mechanism needs to be analysed as part of this broader framing. Clearly establishing the specificities of the tax mechanism, both in terms of the tax itself and calibrating it for impact on health-related objectives is critical. However, the adoption and implementation of the instrument itself must run through government systems and institutions that are tasked with setting policy priorities, collecting and administering taxes and budgeting and allocating resources. The role of these larger system issues becomes even more relevant when there are considerations around earmarking health tax revenues for a particular purpose or institution (e.g. tobacco tax revenues dedicated to fund anti-smoking prevention activities). In this case, the health tax revenues have to interact with broader budgeting processes to ensure the earmark is both feasible and also additional in terms of the revenues it generates. This chapter specifically takes this broader frame to health taxes and considers the key institutional, public financial management (PFM) and health financing factors that can influence policy objectives. In doing so, it delineates those issues that cut across all tax instruments and can be applied to health taxes and those that are specific to health taxes themselves. Importantly, the majority of the issues are not necessarily unique to health taxes, but are critical to consider when looking to introduce or change a health tax.

9.2. General governance aspects of taxation: Strengthening institutions

9.2.1. Taxation and achieving SDGs are closely linked through four pathways

Taxation is critical for countries to be able to meet policy objectives and obligations to citizens. Taxes are clearly critical to fund government services, including health, education and infrastructure, among others, as well as to facilitate inclusive economic growth, reduce poverty and address rising debt levels and other macro-fiscal challenges.[1] However, for many developing countries tax revenue collections remain persistently below 15% of GDP level that has been found to be critical to meet the most pressing developmental needs. It is estimated that several trillions of dollars are needed to invest across all sectors to meet the sustainable development goals (SDGs).[2,3]

As important as taxes are in determining a government's ability to generate funding for government services, revenue generation is not the only reason why taxation matters for achieving the SDGs. The connection between the two can be categorised under four broad pathways[4]:

- Taxes generate the funds that governments use to finance activities in support of the SDGs;
- Taxation affects equity and economic growth;
- Taxes influence people's behaviour and choices, with implications for health and human development outcomes, gender equity and the environment and
- Fair and equitable taxation promotes taxpayer trust in government and strengthens social contracts that underpin development.

These pathways can be applied to how we understand health taxes as well. In terms of revenue generation, countries which instituted or increased health taxes – particularly for tobacco excise tax – revenue gains have in some contexts been non-trivial: for example, in large middle-income countries with high prevalence rates, the tobacco excise revenue can be close to 1% of GDP (e.g. 1.4% of GDP in Turkey and 1% of GDP in Egypt). However, as shown in Chapter 2 of this volume, health tax revenues account for less than 1% of GDP in all income groups in the sample of OECD countries – 0.4% for low-income countries; and 0.8% each for middle- and high-income countries.[a] In looking at these funds in relation to health spending, from purely a magnitude perspective, the authors find that on average, health tax revenues are equivalent to 25% of domestic government health expenditure in low-income countries, 31% in lower-middle-income countries, 23% in upper-middle-income countries and 16% in high-income countries. These relatively high averages reflect the relatively low prioritisation of health within overall government budgets and not necessarily the large magnitude of health tax revenue.[5,6]

In the case of SSB taxes, some early implementers show consistent revenue gains following the implementation of these taxes. In Mexico, for instance, the SSB tax revenue averaged around 0.1% of GDP annually since it was introduced in 2014. Second, these taxes can contribute to overall inclusive growth, equity and welfare. World Bank research shows that these taxes are progressive when second-order effects (reduced medical expenditures and additional years of productive life) are considered.[b] Third, as discussed throughout this book, health taxes present a clear-cut way to

[a] It should be noted that, the sample used for this analysis is not fully complete, especially limited number of low-income countries have this data available – one of key global public good contribution to this field would be to ensure comprehensive database of health tax revenue data by country and product type; and, there is variation by country experiences in terms of health tax revenue to GDP even within country income groups. Take for example, countries in East Asia with high prevalence of tobacco consumption such as Indonesia, where over 95% of excise tax revenues are earned from tobacco products, tobacco excise tax revenue remained stable at just about over 1% of GDP.

[b] See World Bank research utilising country level household survey data analysis on Distributional and Poverty Effect of Tobacco Taxation: Bangladesh, Bosnia and Herzego vina, Chile, Georgia, Indonesia, Moldova, Russia, South Africa, Ukraine, Uzbekistan and Vietnam (Distributional Effects of Tobacco Taxation: A Comparative Analysis) and on the Distributional and Poverty Effect of Sugar Sweetened Beverage Taxation: Kazakhstan.

directly reduce the consumption of products that are detrimental to health by incentivising behaviour change.[c] Fourth, the discussions around earmarking health tax revenue have implications for the social contract with citizens. While this is by no means a straightforward issue and we cover it in detail later in this chapter, there is political value in taxpayers seeing their money going to *some worthwhile use*.

9.2.2. Revenue imperative of the state: How do health taxes fit in?

Health taxes – excise taxes levied on tobacco, alcohol and sugary beverages – serve both health and revenue goals. Chapter 8 discussed in detail the tax design considerations for maximising the effectiveness of health taxes in meeting the goal of reducing consumption of the targeted unhealthy products.

Chapter 2 of this book explained in detail why health taxes need to be embedded within the design and functioning of the broader tax system (as opposed to considering them in isolation); and, how to apply general principles of efficiency; equity; administrative simplicity, transparency and tax certainty; revenue-raising potential; and, consideration of non-tax system factors to health taxes. Country authorities have well-tested tools and approaches at their disposal to adopt this more holistic tax system perspective. One example is Medium-Term Revenue Strategy (MTRS), which is a sustained process of implementation of this tax system reform over time and provides a framework to consider health taxes within a broader and more medium-term perspective of the tax system reform.[d]

---

[c] See Chapter 3 of this book; Allcott H, Lockwood B, Taubinsky D. Should we tax sugar-sweetened beverages? An overview of theory and evidence. *Journal of Economic Perspectives*. 2019; 33(3): 202–227.

[d] Medium-Term Revenue Strategy (MTRS) to tax system reform is a concept put forward by the Platform for Collaboration on Tax (PCT) – a partnership of the IMF, OECD, UN and WBG – designed to support country-led tax reform efforts.

Box 9.1. Medium-Term Revenue Strategy (MTRS)

Currently, 23 countries are at different stages of MTRS.[7] The MTRS starts from the formulation of a high-level road map of tax system reform in a country – extending over 4–6 years. The core elements of an MTRS include 'a social contract in the country on revenue mobilisation goals, a comprehensive reform plan for the tax system, domestic political commitment for sustained implementation of the reform plan, and secured support for capacity development to support the country in overcoming constraints in developing and implementing the MTRS'.[8]

COVID-19 has placed significant fiscal pressures on all countries. The compounded effect of the sharp economic recession; and, tax policy relief measures adopted to respond to the crisis are expected to lead to substantial revenue losses in the short run. The experience from the aftermath of the 2008 Global Financial Crisis across a wide set of countries shows that tax revenues do not recover as quickly as economic growth does. For this reason, 'countries will have to reassess their medium-term projections of expenditure needs and reorient the tax systems reform in light of revised goals, possibly reprioritising their development goals – including the SDGs for 2030. This context underscores more than ever the salience of the MTRS approach in supporting tax system reform going forward'.[7]

How about tax administration capacity? As a tax scholar remarked 'the best tax policy in the world is worth little if it cannot be implemented effectively'.[9] An effective tax administration is where taxpayers meet their tax obligations, in other words, there's a high level of compliance. Efficiency in tax administration refers to minimising the costs per unit of tax revenue collected, in other words, when a tax is efficiently administered it will use minimal resources in relation to the revenues generated. Administration of excise taxes is integrated in the broader tax system of the country and it needs to take account the existing capabilities and capacities of the authorities who administer this overall system. A well-designed health tax keeps administrative and compliance costs as low as possible. Excise taxes are relatively easier taxes to administer (e.g. than Personal Income Tax, or Corporate Income Tax): they are administered on a relatively fewer products; and the task of administering them is relatively simple when these taxes are imposed on large domestic producers and/or imports. Nevertheless, there are still multiple functions involved in their administration such as control over the distribution chain; licensing of all involved in the manufacture, import, distribution and retail sales of the taxed product; and, the monitoring of the product as it moves through the distribution chain.[10] Tax and customs administration-related challenges of implementing health taxes as well as concrete measures countries can take to address them are covered in detail in Chapters 2, 3, and 9.

9.3. Public financing aspects of health taxes: Key considerations to push into the results chain

9.3.1. Efficient expenditure practice perspective for health

Domestic revenues will have a developmental impact (only) if channelled to productive and beneficial public expenditure, an insight particularly holds true when it comes to public spending on health. Empirical studies provide evidence of this for both in high- and low-income country context. An OECD Report suggested that 20% of all health expenditure in OECD countries was wasted and did not contribute to the desired health outcomes.[11] The 2010 *World Health Report* estimated that between 20% and 40% of all resources spent on health are wasted across countries of all income levels.[12] One recent estimate suggests that countries could save as much through efficiency efforts in health, education and infrastructure as they could raise through tax reform.[2] While much of the focus in health financing is on the revenue side, including potentially from earmarked health taxes, it is critical to also consider the expenditure side of the equation to ensure value for money.

Country authorities need to consider health taxes in the bigger frame of overall good-practice expenditure and revenue management strategies. Aligning central budgeting allocations and sector priorities and goals have been a key development challenge, and this is particularly important to go beyond incremental and line-item annual budgeting process. This is where public financial management (PFM) comes in. PFM is system of processes by which government plans, allocates and implements and accounts for its budget (from medium-term budgeting to preparation of an annual budget to its execution). The key objectives of the PFM system are:

- aggregate fiscal discipline – controlling the total budget to ensure that aggregate levels of revenue and public spending are consistent with targets for the fiscal deficit and do not generate unsustainable levels of public borrowing;
- allocative efficiency – planning and executing the budget in a way that public resources are allocated to agreed strategic priorities to meet development objectives;
- and technical efficiency – use budgeted revenues to achieve maximum value for money in the delivery of services.[e]

When PFM arrangements underpinning health service delivery systems are weak, there are no substitute mechanisms for allocating resources to priorities or for ensuring that funds are used for intended purposes.[13] A consistent finding is that good governance has an important role in health

[e] Campos and Pradhan 1996; Schick 1998; PEFA, Public Financial Management, and Good Governance. November 2019.

service delivery: increased public funding of health programs is likely to be more effective in countries with better governance. While links between good PFM systems and health service delivery are positive, it is harder to provide strong empirical evidence on the impact of PFM systems on health, mainly due to limited number of studies and data limitations – quality of PFM systems data, lack of health outcome data at granular level, etc.[35]

PFM systems are organised in line with the budget cycle – budget planning; budget formulation; budget evaluation.

See Table 9.1 which provides a summary of the relevant PFM cycles, related diagnostic tools and elements that are at authorities' disposal for a given cycle; and health tax specific issues.

Table 9.1. PFM cycle and health taxes.

PFM cycle	Tools or elements of the PFM cycle	Health tax specific issues
Goal development	Development plans; Integrated national financing frameworks	– Health taxes' anticipated impact on consumption, health outcomes, revenue potential, industry and welfare impact
Revenue projection/ mobilisation	– Annual tax revenue forecasts – Medium-term revenue strategies (MTRS) – Tax Policy and Tax Administration diagnostics for excise taxes	– Health-related excise tax revenue forecasting – Tax policy design – Identifying bottlenecks in tax and customs administration capacity
Budget planning	Annual and medium-term policy and strategic planning (including medium-term expenditure framework (MTEFs)	Simulations on impact on the health sector budget, government budget

Source: Draws on Refs.[14,15]; Marshalling the Evidence for Health Governance Thematic Working Group Report 2017; and, PFM in Health Toolkit, 2019, WB.

PFM modernisation efforts, especially relevant in the context of health sector, include improvements via multi-year budgeting and program-based budgeting. For example, program-based budgeting looks to increase both flexibility and accountability in the use of public resources.[f]

Box 9.2. Medium-Term Expenditure Frameworks

Since our focus here is health taxes and how they may connect to health financing, it's important to take a step back and start from how governments make developmental plans, and how health taxes may factor in these processes.

Most countries have a process for generating a multi-dimensional and medium- to long-term development plan and map it to a financing plan. For example, a national financing framework sets out relations between a country's overarching development goals and objectives; main sources of financing available to achieve these objectives; and, policies to mobilise, manage and align these resources with national goals.[16]

While the annual budget is the main instrument of fiscal policy, the Medium-Term Expenditure Frameworks (MTEFs) have been a key tool available to country authorities for medium-term planning. 'LMICs have been working on the development of MTEF for decades. Such reforms seek to move from PFM systems focused on annual spending and resource raising plans, strict input control and procedures to those characterised by results-focus, spending accountability and efficient execution'. An earlier synthesis of nine low- and middle-income case studies found that the introduction

[f] Barroy H, Blecher M, Lakin J, eds. *How to Make Budgets Work for Health? A Practical Guide to Designing, Implementing and Monitoring Programme Budgets in Health*. Geneva: World Health Organization, 2022.

of MTEF – in close relation with poverty-reduction strategies – encouraged higher prioritisation and enhanced country ownership and customisation; and improved outcomes for poor and vulnerable groups by linking them to domestic decision-making processes, particularly in health.[g] Often PFM reforms are highly political and take time to implement. Similarly, WHO (2017) argues that not all countries that adopted a medium-term expenditure framework (MTEF), ended up with better alignment of government policies, plans and budgets either because countries applied MTEF without adequately adapting it to their country context, or because they have overlaid the MTEF on the existing budgeting process without adequately linking the two.

Whether the tool utilised is national development financing plan, annual budgeting, or MTEFs, improving alignment between the PFM system, health financing and health system governance requires ongoing dialogue between health and finance authorities and other entities, such as local governments.[13,14]

The long-established and tested PFM tools can help respond to the complex demands of the health sector, but their implementation requires both capacity and ministerial cooperation. While Ministries of Health should take a more active role in engaging with Ministries of Finance in budget processes as well as in PFM reform-related activities to make sure reforms better respond to sector's needs. Such engagement requires capacity and resources. This notion holds true also when it comes to health taxes and any potential health tax earmarking for health sector.

---

[g] Wilhelm VA, Krause P. *Minding the Gaps: Integrating Poverty Reduction Strategies and Budgets for Domestic Accountability*. Washington, DC: World Bank; 2008. © World Bank. https://openknowledge.worldbank.org/handle/10986/6801 License: CC BY 3.0 IGO.

9.4. Earmarking health taxes and health financing

9.4.1. Background on health financing

Public financing in the form of pre-paid, pooled resources is central to making progress towards universal health coverage (UHC) (SDG Goal 3.8).[6] This includes all pre-paid, pooled resources and in most low- and middle-income countries the primary revenue source will be general tax revenue, which can include health tax revenues. Health financing can be particularly complex due to both potentially fragmented revenue sources, as well as inherent uncertainty in the health needs of populations. For example, as demonstrated by the need for exceptional spending measures, when 2020 budgets were set policymakers did not foresee the need for additional funds for the health system response to COVID-19. Added to this is the need for redistribution built into health financing systems. Efficient and sustainable health financing systems require redistribution from young to old, healthy to sick and rich to poor. Therefore, the revenues that are generated and prioritised for the health sector through the budgeting process are just one input into a well-functioning health financing system. Ultimately, those funds need to reach users through service delivery and other channels and be well-coordinated with priorities across the public sector which also impact on health. Therefore, the relationship between allocation of resources for health and achievement of health outcomes is not a one-to-one relationship, and there are many bottlenecks and capacity constraints moving down the results chain.

9.4.2. Earmarking debate

Discussions around the fiscal implications of health taxes often turn the question of earmarking. While there is a logic to tie revenues from health taxes to the health sector itself, the evidence around this practice is mixed and nuanced. As a result, it is important to understand the overall theoretical and practical experiences with earmarking when considering its connection with health taxes.

Earmarking is a public finance term that refers to the practice of designating specific revenues to finance a particular expenditure purpose and can generally come in two forms.[17] Expenditure earmarking involves mandating a certain proportion of general funds be spent for a specific purpose. An example of this was the United Kingdom's mandate that 0.7% of GNI was to be spent on development assistance.[18] Revenue earmarking involves ring-fencing all or a portion of a tax or other revenue source for a particular purpose. Using lottery ticket sales to fund portions of education spending is an example of a revenue earmark.[19] For purposes of this chapter, and the overall discussion around the fiscal implications of health taxes, the focus is on revenue earmarking.

The concept of directly tying revenues to expenditures on a particular program or service is relatively straightforward and is a common practice by governments around the world. However, earmarking revenues is not a singular concept. Rather, there is potential variability associated with the practice of earmarking with respect to both revenues and related expenditures. This variability in the practical application of earmarking has important implications for the debate on the potential consequences of earmarking revenues for the health sector, regardless of whether the revenue source is health taxes or another form of revenue.

In theory, there are generally two forms of revenue earmarking – soft and hard. Soft earmarking is connected with a broad expenditure purpose and greater flexibility in terms of the revenue–expenditure linkage and allocation mechanisms more broadly. Hard earmarking means that a revenue source can only be used for a particular service or programme and the revenue cannot be allocated to any other purpose. In practice, we see that there is often a continuum of earmarking practices that do not fall neatly into 'soft' or 'hard' but rather have some elements of each type.

Table 9.2 summarises the main arguments for and against earmarking. As demonstrated by the legitimate points on both sides, assessing the impact of earmarking, regardless of revenue source and expenditure purpose, is

Table 9.2. Arguments for and against earmarking.

Arguments for earmarking	Arguments against earmarking
Revenue protection: Earmarking revenues may protect resources for a program or service by ring-fencing them from competing political interests and bypassing budgetary constraints	**Budget rigidity:** Earmarking introduces rigidities into the budgetary process that may lead to an inefficient allocation of resources
Efficiency: More closely linking taxation to benefits may increase the efficiency of public expenditure	**Economic distortion:** Earmarking may also lead to distortions in the overall economy
Public support: More closely linking taxation to benefits may decrease public resistance to taxation	**Pro-cyclicality:** Earmarked revenues will be inherently pro-cyclical and therefore susceptible to booms and busts and reduce government flexibility to manage downturns
Accountability: More closely linking taxation to benefits may increase accountability	**Fragmentation**: Separate revenue sources can lead to undue fragmentation both within the health sector as financing drives delivery systems and can also constraint the ability for the health sector to effectively coordinate with other sectors in achieving objectives
Cost awareness: Earmarking revenues can educate people about the cost of a particular program or service	**Decreased solidarity:** Solidarity in financing public services may decrease by defining each individuals' share of a particular service or sector based on revenues contributed
Flexibility: Earmarking may increase the flexibility in how funds can be used (e.g. for health, avoid restrictions in public budget systems that limit the effectiveness of pooling and purchasing arrangements by keeping these funds off-budget)	**Susceptibility to special interests:** Earmarked revenues may be particularly susceptible to the influence of specific interest groups and professional lobbies that do not necessarily align with intended objectives

Source: Cashin et al.[15]

by no means a straightforward process. Proponents of earmarking point to revenue protection, efficiency enhancement, building public support for a new tax, accountability, cost awareness and increase flexibility through off-budget funding arrangements. While opponents point to budget rigidities, economic distortion, procyclicality, increase fragmentation, decreased equity and susceptibility to special interests as all reasons to avoid earmarking. Each of the arguments has validity in certain contexts. In this way, the devil is in the details of precisely how the earmark is designed and implemented and importantly how it fits within the overall fiscal framework of a government. As demonstrated by Cashin et al.[14] there is a wide range of both revenue and expenditure characteristics that will need to be determined when introducing an earmark. As discussed previously in the chapter, how taxation is collected and transferred directly impacts the potential effectiveness of a health tax both from a revenue and health impact perspective. Decisions around expenditure purpose, how closely linked revenues are to actual expenditures and the flexibility with which expenditures can be made are critically important in determining the effectiveness of an earmark from a fiscal perspective.

Even under the circumstances that best practices regarding transparency and accountability are applied to hard earmarked funds, there is no guarantee that this type of earmarking will increase available resources to frontlines. A recent WHO report reviewing experience in Africa estimates that 13 of 26 African countries have an average of more than 15% under-spending of their annual health budget allocations with a deteriorating trend, with most budget execution rates in health decreasing between 2008 and 2016 across African countries.[20] Therefore, in this context, a large share of allocations goes unspent. While this finding is not necessarily tied directly to earmarking, it highlights that overall health financing bottlenecks may be a binding constraint to effectively increasing spending in the health sector, whether it is through earmarked or other revenue sources.

Furthermore, the often time-bound nature of earmarks means that they are not anchored within broader social and political consensus and may hinder authorities' ability to adopt counter-cyclical policy. For example, in the case of health taxes, when consumption of the taxed product decreases, related revenues should also decrease. This can create challenges when expenditure demands are not correlated with the revenue source. For instance, children do not need less education because smoking goes down. In this case, there will be a need to supplement previously earmarking funds from other sources. This is seen in the recent experience with payroll tax earmarking for national health insurance in Estonia. As the population has aged and there are more retirees, there was a need to expand wage-based earmarked contributions with more general revenues that did not rely purely on employment-based sources of revenue.[21] While this change has now been made, it took years of advocacy and legislative efforts. The issues around linking entitlement to contribution in the context of payroll taxation may be distinct from considerations around health taxes, where demand has been shown to be relatively inelastic; however, recent evidence from the implementation of an SSB tax in Mexico shows that responsiveness may vary.[22]

9.4.3. Experience with earmarking and health financing[h]

As calls for 'innovative' or new sources of revenue have increased for the health sector, so too has the interest in earmarked sources of revenues. To respond to this increased interest, recent analysis has worked to build the evidence base around the potential impact of earmarked sources of revenue on health financing and overall fiscal space for health. These findings have direct implications for the discussions around health tax revenues within the broader fiscal framework.

The health sector has a long history of earmarking, with at least 80 countries earmarking revenue sources for the health sector as of 2016.[15] Importantly, the majority of those countries (62) used income or payroll taxes to fund access to healthcare for the population or formal sector works

[h] This section builds heavily from Cashin C, Sparkes S, Bloom D., *Earmarking for Health: From Theory to Practice*. Geneva: World Health Organization; 2017.

in a public scheme. Health tax revenues, coming from tobacco taxes, alcohol taxes or SSB taxes were earmarked for the health sector in 54 countries. There can be many reasons to tie health tax revenues to health sector financing; all of which are not necessarily related to funding decisions.

There have been three studies examining the impact of earmarking in the health sector in 2015, 2016 and 2017 respectively.[15,23,24] Each of these studies considers both the fiscal implications of earmarking for the health sector and the rationale for this type of policy choice. The first examines key lessons that emerge from earmarking tobacco tax revenues in Botswana, Egypt, Iceland, Romania, Poland, the Philippines, Vietnam, Thailand and Peru.[24] The studies consider both revenue and financing-related issues and legislative and political processes. From a fiscal perspective, the studies find that while tobacco taxes have the potential to increase overall government revenues, the actual amount of that is raised is generally small in relation to the overall government health budget. Among the countries studied, funds from earmarked tobacco taxes as a percentage of general government expenditure on health ranged from 0.001% in Poland to 1.3% in Panama.

One outlier that is analysed in both WHO studies is the Philippines. In 2012, a reform significantly increased taxes on both tobacco and alcohol products and earmarked a large portion of the additional revenues (100% of additional alcohol revenues and 85% of additional tobacco tax revenues) for health coverage expansion through the Philippine Health Insurance Corporation (PhilHealth). As shown in Table 9.3 this reform has raised substantial revenues for the health sector, amounting to 1.1% of GDP in 2015, which tripled the Department of Health's budget.[15] Importantly, the Department of Budget and Management has some discretion over the size and timing of allocation for the health sector. In this way, the earmarked funds are subject to the same budgetary processes and discretions as other sources of public funds for the health sector.

Just as it is important to analyse earmarked revenues for the health sector in relation to over public financing for health, it is also important to examine the baseline from which countries are generating health sector

Table 9.3. Earmarked tobacco tax revenues as share of total health expenditure (2013).

Country	Annual funds from tobacco tax earmarked as a percentage of domestic government health expenditure*	Domestic general government health expenditure (% of GDP) (2013)
Botswana	0.08%	4.0
Egypt, Arab Rep.	1.29%	1.4
Iceland	0.08%	6.6
Panama	1.49%	4.1
Philippines	**33.17%**	**1.2**
Poland	0.001%	4.5
Romania	0.00%	4.1
Thailand	1.15%	2.6

*Estimated annual tax revenues taken from 2013 to 2015 based on WHO (2016) and domestic government health expenditure from 2013 from WHO Global Health Expenditure database.

revenues. Table 9.3 compares the share of public expenditure on health that comes from earmarked tobacco taxes, as well as general government expenditure on health as a percentage of GDP. This comparison is important because the size of the denominator – the revenue base in relation to the overall macroeconomic picture – sets the stage for the share of tobacco taxes can ultimately comprise of overall public expenditure on health. As shown subsequently, while the Philippines generates a remarkable share of public expenditure on health from tobacco tax revenues, public expenditure on health as a share of GDP is below average and relatively low in comparison to other countries that earmark tobacco taxes for the health sector. Therefore, the Philippines reform can be seen as potentially redressing underinvestment in health from the public sector. Whereas, revenues from Iceland's tobacco tax contributed a relatively small portion of domestic government expenditure on health but a relatively large share of GDP is dedicated to government health expenditure.

Many countries and sub-national entities that earmark health tax revenues for the health sector do so in a targeted way. This can be considered as a tight revenue–expenditure linkage. For instance, in 1998, the State of California introduced earmarking of its revenues from its tobacco tax to directly its tobacco control education campaign.[25] Similarly, Thailand earmarks tobacco and alcohol taxation for its ThaiHealth Promotion Fund, which is responsible for public health education campaigns and programmes to combat the harmful use of alcohol, tobacco, unhealthy diets and sedentary behaviour.[26] This type of hard earmarking, with a strong benefits rationale,[i] whereby health system costs to curb unhealthy behaviour are paid for by those consuming the unhealthy products, may be less prone to fungibility issues and can lend themselves to transparency and accountability. As Bird[23] highlights, this form of earmarking can be viewed as 'marrying sin and virtue' in a way by taxing the 'bad' and doing 'good' with the proceeds from the tax.

9.4.4. Earmarking and public financial management

The interface between earmarking and PFM systems comes in different forms. On the one hand, earmarking is sometimes pursued as a way to match funds with policy priorities when there is a perceived shortcoming in the budgeting process. For example, if there is a concern that an important issue (e.g. tobacco control measures) is not funded and there is traction in the government to operationalise that priority through a new funding mechanism. In this case, earmarking does not replace the priority setting mechanism and rather operationalises a priority through an identified funding source. An earmarked source of revenues with a tight expenditure purpose can also lend itself to monitoring and accountability as it is easier to track funds and assess their impact against stated objectives.

Earmarking may be helpful to facilitate expenditure management when routine PFM systems are too weak or too rigid. For example, the Thai Health Promotion Funds sits as a semi-autonomous agency that is not directly answerable to the Ministry of Health in part because it does

[i] Refers to the benefits principle of taxation which argues that taxes should be borne by those who benefit the most from the associated expenditure.

not have to rely on it for budget allocations. Similarly, the Ghana National Health Insurance Agency (NHIA) is financed in part from both earmarked payroll and VAT revenues and sits as an extra-budgetary agency. While the revenue source is not health taxes, the same governance structure and PFM issues may apply. Beyond budget prioritisation, this type of financing arrangement may circumvent deficiencies in the overall PFM system that might delay the release of funds. However, in the case of Ghana, issues related to releasing earmarked revenues from the Ministry of Finance to the NHIA have led to long delays in claims payments to providers. Due to a mistrust by finance authorities in the capacity and efficiency of the NHIA, finance authorities have withheld the transfer of earmarked VAT revenues to NHIA. As a result, the NHIA has not been able to pay claims in a timely manner to providers which can lead to increased user charges to patients or even decreased access.

While this form of bypassing the regular budgeting process can be expedient, it can also affect efficiency and effectiveness of PFM systems at each stage of the budget cycle by introducing rigidities and exacerbating inefficiencies.[15] For example, earmarking can worsen fragmentation or funds and hence limit pooling. This in turn can limit redistribution and impact on equity and financial protection objectives. For example, in Gabon two earmarked taxes were introduced to fund health insurance coverage for low-income groups. The funds for these groups were not pooled with funds for other income groups, which limited the redistributional impact and also created duplicative processes.[27]

Earmarking can be particularly problematic from a PFM perspective in the case that appropriate safeguards are not introduced proactively. Some of the potential pitfalls include bypassing or reduced parliamentary supervision; lack of annual and other reviews associated with the established budget process; potentially bypassing central treasury account; and, associated transparency and governance issues of parallel funds that are not under the purview of overall budget scrutiny.

In general, just as any earmarked source of revenue needs to be assessed in relation to overall government and health sector financing, it also needs to be examined in the context of overall PFM arrangements. Not taking into account these underlying systems can directly constrain the policy objectives of the earmark.

9.4.5. Key consideration and lessons in designing effective earmarking policies

While the evidence around earmarking from a health financing perspective can be mixed, there are some key considerations and lessons that have emerged in terms of adopting and designing effective earmarking policies. Importantly, the various country analyses have shown that the introduction or increase of health taxes is more politically acceptable when their revenues are earmarked for the health sector or for a particular objective or agency within the health sector. Given the evidence around the potential health benefits of health taxes,[28,29] a careful balance needs to be struck between promoting earmarking, while also being realistic about its potential fiscal impact.

Based on these reviews, several key lessons emerge in terms of how to design earmarks effectively from a health financing perspective. Through this careful design process, both the possible pros and cons of earmarking can be taken into consideration and managed. First, revenue sources should be balanced with expenditure purposes through soft earmarking. Through a softer approach, the earmark can help to advance a health sector priority (i.e. introduce health taxes) without introducing undue rigidities, inefficiency or economic distortions. In this way, the earmarked source of revenues continues to be allocated through standard budgeting and priority-setting processes. However, by defining the expenditure purpose in a relatively specific way, the results of spending can be tracked and potential for fungibility (the reduction of other revenue sources to compensate for the earmarked source) can be decreased.

This form of soft earmarking can also help both budget and health authorities to adjust spending priorities as needs on the sector shift, as starkly demonstrated by COVID-19. Built-in 'release valves' allow a certain share of revenues to be reallocated as new priorities emerge. Ghana, the Philippines and Estonia all have taken advantage of the flexibility for earmarked sources of revenue for the health sector built into legislation.

As stressed by Bird,[30] this form of earmarking can potentially lead to the establishment of an expenditure floor, it does not necessarily lead to additional revenues for the health sector. The simple reason is that money is fungible and therefore as long as there are other sources of revenues that are allocated for an expenditure purpose earmarking may not lead to increased spending. This general finding bears out in country experiences, as well, with very few cases of real, long-term sustainable increases in funding for the health sector materialising.[15,23]

Second, strong PFM and governance systems are critical to ensuring an earmark can meet its intended spending objective. As shown in Ghana and Indonesia undue delays and a lack of transparency in terms of allocation mechanisms can work against and even distract from overall health financing objectives. They are also often channelled to extra-budgetary funds that do not have the same accountability as general government revenues.

See Table 9.4 which provides a summary of the key PFM cycles, related diagnostic tools and elements that are at authorities' disposal for a given cycle; and earmarking related considerations related to health taxes.

Third, earmarking should involve a clear time horizon, after which it is reviewed and subject to reapproval. Ultimately, earmarking is inherently linked to policy priorities in that it links funding to a priority at a moment in time. These priorities and needs might shift over time. The re-approval can also help in the case that financing objectives are not met. This was the case in Gabon when its mobile phone tax levy earmark was abolished after 10 years of implementation, in part because associated revenues were not sufficient for the intended expenditure purpose.[27] Therefore, a review process is important to address efficiency concerns related to shifting priorities, needs and macro-fiscal contexts. This review process is particularly important in the case of health taxes, where the objective of introducing the tax is to reduce the consumption of the relevant product.

Table 9.4. PFM cycle and earmarking issues.

PFM cycle	Tools or elements of the PFM cycle	Earmarked health tax revenues specific issues
Goal development	– Development plans – Integrated national financing frameworks	– Whether to revenue earmark a health tax or not? If yes, what portion of it to earmark? – Decision on expenditure purpose. – How does the policy/program funded with earmarked resources fit with the national development objectives? – Decisions on earmark modality: soft versus hard earmark.
Revenue projection/ mobilisation	– Annual tax revenue forecasts – Medium-term revenue strategies (MTRS) – Tax Policy and tax administration diagnostics for excise taxes	– Does earmarking improve health equity by channelling revenues from health taxes to services needed by the poor? – Can the earmark help to garner public support or forge alliances with government/non-government authorities? – What is the marginal revenue that can be raised through the earmarked source?
Budget planning	– Policy and strategic planning (medium-term expenditure framework (MTEFs)	– Will the earmark improve or impede the efficiency of budget allocations? Or is it neutral? – How does the earmarked revenue match with expenditure purpose need?

(Continued)

Table 9.4. *(Continued)*

PFM cycle	Tools or elements of the PFM cycle	Earmarked health tax revenues specific issues
Budget prioritisation	– Expenditure policy prioritisation	– Is a release valve or contingency option in place to reallocate earmarked funds if other urgent needs or priorities arise? – How does the earmark interact with other sources of revenue? – Is the earmark time-bound or linked to a health outcome after which it falls away?
Budget formulation How public spending priorities are determined and funds are allocated	– Accounting standards/budget classification – Program-based budgeting – Improvements to line item/input budgeting if this is more suitable given country's PFM capacity	– Does the earmark add to the fragmentation of funding flows? – Are mechanisms in place to ensure efficient spending of earmarked revenues? – Can earmarked revenues be spent flexibly within the expenditure purpose, or are restrictions in place related to line-item budgets or other PFM rules? – Can unspent earmarked revenues be carried forward into the next fiscal year?

Table 9.4. *(Continued)*

PFM cycle	Tools or elements of the PFM cycle	Earmarked health tax revenues specific issues
Budget execution How budgets are used and providers of services and goods are paid	– Treasury operations – IFMIS – Procurement – Strategic purchasing – Results based financing	– Will the funds flow through the treasury or consolidated fund into an extrabudgetary fund, or will they go directly to an implementing agency? – How to ensure earmarked fund flows will not be delayed? – Will the institution that receives the earmarked revenues have the absorptive capacity to spend the funds? Will a waterfall account be created so that revenues generated in excess of expenditure needs, flow into another account or the consolidated fund?
Budget evaluation How public spending is accounted for	– Monitoring and reporting – Internal controls and internal Audit—Financial reporting (use of IPSAS); performance reporting; fiscal transparency; – Open government initiatives – External audit and parliamentary oversight – PFM oversight through media and civil society	– Can earmarked revenues be accounted for at every step, from collection to expenditure? – How will the institution that spends the earmarked revenues be accountable for results or outcomes?

Source: Draws on Refs.[14,15]; Marshalling the Evidence for Health Governance Thematic Working Group Report 2017; and, PFM in Health Toolkit, 2019, WB.

Finally, and most importantly, the key message coming from the evidence base around earmarking health tax revenues for health financing purposes is to not lose sight of the whole picture. This is both in terms of overall financing for the health sector and the overall PFM system. From a health financing perspective, these revenues can help boost revenues, but from a system-level perspective they are generally marginal in relation to general government revenues. As a result, they can be subject to fungibility, whereby one revenue source increases as another is decreased. Additionally, overall weaknesses in tax administration and public financial management systems will also pertain to health taxes. Therefore, these revenues, along with overall government revenues, can also suffer from low budget execution rates, delays in disbursements and a lack of transparency in allocation processes. In this case, underlying systems will need to be strengthened either in conjunction with or prior to considering earmarking.

9.5. The earmarking interface between health and finance

While earmarking policies are ultimately within the purview of finance authorities, they require active engagement with the sector that is supposed to receive the revenues. In the case of health taxes, this engagement between health and finance authorities becomes all the more critical because of the health objective of the tax itself, as well as the potential to dedicate revenues to health sector priorities. These dynamics can either facilitate or hinder tax adoption based on the specific context and relevant interests at play. The position, power and influence of stakeholders with vested interests can determine the trajectory of a reform.[31] This section considers this interaction between health and finance authorities. These intra-governmental politics are often quite distinct from the technical specificities of the earmark itself. In some cases, the introduction of an earmark can help to align interests between health and finance authorities, all while garnering public support for the introduction of a new tax.[15]

The relationship between health and finance authorities often depends on the specific design of the tax, including whether the earmark is hard or soft and the expenditure purpose of that tax. Earmarking health taxes has also been identified as a mechanism for increasing cross-government support in some contexts.[24] As demonstrated in both France[32] or Mexico,[33] there is often alignment between the health and general revenue-raising objectives of these taxes. In both countries, SSB taxes were introduced at times of fiscal stress where finance authorities were eager to find new sources of revenues. In this context, the health sector's objective of reducing the consumption of unhealthy products helps to also bring in general government revenues. Given the taxation function sits within the ministry of finance's purview, this alignment of objectives can be particularly critical in the face of strong opposition and financial influence of the affected industries.

However, the case of earmarking can bring in additional complications in this dynamic between finance and health. As discussed in the previous section, hard earmarking introduces rigidities and possible inefficiencies into the budget process and works against the principle that public spending should be determined by policy decisions and not by the revenue raised by a specific tax.[34] Therefore, health authorities need to consider the positions of ministries of finance as they work to promote health taxes as a health intervention.

As demonstrated by Cashin et al.,[15] the adoption of earmarks often happens at a time when health and finance authorities have aligned objectives. However, earmarking can also help to get public support for a new tax. In both the Philippines and Vietnam, despite opposition from industry groups, having the source of funds be a tobacco tax helped to garner support.[15] The combination of these factors means that earmarking can be politically expedient to demonstrate a visible commitment to a population policy or programme while introducing a new tax, which is often politically unpopular. However, aligning the interests of finance authorities often necessitates a soft earmarking approach, whereby there is still some allocation discretion and flexibilities. The issue becomes how to take advantage of this alignment for political purposes, without the health sector losing sight of advocacy with finance authorities for sustained increases in allocations. In this way, the politics of adopting earmarking health tax revenues should be decoupled with the politics of the implementation of that earmark. This implementation process can lead to decreased allocations from other sources of revenue and even a net reduction in revenues for health sector.[23]

The approach taken in both Vietnam and Thailand to earmark contributions from tobacco and/or alcohol taxation into special funds to finance anti-smoking and overall health promotion activities is another way to align interests. In both cases, the funds are kept as off-budget entities that are under the purview of the Ministry of Finance.[15] Therefore, while they are not subject to routine budgeting processes, they also have a separate board structure to manage the funds. Non-governmental organisations have been an important partner in both countries in terms of advancing the health tax reforms and in promoting the Thai Health Promotion Fund and the Vietnam Tobacco Control Fund.

These experiences point to the importance of active engagement between health and finance authorities in the development and eventual adoption and implementation of earmarking policies. Budget allocations and the overall PFM system are the responsibility of finance authorities; however, there is space for possible policy solutions that consider the interests of both sets of government stakeholders.

Key messages

- As health taxes are part of larger tax systems, policies and administrations, the design and implementation of these taxes should be analysed within the context of countries' overall tax and governance systems. Part of these public financing issues includes how the revenue from health taxes is ultimately allocated and used.
- As of 2017, at least 80 countries earmarked a specific source of revenues for health. Although many of these country examples

involve earmarking payroll or income taxes to fund healthcare, they also represent at least 54 countries that earmark all or a portion of tobacco, alcohol or sugar-sweetened beverage (SSB) taxation for the health sector.

- Despite their prevalence, care must be exercised to help ensure that these earmarks bring a sustained net increase in revenue for the sector and address issues related to fungibility of funds, and that earmarking does not create rigidities and inefficiencies.
- The specificities of earmarking vary greatly in practice and range from a spectrum of soft to hard. From a political economy perspective, soft earmarking has helped to advance the adoption of new health taxes in some settings as having a tight revenue-expenditure link can boost public support for health taxes.
- In general, the closer the practice is to standard budget process, where revenues are matched with political priorities and population needs, the more effective it is.

References

1. Junquera-Varela FR, Verhoeven M, Shukla GP, Haven B, Awasthi R, et al. *Strengthening Domestic Resource Mobilization: Moving from Theory to Practice in Low- and Middle-Income Countries*. Washington, DC: World Bank; 2017.
2. Gaspar V, Amaglobeli D, Garcia-Escribano M, Prady D, Soto M. *Fiscal Policy and Development: Human, Social, and Physical Investments for the SDGs*. Washinton, DC: International Monetary Fund; 2019.
3. UNCTAD. *Trade and Development Report*. New York: United Nations; 2014.
4. Platform for Collaboration on Tax, editor Taxation & SDGs. *First Global Conference of the Platform for Collaboration on Tax*. New York; 2018.
5. Tandon A, Cain J, Kurowski C, Dozol A, Postolovska I. From slippery slopes to steep hills: Contrasting landscapes of economic growth and public spending for health. *Social Science & Medicine*. 2020; 259: 113171.
6. Barroy H, Vaughan K, Tapsoba Y, Dale E, Van de Maele N. *Towards Universal Health Coverage: Thinking Public*. Geneva: World Health Organization; 2017.
7. Platform for Collaboration on Tax. PCT Progress Report 2020. New York; 2020.
8. Platform for Collaboration on Tax. PCT Progress Report 2018–2019. New York; 2019.
9. Bird RM. Administrative dimensions of tax reform. *Asia-Pacific Tax Bulletin*. 2004; 10(3): 134–150

10. Chaloupka FJ, Powell LM. *Using Fiscal Policy to Promote Health: Taxing Tobacco, Alcohol, and Sugary Beverages.* Background Paper for the Task Force on Fiscal Policy for Health. New York: Bloomberg Philanthropies; 2018.
11. Gautam A. Tackling wasteful spending on health. Paris: OECD; 2017.
12. World Health Organization. *The World Health Report – Health Systems Financing: The Path to Universal Coverage.* Geneva: World Health Organization; 2010.
13. World Bank. *FinHealth: PFM in Health Toolkit.* Washington, DC; 2019. https://www.pfm4health.net/_files/ugd/18961e_ae49d69d8534407990bc858320bbba74.pdf.
14. Cashin C, Bloom D, Sparkes S, Barroy H, Kutzin J, O'Dougherty S. *Aligning Public Financial Management and Health Financing.* Geneva: World Health Organization; 2017. Contract No.: Health Financing Working Paper No. 4.
15. Cashin C, Sparkes S, Bloom D. *Earmarking for Health: From Theory to Practice.* Geneva: World Health Organization; 2017.
16. Inter-agency Task Force on Financing for Development. *Financing for Sustainable Development Report.* New York: United Nations; 2019.
17. Buchanan JM. The economics of earmarked taxes. *Journal of Political Economy.* 1963; 71(5): 457–469.
18. Manji A. The International Development (Official Development Assistance Target) Act 2015: legislative spending targets, poverty alleviation and aid scrutiny. *The Modern Law Review.* 2016; 79(4): 655–677.
19. Stivender CO, Gaggl P, Amato LH, Farrow-Chestnut TE. The impact of education earmarking on state-level lottery sales. *The BE Journal of Economic Analysis & Policy.* 2016; 16(3): 1473–1500.
20. Barroy H, Kabaniha G, Boudreaux C, Cammack T, Bain N. *Leveraging Public Financial Management for Better Health in Africa: Key Bottlenecks and Opportunities for Reform.* Geneva: World Health Organization; 2019.
21. Habicht T, Reinap M, Kasekamp K, Habicht J, van Ginneken E, Webb E. The 2017 reform to improve financial sustainability of national health insurance in Estonia: Analysis and first lessons on broadening the revenue base. *Health Policy.* 2019; 123(8): 695–699.
22. Colchero MA, Guerrero-López CM, Molina M, Rivera JA. Beverages sales in Mexico before and after implementation of a sugar sweetened beverage tax. *Plos One.* 2016; 11(9): e0163463.
23. Bird RM. *Tobacco and Alcohol Excise Taxes for Improving Public Health and Revenue Outcomes : Marrying Sin and Virtue?* Washington, DC: The World Bank; 2015.
24. World Health Organization. *Earmarked Tobacco Taxes: Lessons Learnt from Nine Countries.* Geneva: World Health Organization; 2016.
25. Novotny TE, Siegel MB. California's tobacco control saga. *Health Affairs.* 1996; 15(1): 58–72.
26. Pongutta S, Suphanchaimat R, Patcharanarumol W, Tangcharoensathien V. Lessons from the Thai health promotion foundation. *Bulletin of the World Health Organization.* 2019; 97(3): 213.

27. Aboubacar I, Essono M, Mailfert M, Barroy H. *Health Financing and Budgeting Reform in Gabon: Progress and Challenges on the Road to Universal Health Coverage.* Geneva: World Health Organization; 2020.
28. Blakely T, Cleghorn C, Mizdrak A, Waterlander W, Nghiem N, Swinburn B, et al. The effect of food taxes and subsidies on population health and health costs: A modelling study. *The Lancet Public Health.* 2020; 5(7): e404–e413.
29. Basto-Abreu A, Barrientos-Gutiérrez T, Vidaña-Pérez D, Colchero MA, Hernández-F M, Hernández-Ávila M, et al. Cost-effectiveness of the sugar-sweetened beverage excise tax in Mexico. *Health Affairs.* 2019; 38(11): 1824–1831.
30. Bird, Richard M. Tobacco and Alcohol Excise Taxes for Improving Public Health and Revenue Outcomes : Marrying Sin and Virtue? Policy Research Working Paper; No. 7500. 2015. World Bank, Washington, DC. © World Bank. https://openknowledge.worldbank.org/handle/10986/23464 License: CC BY 3.0 IGO. http://hdl.handle.net/10986/23464.
31. Sparkes SP, Bump JB, Özçelik EA, Kutzin J, Reich MR. Political economy analysis for health financing reform. *Health Systems & Reform.* 2019: 5(3): 183–194.
32. Le Bodo Y, Etilé F, Gagnon F, De Wals P. Conditions influencing the adoption of a soda tax for public health: Analysis of the French case (2005–2012). *Food Policy.* 2019; 88: 101765.
33. James E, Lajous M, Reich MR. The politics of taxes for health: an analysis of the passage of the sugar-sweetened beverage tax in Mexico. *Health Systems & Reform.* 2020; 6(1): e1669122.
34. Wilkinson M. Paying for public spending: Is there a role for earmarked taxes? *Fiscal Studies.* 1994; 15(4): 119–135.
35. Goryakin Y, Revill P, Mirelman A, Sweeney R, Ochalek J, Suhrcke M. *Public Financial Management and Health Service Delivery: A Literature Review.* London; 2017.

https://doi.org/10.1142/9781800612396_0012

Special Focus 3

Managing the Politics of Earmarked Health Taxes

Katherine Smith* and Mark Hellowell†

SF 3.1. Introduction

The public health interest in health taxes has largely focused on their ability to raise the cost of manufacturing, distributing, selling and/or consuming such products, reducing their consumption. However, there is increasing interest in using such taxes to mobilise additional government revenues to fund investments and programmes that contribute to health systems goals. For example, a recent report by the World Bank found that the large financing gap for Universal Health Coverage (UHC) in low- and lower-middle-income countries (LMICs) (now exacerbated by the economic effects of the COVID-19 pandemic), could be mitigated by tax increases on tobacco, alcohol, and sugar-sweetened beverages (SSBs).[1] The World Bank authors estimate that tax increases that raise the retail prices of these products by 50% could generate additional revenues of approximately $24.7 billion in 54 LMICs by 2030. If allocated to the health sector at a level of 50%, the excise tax increases would lower the estimated financing gap by $2.9 billion in

* University of Strathclyde, UK.

† University of Edinburgh, UK.

low-income countries and $6.6 billion in lower-middle-income countries (as well as reducing future costs by curbing the growth of non-communicable disease (NCD) burdens). However, this effect depends on the taxes being 'earmarked' – that is, allocated to specific purposes, a process alternatively called 'hypothecation'.

Our starting point in this contribution is to recognise that public support for new or increased consumption taxes is generally low, and yet, to be initiated and sustained over time, new health tax policies require sufficient support from citizens, policymakers and other stakeholders. Research across multiple contexts, and multiple specific taxes, suggests that the level of support is often higher when credible commitments are made to earmark the related funds for activities that are highly valued by the population.[2] Building on this understanding, we consider how the process of earmarking can impact, and has impacted, on the political feasibility and sustainability of health tax policies. Specifically, we seek to understand the perspectives of a range of stakeholders on health taxes and how these might be influenced by earmarking. In addition to members of the general public, who can be offered opportunities to engage with policy discussions about new tax proposals via consultations – or even, in some cases, direct votes on proposals – there exist multiple non-governmental and commercial sector actors with strong views about, and interests in, health taxes generally and, more specifically, the earmarking of such taxes. As this contribution shows, these actors often work hard to ensure that political and media discussions are influenced by their views and interests (see Refs.[2,3]). Finally, where cross-government support for earmarking is required, it is important to consider the views of policymakers beyond health and finance on earmarking health taxes (a rather smaller literature – see Ref.[2]).

Since it would be impossible to thoroughly review the available research literatures on the range of perspectives with respect to the earmarking of health taxes, this section identifies key insights regarding the views and interests of: (i) members of the public; (ii) policymakers and (iii) commercial sector actors. The third section focuses primarily on tobacco industry actors since these activities are most comprehensively covered in the literature, but it also touches on the more limited literature examining the views of food, beverage and alcohol industry actors. It is notable that this contribution does not explore the views of civil society actors on earmarking in any detail. The reasons for this are that, although existing literature explores the role of these groups in efforts to promote the use of health taxes (which, as Chapter 13 sets out, can be crucial), there is a dearth of research exploring the perspectives of civil society actors on earmarking health taxes. In the contribution conclusion, we reflect on the potential reasons for, and importance of, this current knowledge gap.

SF 3.2. Public support for 'earmarked' health taxes

While public preferences vary by context and by specific tax proposal (e.g. while there is some evidence that the public can be supportive of SSB taxes in some contexts, support for new or increased consumption taxes in general is low – see Refs.[4–7]). However, there is remarkably consistent evidence that public support, across contexts, is higher when credible commitments are made to earmark funds for specified health objectives and related activities, such as subsidising healthier foods,[7] targeting child obesity,[8] providing support to smokers who want to quit,[9] and expanding access to free or subsidised health care in contexts where UHC has not been achieved.[10] Indeed, studies of proposals to raise tobacco taxes have found that public support tends to increase when such proposals include a commitment to earmark tobacco tax increases for health-related spending – evidence here comes from Germany,[11] Greece,[12] Indonesia,[13] New Zealand,[14] the Philippines,[10] the United Kingdom,[15] the United States[16,17] and Taiwan,[18] among others.

There are multiple reasons why 'earmarking' might increase public support for health taxes (although understanding people's rationales for favouring health taxes that are earmarked is much less well researched).

In the absence of earmarking, there is an inherent disconnection between the payment of taxes and the allocation of funds to specific objectives and activities, which can create or exacerbate concerns that public spending priorities are misaligned with public preferences. Earmarking can provide a way of addressing such concerns by ensuring that funds are allocated towards activities that command broad public support, thereby increasing a sense among countries' citizens that they 'have a say' in decisions about how public money is spent,[18] and strengthening the ethical case for taxation (e.g. an argument that it is right for consumers of health-damaging products to contribute more tax to support health care was effectively deployed by officials of the Romanian Ministry of Health to support an earmarked tobacco tax increase – see Ref.[19]). Earmarking health taxes can also enable policymakers to respond to considerable public concerns about the regressive nature of consumption taxes that pertains in many country contexts (i.e. the possibility that they will increase the tax burden of those on low incomes) (e.g. Refs.[20–24]), via commitments to direct spending towards those most affected by the health effects of the taxed product, or towards the poorest, and/or other vulnerable social groups.[22,25]

On the other hand, while earmarking can generate a strong signal to the public that new or increased taxes will be used to fund activities in accordance with public preferences, in practice, funds may not always be earmarked to the extent that was initially claimed, leading to a loss of trust in and public support for the tax.[26,27] Because money is 'fungible' (i.e. any unit of a given currency is ultimately substitutable for any other), it is difficult to trace the connection between specific revenue streams and specific activities. Unless a specific revenue stream is the *only* source of funding for a specific area of expenditure (which is neither feasible nor desirable in most cases – see Ref.[10]), increased revenues from a specific source can be offset by reducing revenues from other sources, leading to no overall increase. We call this the accountability problem. Where steps are not taken to address this problem (e.g. through assiduous monitoring – ideally by an independent entity such as a supreme audit institution), actors opposed to the tax may use such lacunae in financial accountability to undermine public support.[3]

Moreover, it is important to note that decisions to earmark revenues from a proposed tax or tax increase do not *guarantee* a high level of public support, since this form of accountability is far from the only factor shaping public opinion (mass media coverage and counter-lobbying by corporate interests being notable others – see, e.g. Refs.[27–29]). There may also, in some contexts, be institutional factors that offset, or outweigh, the political benefits of earmarking health taxes. For example, in recent years, a number of city authorities in California have run referenda on new SSB taxes. One of the challenges faced by advocates of such taxes is that while new taxes can pass with a simple majority, earmarked commitments require a two-thirds majority.[30] In such cases, the political analysis of earmarking becomes more complicated, and less favourable overall. In other words, while advocates of SSB taxes might believe that earmarking will increase public support for the SSB tax, for reasons described previously, they may be unclear as to whether this increase will be sufficient to achieve the two-thirds majority required for an earmarked tax proposal to pass. Empirically, the result has differed across Californian cities; in some cases leading to new SSB taxes being passed, while in others proposals have been rejected.[30]

SF 3.3. Government support for 'earmarked' health taxes

The literature exploring policymakers' perspectives on the earmarking of health taxes is more limited and there are contrasting conclusions. Research suggests that government officials are often wary about the idea of earmarking health taxes for specific spending purposes. In addition, policymakers may be subject to formal restrictions on earmarking (e.g. Ref.[17]) or may simply believe that policy buy-in would be too low to warrant pursuing. An interview-based study in Saudi Arabia, for example, found that neither policy officials from the health or finance sectors felt there was any appetite for earmarking the revenue from a new SSB tax for health-related spending, attributing this to the lack of precedent for earmarking.[31] Similarly, a study of Israeli policy stakeholders on the prospect of new taxes on SSBs and unhealthy snacks revealed strong opposition to earmarking among Ministry of Finance officials, to the extent that many other stakeholders believed earmarking was not a realistic prospect.[32] Likewise, a US study of efforts to pass a new alcohol tax in three states found that, although legislators acknowledged that public support was likely to increase if commitments were made to earmarking revenues for health spending, their clear preference was for the revenue to go to the general budget.[33]

This reflects resistance among public officials to proposals for earmarking taxes (more broadly) on the basis that it deprives public officials of crucial flexibility in public spending.[34] Indeed, while policymakers working within ministries and departments focusing on health may support earmarking taxes for health spending, officials within finance ministries are generally likely to oppose such commitments and their impacts on the flexibility of budgetary arrangements.[35] However, research exploring such perspectives on proposals to implement SSB taxes in the United States (which were subject to voter ballots) found that most respondents viewed commitments to reinvest accrued revenues into health-related activities as a persuasive argument in favour of such taxes.[36] In addition, the majority of respondents believed public support would be lower when policymakers failed to specify how revenues from proposed health taxes would be spent.[36] Overall, this suggests that, where there is both (a) a precedent for earmarking health taxes and (b) high levels of citizen engagement in decisions about the taxes (e.g. via consultation or even voting), policymakers that support such taxes should view earmarking as strategically attractive (or even necessary).

The earmarking of health taxes has also been identified as a promising mechanism for increasing the degree of cross-departmental government support in some contexts.[2] For example, a tax on unhealthy food products introduced in French Polynesia in 2002 enjoyed extremely broad ministerial support, a finding attributed to the use of the tax to co-finance a broad range of public health and cultural, educational and youth-focused initiatives, which benefitted 7 of the 17 ministers in government.[37] In addition, our work with country governments in several LMICs has shown how Ministries of Finance often seek guarantees from other ministries that new revenue streams have been identified before new intervention areas and activities will be supported. For instance, to obtain support from Ministries of Finance for new (or expanded) National Health Insurance Funds (often a key part of UHC efforts in LMICs), ministries that support such proposals are often required to identify a specific revenue stream that will be used to fund or co-fund the necessary budgetary commitments. In such cases, earmarked health taxes are often viewed by Ministries of Finance as feasible and a more economically desirable option than potential alternatives such as (highly distortionary) taxes on payroll/salaries.

The combination of (a) the strategic value (for attracting public support) of *claiming* that the revenue from new health taxes/tax increases will be dedicated to health spending with (b) the accountability problem and (c) strong pressures to 'flex' public spending allocations over the political and economic cycles, helps explain the existence of several cases in which commitments to earmarking health taxes for specific purposes have been made but not honoured. Indeed, there are multiple case studies in the literature on US state-level tobacco tax increases which were passed by public ballot on the basis that the revenue would be used for particular purposes but for which evidence suggests revenues were subsequently diverted (e.g. Refs.[38–40]). Similarly, an analysis of a Scottish Government tax on large retailers selling alcohol and tobacco found that, despite efforts by policymakers to frame the new tax as one that would be dedicated to health-related purposes, in fact 'the revenue raised from the Supplement was not meaningfully hypothecated – and indeed it seems likely that there was never any intention to formally hypothecate for health purposes' (Ref.[26], p. 825). Where divergences between stated revenue-spending intentions and actual revenue spending occur, this may undermine public support for existing or future health taxes, and create lobbying opportunities for interests opposed to the implementation or maintenance of such taxes.[3,27]

SF 3.4. Commercial sector opposition to 'earmarked' health taxes

As Chapter 12 sets out, multiple commercial sector actors have a potential interest in proposals to earmark health taxes, including those whose profits may be impacted by the taxes (e.g. unhealthy commodity industries, such as tobacco, alcohol and ultra-processed food manufacturers and retailers) and those who may benefit from commitments to invest accrued revenues on health (e.g. health and social care providers and pharmaceutical companies). In this section, we focus on the available literature concerning the perspectives of actors working for unhealthy commodity industries on health taxes. This is a rather imbalanced literature which, until recently, was dominated by analyses of transnational tobacco company perspectives. This reflects the fact that litigation cases in the United States have require tobacco companies to place some of their internal documents into the public domain, providing a resource to researchers seeking to analyse and understand commercial sector perspectives on a wide range of policy issues.[41]

A systematic review of the literature concerning tobacco industry efforts to influence tobacco tax policies found that tobacco companies work hard to prevent significant tobacco excise increases – and that they are particularly aggressive in opposing proposals for taxes that are 'earmarked' for tobacco control or spending on other health-related objectives or activities.[3] The review identified 17 studies, all focusing on the United States, concerning proposals for tax increases in which officials had made commitments to earmark the revenue for health-related programmes. In all cases, tobacco companies worked to oppose these proposals (most of which involved direct public ballots/votes), often successfully. The review found that such actors make use of the accountability problem outlined previously. Indeed, the most commonly identified industry argument in these studies was that earmarked funds would be used in ways which the public did not support and/or which differed from those described in the original proposal.[3] Specifically in the US context, the industry has argued that tobacco taxes would be misused to subsidise healthcare for poorer groups, which the industry sometimes framed as a diversion of funds to 'greedy' doctors, hospitals, healthcare companies, insurers and/or community health activists. Such efforts were helped by the fact that healthcare and health insurance organisations often *wanted* to divert the funds and by the fact the tobacco industry sometimes worked with such actors to try to *achieve* such diversions (e.g. Refs.[38–40]). This not only limited the availability of resources for tobacco control efforts (for which funds had originally been earmarked) but also provided evidence to support the tobacco industry's arguments that earmarking commitments would not be honoured.

There has recently been an increase in studies exploring the perspectives of food and beverage company actors on health taxes, in the context of widespread policy experimentation with SSB and food taxes (see Ref.[2] and Chapter 13 in this book). However, while this literature charts strong food and beverage company opposition to proposals for taxes on their products (see Ref.[42]), we could not identify any specific analysis of perspectives on, or responses to, proposals for earmarking such taxes. The literature exploring alcohol industry perspectives on health taxes is even more limited. This suggests we currently know very little about broader commercial perspectives on earmarking health taxes. However, given the evidence (discussed in this contribution) that earmarking increases public support for health taxes, combined with the extensive evidence of unhealthy commodity industry opposition to health taxes (as set out in Chapter 13), it would be not be surprising to find that the tobacco industry's opposition to earmarking extended to other unhealthy commodity industries.

SF 3.5. Conclusion

Existing literature shows that commitments to earmarking health taxes for specific purposes (especially health purposes, such as funding UHC, health system strengthening or preventive public health services), can increase public and political support for such policies.[4,37,43,44] For precisely this reason, tobacco industry actors have actively opposed earmarking principles and questioned the legitimacy of the associated commitments. In doing so, such actors have aimed to undermine the degree of public and political support by raising the connection between taxes paid and the socially valuable interventions and activities that they enable. For these reasons, we argue that earmarking is a process that should command the interest and support of the public health community (e.g. non-governmental organisations, researchers and practitioners). Yet, the dearth of research exploring the views of public health actors on earmarking health taxes, combined with at least two case studies in which the absence of public health support has been noted as a factor in the failure of the taxes to be sustained,[27,29] suggests efforts are needed to encourage and facilitate such engagement.

Earmarking is something that can help to offset and counter the influence of industry interests with regard to the initiation and sustainability of health taxes. However, this is only the case where governments are able to set out credible mechanisms for abiding by their earmarking commitments once these taxes have been implemented. Failure to do so has provided a lobbying focus for commercial actors (and others) opposed to health taxes, undermining public and political support for them. The public health community may therefore wish to both promote earmarking in principle, and also advocate to ensure that commitments to earmarking health taxes are feasible and honoured in practice. There is currently little evidence of such support. Meanwhile, as we outline in this contribution, analyses of US tobacco tax increases found that some health and medical actors had even worked with commercial actors to divert the revenue of tobacco tax increases away from original commitments, unwittingly providing evidence to undermine public confidence in future proposals for earmarked health taxes.

References

1. World Bank Group. *High-Performance Health Financing for Universal Health Coverage: Driving Sustainable, Inclusive Growth in the 21st Century*, 2019, https://openknowledge.worldbank.org/handle/10986/31930.
2. Wright A, Smith KE, Hellowell M. Policy lessons from health taxes: a systematic review of empirical studies. *BMC Public Health*. 2017; 17: 583.
3. Smith KE, Savell E, Gilmore AB. What is known about tobacco industry efforts to influence tobacco tax? A systematic review of empirical studies. *Tobacco Control*. 2013; 22(2): 144–153.
4. Barry C, Niederdeppe J, Gollust S. Taxes on sugar-sweetened beverages: Results from a 2011 national public opinion survey. *American Journal of Preventative Medicine*. 2013; 44: 158–163.
5. Beeken R, Wardle J. Public beliefs about the causes of obesity and attitudes towards policy initiatives in Great Britain. *Public Health Nutrition*. 2013; 16: 2132–2137.
6. González-Zapata LI, Alvarez-Dardet C, Millstone E, Clemente-Gómez V, Holdsworth M, Ortiz-Moncada R, et al. The potential role of taxes and subsidies on food in the prevention of obesity in Europe. *Journal of Epidemiology and Community Health*. 2010; 64: 696–704.
7. Morley B, Martin J, Niven P, Wakefield M. Public opinion of food-related obesity prevention policy initiatives. *Health Promotion Journal of Australia*. 2012; 23: 86–91.
8. Donaldson EA, Cohen JE, Rutkow L, Villanti AC, Kanarek NF, Barry CL. Public support for a sugar-sweetened beverage tax and pro-tax messages in a Mid-Atlantic US state. *Public Health Nutrition*, 2015; 18: 2263–2273.
9. Chaloupka F. *Tobacco Control Lessons Learned: The Impact of State and Local Policies*. Research Paper Series, No. 38, ImpacTeen, University of Illinois at Chicago: Chicago, USA; 2010.
10. Cashin C, Sparkes S, Bloom D. *Earmarking for Health: From Theory to Practice*. Department of Health Systems Governance and Financing Health Systems and Innovation, World Health Organization. Geneva, Switzerland; 2017. https://apps.who.int/iris/bitstream/handle/10665/255004/9789241512206-eng.pdf.
11. Hanewinkel R, Isensee B. Opinion on tobacco tax increase: factors associated with individuals' support in Germany. *Health Policy*. 2008; 86(2–3): 234–238.
12. Vardavas CI, Filippidis FT, Agaku IT, et al. Tobacco taxation: The importance of earmarking the revenue to health care and tobacco control. *Tobacco Induced Diseases*. 2012; 10: 21.
13. Thabrany H, Laborahima Z. People's support on sin tax to finance UHC in Indonesia. *Journal Ekonomi Kesehatan*. 2016; 1: 1.

14. Wilson N, Weerasekera D, Edwards R, Thomson G, Devlin M, Gifford H. Characteristics of smoker support for increasing a dedicated tobacco tax: National survey data from New Zealand. *Nicotine & Tobacco Research.* 2010; 12(2): 168–173.
15. Sussex J, Burge P, Lu H, Exley J, King S. Public acceptability of health and social care funding options. The Health Foundation, 01/05/22. https://www.health.org.uk/sites/default/files/upload/publications/2019/Public%20acceptability%20of%20health%20and%20social%20care%20funding%20options_0.pdf.
16. Nicholl J. Tobacco tax initiatives to prevent tobacco use. *Cancer.* 1998; 83: 2666–2679.
17. Chainani AA. *Sugar-Sweetened Beverage Taxes: Learning from Passage and Failure in California Cities.* University of the Sciences in Philadelphia, ProQuest Dissertations Publishing, 2019. 13859719.
18. Lin T-F, Chan Y-S, Chen J. Awareness of tobacco tax policy and public opinion on tobacco tax reform in Taiwan. *Asian Pacific Journal of Health Economics and Policy* 2020; 3: 2–14.
19. WHO. *Earmarked Tobacco Taxes: Lessons Learnt from Nine Countries.* Geneva: WHO; 2016, https://apps.who.int/iris/bitstream/handle/10665/206007/9789241510424_eng.pdf#.
20. Allais O, Bertail P, Nichle V. The effects of a fat tax on French households' purchases: A nutritional approach. *American Journal of Agricultural Economics.* 2010; 92: 228–245.
21. ECORYS. *Food Taxes and Their Impact on Competitiveness in the Agri-Food Sector: Final Report.* Rotterdam: ECORYS; 2014.
22. Hirono KT, Smith KE. Australia's $40 per pack cigarette tax plans: The need to consider equity, *Tobacco Control.* 2018; 27: 229–233.
23. Hoek J, Smith K. A qualitative analysis of low income smokers' responses to tobacco excise tax increases. *International Journal of Drug Policy.* 2016; 37: 82–89.
24. Shill J, Mavoa H, Allender S, Lawrence M, Sacks G, Peeters A, et al. Government regulation to promote healthy food environments – A view from inside state governments. *Obesity Reviews.* 2012; 13: 162–173.
25. Madden, D. The poverty effects of a "fat-tax" in Ireland. *Health Economics.* 2015; 24: 104–121.
26. IARC (International Agency for Research on Cancer). *IARC Handbooks of Cancer Prevention Volume 14: Tobacco Control: Effectiveness of Tax and Price Policies for Tobacco Control.* Lyon: World Health Organization; 2011.
27. Hellowell M, Smith KE, Wright A. Hard to avoid but difficult to sustain: Scotland's innovative health tax on large retailers selling tobacco and alcohol. *Milbank Quarterly.* 2016; 94: 800–831.
28. Bodker M, Pisinger C, Toft U, Jorgensen T. The rise and fall of the world's first fat tax. *Health Policy.* 2015; 119: 737–742.
29. Vallgårda S, Holm L, Jensen JD. The Danish tax on saturated fat: Why it did not survive. *European Journal of Clinical Nutrition.* 2015; 69: 223–226.
30. Marriott R, Price Dillard J. Sweet talk for voters: A survey of persuasive messaging in ten U. S. sugar-sweetened beverage tax referendums. *Critical Public Health.* 2021; 31(4): 477–486.

31. Alsukait R, Bleich S, Wilde P, Singh G, Folta S. Sugary drink excise tax policy process and implementation: Case study from Saudi Arabia. *Food Policy.* 2020; 90: 101789.
32. Tamir O, Cohen-Yogev T, Furman-Assaf S, et al. Taxation of sugar sweetened beverages and unhealthy foods: A qualitative study of key opinion leaders' views. *Israel Journal of Health Policy Research.* 2018; 7: 43.
33. Ramirez RL, Jernigan DH. Increasing alcohol taxes: analysis of case studies from Illinois, Maryland, and Massachusetts. *Journal of Studies on Alcohol and Drugs.* 2017; 78(5): 763–769.
34. Stowers GN. Earmarking as a strategy against budgetary constraints: San Francisco's Children's Amendment. *Public Budgeting & Finance.* 1995; 15: 68–85.
35. Thow AM, Downs SM, Mayes C, Trevena H, Waqanivalu T, Cawley J. Fiscal policy to improve diets and prevent non-communicable diseases: From recommendations to action. *Bulletin of the World Health Organization.* 2018; 96(3): 201–210.
36. Jou J, Niederdeppe J, Barry CL, Gollust SE. Strategic messaging to promote taxation of sugar-sweetened beverages: Lessons from recent political campaigns. *American Journal of Public Health.* 2014; 104(5): 847–853.
37. Thow AM, Quested C, Juventin L, Kun R, Khan AN, Swinburn B. Taxing soft drinks in the Pacific: implementation lessons for improving health. *Health Promotion International.* 2011; 26: 55–64.
38. Balbach ED, Traynor MP, Glantz SA. The implementation of California's tobacco tax initiative: The critical role of outsider strategies in protecting proposition 99. *Journal of Health Politics, Policy and Law.* 2000; 25: 689–715.
39. Begay ME, Traynor M, Glantz SA. The tobacco industry, state-politics, and tobacco education in California. *American Journal of Public Health.* 1993; 83: 1214–1221.
40. Traynor MP, Glantz SA. California's tobacco tax initiative: The development and passage of Proposition 99. *Journal of Health Politics, Policy and Law.* 1996; 21: 543–585.
41. Collin J, Lee K, Gilmore AB. Unlocking the corporate documents of British American Tobacco: An invaluable global resource needs radically improved access. *Lancet.* 2004; 363: 1746–1747.
42. Du M, Tugendhaft A, Erzse A, Hofman KJ. Sugar-sweetened beverage taxes: Industry response and tactics. *The Yale Journal of Biology and Medicine,* 2018; 91(2): 185–190.
43. Julia C, Méjean C, Vicari F, Péneau S, Hercberg S. Public perception and characteristics related to acceptance of the sugar-sweetened beverage taxation launched in France in 2012. *Public Health Nutrition.* 2015; 18: 2679–2688.
44. Somerville C, Marteau TM, Kinmonth AL, Cohn S. Public attitudes towards pricing policies to change health-related behaviours: A UK focus group study. *European Journal of Public Health.* 2015; 25: 1058–64.

https://doi.org/10.1142/9781800612396_0013

Chapter 10

Monitoring and Measuring Health Taxes

Rosa Carolina Sandoval*, Maxime Roche*, Anne-Marie Perucic†, Miriam Alvarado‡, Itziar Belausteguigoitia§, Luis Galicia¶, and Guillermo Paraje||

We draw from the well-established global monitoring of tobacco taxes by the World Health Organization and provide a proposed similar approach to develop new – or adapt existing – monitoring tools for taxes on alcoholic beverages and sugar-sweetened beverages (SSBs). Since 2008, the periodical and global monitoring of tobacco tax levels, prices, affordability and additional tax structure and tax administration information has enabled standardised comparisons across countries and over time, informed policymaking and institutional opportunities or barriers to apply tobacco taxes, led to defining best practices in the design of such taxes, and provided powerful tools for advocacy, especially with ministries of finance to promote fiscal and health policy coherence. Monitoring taxes on alcoholic beverages and SSBs

* Pan American Health Organization, USA.

† World Health Organization, Switzerland.

‡ University of Cambridge, UK.

§ University of Lancaster, UK.

¶ Ministry of Health of Uruguay, Uruguay.

|| Universidad Adolfo Ibáñez, Chile.

in a similar way would require adjusting the methodology used to monitor taxes on tobacco products to the unique characteristics of these beverages – namely the fact that these products are more diverse than tobacco products in terms of product types consumed, and in volume sizes and content. In addition to collecting data on the tax structure, tax rates, tax bases and nominal retail prices on several different beverage types, monitoring taxes on alcoholic beverages and SSBs would require information on beverage volume sizes and sugar content and alcohol concentration. A balance would need to be reached between characterising the diversity of global or regional consumption patterns, ensuring the standardisation and precision of the indicators, and limiting the data requirements from national authorities. While institutional considerations are to be considered in expanding the global routine monitoring systems for taxes on alcoholic beverages and SSBs, there are lessons to be learned and potential synergies from the experience monitoring tobacco taxes. The successful monitoring of taxes applied on these three unhealthy products would play a great role in promoting global action and driving progress to reduce the burden of non-communicable diseases.

10.1. WHO mandates and the importance of monitoring and measuring health taxes

Non-communicable diseases (NCDs) – mainly cardiovascular diseases, cancers, chronic respiratory diseases, and diabetes – are the biggest cause of death worldwide. More than 40 million people die annually from NCDs (71% of global deaths), including 15 million people who die prematurely before the age of 70. More than 85% of these premature deaths occur in low- and middle-income countries and could have largely been prevented.[1] Worldwide, the cost of the four main NCDs has been estimated to be USD 3.8 trillion in 2010 and is projected to increase to USD 7 trillion by 2030.[2] Most NCDs are linked to four common risk factors, namely tobacco use, harmful use of alcohol, unhealthy diet and physical inactivity.

To strengthen national efforts to address the burden of NCDs, the 66th World Health Assembly – the decision-making body of the WHO comprised of delegations from all WHO Member States – endorsed the WHO Global Action Plan for the Prevention and Control of NCDs 2013–2020 (WHO Global Action Plan). The WHO Global Action Plan recognises the critical importance of reducing the levels of exposure of individuals and populations to common risk factors of NCDs. It provides a menu of policy options, which includes increasing excise taxes on tobacco products and alcoholic beverages, identifying them as part of the NCD 'best-buy' interventions[a] – most cost-effective and feasible interventions to implement to prevent and control NCDs.[3] In addition, in 2017, the 70th World Health Assembly endorsed the Updated Appendix 3 of the WHO Global Action Plan including 'reducing sugar consumption through effective taxation on sugar-sweetened beverages (SSBs)'[b] as a cost-effective intervention in its menu of recommended policy options.[4]

The consumption of tobacco, alcoholic beverages and SSBs has been shown to be associated with increases in the incidence of NCDs, which in turn lead to increased medical costs, loss of productivity and other negative health-related and social costs – that is, externalities.[5] Excise taxes allow policymakers to target and raise the relative price of selected products, making them less affordable than other goods and services in the economy in order to discourage their purchase. The rationale and empirical evidence in support of introducing or increasing excise taxes on tobacco, alcoholic beverages and SSBs have been well documented.[6–9] Introducing or increasing excise taxes on these products, if substantial enough, is an effective intervention that can contribute to correcting the above-mentioned

---

[a] The 16 interventions considered by WHO, in the Updated Appendix 3 of the WHO Global Action Plan, to be NCD 'best-buy' interventions were those with an average cost-effectiveness ratio of ≤ I$100/DALY averted in low- and lower-middle-income countries. Source: https://apps.who.int/iris/bitstream/handle/10665/259232/WHO-NMH-NVI-17.9-eng.pdf.

[b] Sugar-sweetened beverages include all types of beverages containing free sugars, such as carbonated or non-carbonated soft drinks, fruit or vegetable juices and drinks, liquid and powder concentrates, flavoured water, energy and isotonic drinks, ready-to-drink tea, ready-to-drink coffee and flavoured milk drinks. Source: https://www.who.int/news-room/fact-sheets/detail/healthy-diet.

externalities. It has been described as a triple win for governments, as it (1) improves population health, (2) has the potential to reduce long-term healthcare costs and (3) generates revenue.[5]

In order to drive progress in the prevention of NCDs and provide the foundation for advocacy, raising awareness, reinforcing political commitment and promoting global action to tackle these deadly diseases, it is important to monitor effective prevention policies such as health taxes. Indeed, such monitoring can play a critical role in ensuring that policy-making is informed and fostering the effective design and implementation of health taxes. Monitoring is key to the WHO to provide technical cooperation to its Member States.

Although the WHO monitors tobacco taxes, prices and affordability with standardised quantitative indicators calculated every other year starting 2008 for all WHO Member States, comparable measures for alcoholic beverages and SSBs are not available.[10,11] Developing such indicators, as well as complementary qualitative tax structure and tax administration indicators, is necessary to monitor effective tax policies recommended in the WHO Global Action Plan, as well as for analysing trends, establishing best practices and helping countries achieve both the WHO Global Action Plan and the United Nations (UN) Sustainable Development Goals targets.

Consequently, there are lessons to be learned from monitoring tobacco taxation that could be applied to alcoholic beverages and SSBs. Indeed, the experience of measuring and monitoring tobacco tax levels, prices, affordability and additional tax structure and tax administration information has highlighted the following benefits:

(a) allowing to characterise prices, affordability, the tax structure, the tax administration and existing levels of excise taxation in a way that can inform institutional opportunities or barriers to apply excise taxes with a health rationale;
(b) enabling standardised comparisons across countries and over time;

(c) establishing best practices in the design of health taxes and a benchmark level for policy implementation;
(d) providing powerful tools for advocacy, especially with ministries of finance.

This chapter intends to draw lessons from WHO tobacco taxes measuring and monitoring and aims to provide a proposed similar approach to measure and monitor taxes applied to alcoholic beverages and SSBs. To meet these goals, the chapter starts by describing the current WHO global monitoring framework of health taxes and its governance (Section 10.2). Afterwards, it moves to its core by discussing the importance of counting with a standardised and comparable indicator to measure the level of taxation applied to tobacco products and the lessons learned from this experience to develop such indicator for alcoholic beverages and SSBs (Section 10.3). Following a similar structure, it then details other price, affordability and tax structure and tax administration indicators currently monitored for tobacco products and the relevance of collecting and reporting similar information for alcoholic beverages and SSBs (Section 10.4). Finally, the chapter closes with institutional considerations (Section 10.5) and a general conclusion (Section 10.6).

10.2. WHO current global monitoring of health taxes

Following the Political Declaration on NCDs adopted by the 2011 UN General Assembly,[c] the WHO developed the Global Monitoring Framework on NCDs. Adopted by the 66th World Health Assembly in 2013, as part of the WHO Global Action Plan, it tracks and reports progress on the attainment of 9 selected global targets and 25 indicators aimed to prevent and control the four main NCDs (NCD4), requiring the implementation of actions against

[c] Resolution A/RES/66/2 available at: https://digitallibrary.un.org/record/720106?ln=en.

the common risk factors for NCD4 (tobacco use, harmful use of alcohol, insufficient physical activity, unhealthy diet) and strengthening national health system responses.[d]

The nine targets particularly include a relative reduction of 30% of tobacco use, 10% of harmful use of alcohol, and no increase in diabetes and obesity. The 25 indicators measure the attainment of these targets in terms of mortality and morbidity, NCD risk factors prevalence and national health system responses. It is expected that by reaching these targets a decrease on the premature mortality on NCD4 could be reflected.

The WHO Non-communicable Diseases Progress Monitor was developed in response to the request made by the 2014 UN General Assembly[e] to complement the WHO Global Monitoring Framework on NCDs by tracking the implementation of the measures included in the WHO Global Action Plan, particularly the 'best buy' interventions to reduce risk factors for NCDs, which include increasing excise taxes on tobacco products and alcoholic beverages but initially did not include SSBs. It assesses country-level progress through a consistent and standardised monitoring.[12]

Regarding tobacco products, the implementation of measures to reduce their affordability by increasing excise taxes and prices are tracked via indicator 5A. It monitors tobacco taxes through a standardised tax share indicator, which is comparable across countries and over time, for all WHO Member States. This indicator is calculated every two years for the production of the *WHO Report on the Global Tobacco Epidemic* (also known as Global Tobacco Control Report and hereafter referred to as GTCR),[13] which, among other tobacco control policies, monitors taxes in line with Article 6 of the WHO Framework Convention on Tobacco Control establishing that price and tax measures are an effective and important means of reducing tobacco consumption. The tobacco tax share indicator

---

[d] Source: https://www.who.int/teams/ncds/surveillance/monitoring-capacity/gmf.

[e] Resolution A/RES/68/300 available at: https://documents-dds-ny.un.org/doc/UNDOC/GEN/N13/457/45/PDF/N1345745.pdf?OpenElement.

represents the proportion of the final retail price of a 20-cigarette pack of the most sold brand corresponding to indirect taxes (value-added tax (VAT) or sales taxes, excise taxes, import duties and other indirect taxes levied). Indicator 5A is considered fully achieved if a country's tobacco tax share indicator is above 75%.

In comparison, excise taxes on alcoholic beverages are monitored through qualitative characteristics, where indicator 6C of the WHO Non-communicable Diseases Progress Monitor is considered fully achieved if excise taxes on the three main types of alcoholic beverages (beer, wine and spirits) are implemented, no tax incentives or rebates for production of alcoholic beverages are applied and an adjustment for inflation of the level of taxation is implemented.[12] The source for indicator 6C is the WHO Global survey on progress on SDG health target 3.5.[14]

In the case of SSB excise taxes, while they represent an effective intervention to prevent NCDs, the measure was not initially added to the list of 'best buys' interventions in the WHO Global Action Plan when it was approved in 2013, and therefore, not included in the WHO Non-communicable Diseases Progress Monitor. It was, however, later added to the menu of policy options in Appendix 3 of the WHO Global Action Plan approved in 2017, when this one was updated in preparation to the third UN High-level Meeting on NCDs in order to take into consideration the emergence of new evidence of cost-effectiveness and the issuance of new WHO recommendations.[4]

Table 10.1 displays the current status of WHO global monitoring tools for taxes on tobacco, alcoholic beverages and SSBs.

In the case of alcoholic beverages, tax data are collected through the WHO Global survey on progress on SDG health target 3.5, which tracks alcohol consumption, monitoring and policy responses. This instrument collects partial information on taxes applied to alcoholic beverages but does not collect information on nominal prices or tax bases. The data collected allow for describing the type of taxes applied to alcoholic beverages and obtaining limited tax policy information on whether amount-specific

Table 10.1. Current WHO global tobacco, alcohol and SSB tax policy monitoring tools.

	Tobacco	Alcohol	SSB
Tool / Information collected	**WHO Rreport on the Global Tobacco Epidemic:** tracks implementation of MPOWER tobacco control measures	**WHO Global Survey on Progress on SDG Health Target 3.5:** tracks consumption, monitoring and policy responses	**WHO Global Nutrition Policy Review:** tracks implementation of nutrition policies and programmes **WHO NCD Country Capacity Survey:** tracks implementation of the WHO Global Action Plan
Ask whether taxes are applied to these products	Yes	Yes	Yes
Collect information establishing types of taxes applied	Yes	Yes	No
Collect information on tax rates and base	Yes	No (only on rates)	No
Collect information on tax legislation	Yes	Yes	Yes
Collect information on nominal prices	Yes	No	No
Calculate a comparable and standardised tax share indicator (portion of the retail price accounted for by indirect taxes)	Yes	No	No
Calculate a comparable and standardised affordability indicator	Yes	No	No

Sources: Pan American Health Organization. Meeting report: 'Meeting to Develop a Standardised Tax Share Indicator for Alcoholic and Sugar-Sweetened Beverages', 24–25 July 2018, Washington D.C. Pan American Health Organization; 2019; World Health Organization. *Noncommunicable Diseases Progress Monitor 2020*. Geneva: World Health Organization; 2020.

excise taxes are adjusted regularly for inflation or another economic indicator, whether a minimum price policy is applied and whether any tax rebates or subsidies for the production of alcoholic beverages are applied. However, this survey instrument does not allow for the calculation of a standardised tax share or affordability indicator. The data and information collected are reported in the WHO Global status report on alcohol and health[15] and the WHO Global Information System on Alcohol and Health database.[f]

In the case of SSBs, the information collected does not allow for the calculation of a standardised tax share or affordability indicator. The WHO NCD Country Capacity Survey, which monitors country progress on their NCD commitments, asks WHO Member States whether they apply excise taxes on SSBs.[16] Tax data are also collected through the WHO Global Nutrition Policy Review Survey, which tracks the implementation of nutrition policies and programs.[17] Neither survey collects any information on nominal prices. Although both surveys ask respondents if excise taxes are applied on SSBs in their respective countries, they do not collect information on either the type, structure, base or rate of these taxes. Nevertheless, excise tax legislation in place in WHO Member States is collected and available through the WHO Global database on the Implementation of Nutrition Action repository.[g]

Existing global monitoring tools do not allow for tracking progress on tax policies in a comparable manner across the three groups of products. In order to effectively monitor tax policies on alcoholic beverages and SSBs, it will be necessary to develop new – or adapt existing – monitoring tools to collect information analogous to that collected for tobacco taxes, that is, (1) characteristics of the tax structure; (2) tax rates and bases; (3) nominal retail prices and (4) additional tax administration information.

---

[f] WHO Global Information System on Alcohol and Health (GISAH). Available from: https://www.who.int/data/gho/data/themes/global-information-system-on-alcohol-and-health.

[g] WHO Global database on the Implementation of Nutrition Action (GINA). Available from: https://www.who.int/nutrition/gina/en/.

10.3. Counting with a standardised tax share indicator

10.3.1. The tobacco experience

The implementation of tobacco taxes is tracked and published biennially in the GTCR as part of the monitoring framework of the MPOWER[h] tobacco policy package. Through this monitoring framework, the WHO tracks if countries apply taxes on tobacco products, the type of taxes applied, the base and rate of these taxes and additional tax structure and tax administration information. It also collects data on nominal prices of tobacco products and calculates a tax share indicator. This standardised indicator, defined as the share of indirect taxes (VAT or sales taxes, excise taxes, import duties and other indirect taxes) in the price of a 20-cigarette pack of the most sold brand, allows comparisons of levels of taxes across countries and over time. It has been calculated biennially since 2008, with data available for more than 185 countries.

In a simplistic way, the tobacco tax share indicator informs whether the price of cigarettes is comprised mostly by production costs and the manufacturer's or importer's and distributors' profits or by indirect taxes. Figure 10.1 provides an example of this decomposition of the price of cigarettes globally per income level. As of 2018, it shows that, globally, total taxes represent 60.8% of the final retail price of a 20-cigarette pack of the most sold brand, with great heterogeneity between countries' income groups. Along with prices, the share of total taxes and excise taxes in the price of cigarettes are higher in high-income countries.

---

[h] An acronym for six selected tobacco control interventions, each of which reflects one or more provisions of the WHO Framework Convention on Tobacco Control (WHO FCTC): Monitor tobacco use and prevention policies; Protect people from tobacco smoke; Offer help to quit tobacco use; Warn about the dangers of tobacco; Enforce bans on tobacco advertising, promotion, and sponsorship; and Raise taxes on tobacco.

Fig. 10.1. Weighted average retail price and taxation (excise and total shares) of the most sold brand of cigarettes, in 2018.

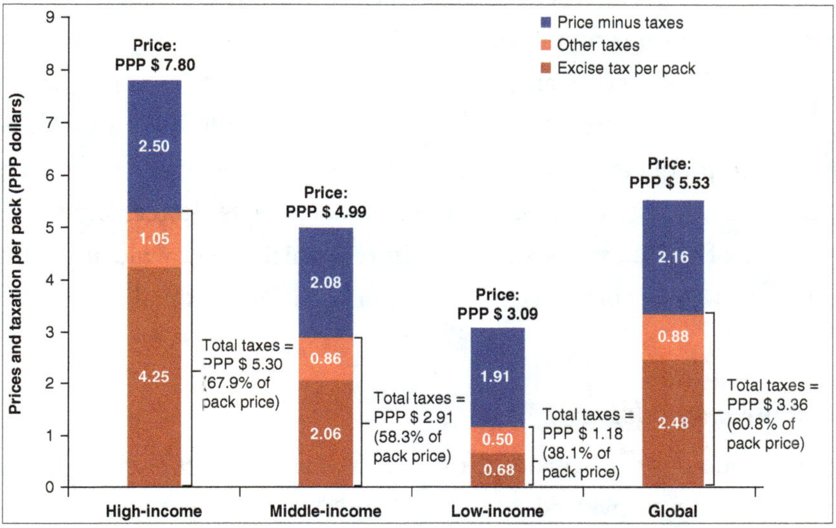

Source: World Health Organization. *WHO Report on the Global Tobacco Epidemic, 2019: Offer Help to Quit Tobacco Use.* Geneva: World Health Organization; 2019, p. 109.

Note: Averages are weighted by WHO estimates of number of current cigarette smokers ages 15+ in each country in 2017. Prices are expressed in Purchasing Power Parity (PPP) adjusted dollars (international dollars) to account for differences in purchasing power across countries. Based on 53 high-income, 97 middle-income and 28 low-income countries with data on prices of the most sold brand, excise and other taxes and PPP conversion factors.

Data collection

Data collection for the calculation of the tobacco tax share focuses mainly on cigarettes as the most consumed tobacco product globally. Nevertheless, other tobacco products are prevalent in certain parts of the world (such as bidis and smokeless tobacco in Bangladesh and India, shisha in the Eastern Mediterranean region, etc.) and studies have shown that substitution may occur between tobacco products type as a consequence of changes in taxes and prices.[18] Therefore, efforts are made by the WHO to collect tax and price information on other tobacco products.

In order to build the tobacco tax share indicator, the WHO collects data on prices and tax rates, bases and structures. The nominal price data collection involves ministries of finance and regional data collectors. Prices are collected for the most sold brands, which are identified using information collected in previous rounds of data collection, WHO's direct work with a number of ministries of finance on tax policy and secondary data from private data analytics providers. The tax data collected focus on indirect taxes levied on tobacco products and are collected through contact with ministries of finance and other sources, including tax law documents, decrees and official schedules of tax rates, bases and structures, which are downloaded from ministerial websites or from databases such as the IMF or the World Bank.[19]

A simple methodology

The methodology to calculate the tobacco tax share indicator is fairly simple and enables an intuitive understanding. It involves dividing the total amount of indirect taxes by the final retail price of a 20-cigarette pack of the most sold brand.[i] This methodology, developed by the WHO, is well-established and has successfully allowed the calculation of this indicator for all WHO Member States biennially since 2008.

Calculating the amount of VAT or sales tax and amount-specific excise taxes – type of excise taxes based on the quantity, weight, volume, sugar content or alcohol concentration of a product – to be paid on a pack of cigarettes is fairly straightforward. In most countries, the VAT rate is applied to the VAT-exclusive retail price and amount-specific excise taxes are defined per number of sticks of cigarettes (e.g. $0.10 per stick) or per kilogram.

On the other hand, calculating the amount of ad valorem excise taxes – type of excise taxes based on a percentage of the value of a product – is more challenging. Although ad valorem excise taxes on locally produced cigarettes are applied and statutorily reported as a percentage of a product's value, the base for this value (e.g. retail price, retail price excluding VAT or producer

---

[i] The tobacco tax indicator is defined as follows:

$$\text{Tobacco tax share} = \frac{\text{Excise taxes + Import duties + VAT or sales tax + Other indirect taxes}}{\text{Final retail price}}$$

price) may differ between countries, such that simply comparing reported statutory ad valorem excise tax rates between countries without taking into account the base on which they apply would lead to biased results. In the case of countries where the tax base is set early in the value chain, such as the producer price, when not provided by countries, the estimation of the tax base is not as straightforward and some assumptions have to be taken. To make things simple and intuitive, the WHO calculates the tax base assuming zero retailer's and wholesaler's profit margins (or mark-up) as these margins are assumed to be very small; this way, ad valorem excise taxes are not underestimated.[19] Country-specific information on these margins is rarely available.

In the case of imported cigarettes, ad valorem excise taxes are typically applied on a base that includes the CIF value[j] and, in most countries, import and custom duties, but not the importer's profit. Assuming the importer's profit margin to be zero would not be realistic and would overestimate the base, and, as a consequence, overestimate the amount of ad valorem excise taxes. Therefore, the WHO calculates the base either based on CIF value information provided by countries or using secondary sources such as the UN Comtrade database.[k] The amounts of import duties and other indirect taxes (other than excise, VAT and import duties), when not amount-specific, are calculated using the same methodology, either based on CIF value information provided by countries or using secondary sources.

While the methodology to calculate the tobacco tax share indicator is reasonably simple and the indicator can be calculated in a relatively short period of time – the process usually takes 8–12 months for all WHO Member States – it can be used to produce rich insights about the use of taxation as a tool to change prices and affordability and in turn consumption. More detail on this methodology can be found in Technical Note III of the GTCR.[19]

---

[j] Cost, Insurance, and Freight (CIF) value is the value of unloaded consignment paid by a seller to cover the costs, insurance, and freight against the possibility of loss or damage to a buyer's order while it is in transit. The CIF value is used in most countries as the base for import duties and ad valorem excise taxes on imported products.

[k] The United Nations Comtrade database is a global trade database providing exports and imports statistics by countries and harmonized tariff codes. Available from: https://comtrade.un.org/.

Lessons learned from the tobacco tax share indicator

An informative indicator

The tobacco tax share indicator – and another set of useful data and indicators described in Section 10.4 of this chapter – provides a baseline assessment of the current tobacco taxes in place. It has been proven to be a very useful tool to communicate the status of the implementation of tobacco taxes, their evolution and how they vary across countries. It has also been instrumental in substantially increasing the knowledge about different tobacco tax designs around the world and determining best practices.

The indicator informs WHO Member States how close they are to achieving the best-practice threshold on tobacco taxes established by the WHO (total indirect taxes accounting for at least 75% of the retail price[l]). It has also shed light into best practices in tax policy design to achieve the objective of making tobacco products less affordable and addressing the ultimate goal of reducing their consumption.

Each country's tax structure is analysed in order to calculate the indicator. As can be seen in Table 10.2, the tobacco tax share indicator is reported with granular information on each of its components: the specific excise tax share, the ad valorem excise tax share, the VAT or sales tax share, the import duties share and the other taxes share.

Below is an example of clear areas for improvement that could be identified from Table 10.2:

- There is an opportunity to improve tobacco tax structures. Indeed, while best practices indicate that amount-specific excise taxes are better positioned to increase prices and reduce the affordability of tobacco products,[20] Bangladesh and Vietnam only use ad valorem excise taxes and China, Egypt, Italy and Turkey have mixed excise tax systems mostly relying on ad valorem excise taxes.

[l] This percentage is the benchmark for application of the measure at the highest level regarding the implementation of the MPOWER tobacco control measures.

- There is an opportunity to increase tobacco taxes to further reduce affordability: Only Brazil, Egypt, Italy and Turkey, out of the 15 largest cigarette consuming countries (consumption in absolute terms), in 2018, have a total tobacco tax share higher than the 75% WHO threshold for application of the measure at the highest level.

Finally, Table 10.2 shows that some countries might have a high excise tax share (sum of the specific and ad valorem excise shares) or total tax share, such as Bangladesh, Brazil or the Philippines, but low prices, as compared in international dollars (at purchasing power parity). This demonstrates the importance to monitor other affordability and price indicators to better capture each country's situation regarding tobacco taxation.

A standardised and comparable indicator across countries and over time

Although additional data, such as on market share and consumption patterns (not provided by the GTCR or any other WHO database), prevalence (provided by the GTCR) and deeper economic analysis are needed to further capture each country's particular situation, the data provided by the GTCR serve as a key starting point and enable comparison of taxation policies across countries and over time. Such comparisons are made possible, in light of the heterogeneity of tax structures, by the use of a standardised methodology and the collection of tax and price data at the same point in time in all WHO Member States.

Even if in producing repeated iterations of the tobacco tax share indicator, there is an inherent tension between updating methods to reflect latest understanding or newly available data and maintaining comparability in methods over time, the methodology needs to remain standardised, consistent and transparent. Nevertheless, it is worth noting that the WHO not only updates data for the most recent year of the tobacco tax share biennially, but retrospective corrections are also made for past years if, during the time data are collected, mistakes or misreported information are discovered.

Table 10.2. Taxes and retail prices of the most sold brand of cigarettes in the 15 largest consuming countries (consumption in absolute terms), in 2018.

2018										
	Brand				Taxes as a % of Price of the Most Sold Brand					
Country	**In Reported Currency**	**Currency Reported***	**International Dollars (At Purchasing Power Parity)**	**In US$ at Official Exchange Rates**	**Specific Excise**	**Ad Valorem Excise**	**Value Added Tax/ Sales Tax**	**Import Duties**	**Other Taxes**	**Total Tax†**
Bangladesh	80.00	BDT	2.53	0.96	0.00%	56.00%	15.00%	0.00%	0.00%	**71.00%**
Brazil	5.00	BRL	2.45	1.33	30.00%	10.00%	32.00%	0.00%	10.97%	**82.97%**
China	14.07	CNY	4.02	2.06	1.14%	34.90%	13.79%	0.00%	5.90%	**55.73%**
Egypt	16.00	EGP	4.68	0.90	27.19%	50.00%	0.00%	0.00%	0.00%	**77.19%**
Germany	6.40	EUR	8.25	7.51	30.69%	21.69%	15.97%	0.00%	0.00%	**68.35%**
India	190.00	INR	10.51	2.77	28.92%	2.30%	21.88%	0.00%	0.95%	**54.04%**
Indonesia	26,250.00	IDR	6.21	1.82	49.45%	0.00%	9.10%	0.00%	0.00%	**58.55%**
Italy	5.50	EUR	7.49	6.45	7.01%	51.00%	18.03%	0.00%	0.00%	**76.04%**
Japan	440.00	JPY	4.45	3.97	55.65%	0.00%	7.41%	0.00%	0.00%	**63.06%**
Philippines	57.75	PHP	3.14	1.08	60.61%	0.00%	10.71%	0.00%	0.00%	**71.32%**
Republic of Korea	4,500.00	KRW	5.28	4.02	64.76%	0.00%	9.09%	0.00%	0.00%	**73.85%**
Russian Federation	125.00	RUB	5.31	1.99	27.49%	15.00%	15.25%	0.00%	0.00%	**57.74%**
Turkey	13.50	TRY	8.54	2.76	3.11%	63.00%	15.25%	0.00%	0.00%	**81.37%**
United States of America	6.86	USD	6.86	6.86	37.76%	0.00%	5.19%	0.00%	0.00%	**42.96%**
Vietnam	20,000.00	VND	2.57	0.87	0.00%	29.75%	6.97%	0.00%	0.00%	**36.72%**

*According to International Organization for Standardization, ISO 4217 currency names and code elements.

†Total tax includes excise taxes, import duties, value-added tax/sales tax and other taxes as applicable.

Source: World Health Organization. *WHO Report on the Global Tobacco Epidemic, 2019: Offer Help to Quit Tobacco Use*. Geneva: World Health Organization; 2019 (Appendix VII, Table 9.1).

A useful tool for advocacy

In general, excise taxes represent a relatively small percentage of total tax revenues. Ministries of finance tend not to be aware of how their tax structure and tax burden compare with other countries or that there is usually much room for excise tax design adjustments as to improve performance and contribute to fiscal and health goals. In this regard, the tobacco tax share indicator is an effective advocacy tool by allowing the monitoring of taxes over time and global, regional and cross-country comparisons.

For example, in Colombia, during a process aiming at increasing excise taxes on tobacco products in 2016, the Ministry of Health and Social Protection compared the tobacco tax share of Colombia with the regional average and the average in high income countries, and used this comparison to make the case and demonstrate that there was room for increasing excise taxes and contributing to health and development goals while having a sound fiscal policy.[21]

The WHO, as well as ministries of health and civil society organisations, has extensively used the tobacco tax share indicator when engaging with different sectors of government on tobacco tax policy to show where their country stood and how their tax policies could be improved. While improving the monitoring of the implementation of tobacco taxes, the tobacco tax share has also provided both policymakers and advocates with relevant arguments to push for tobacco tax increases at country level.

Limitations of the tobacco tax share indicator

In a lot of countries, national average nominal price data for cigarettes are not available and calculating such average nominal price for the purpose of the GTCR would represent an extensive data requirement. Instead, in these countries, price data are collected in one city, typically the capital or the largest city and might not be representative of cigarette prices nationwide. The WHO uses the price of the most sold brand to calculate the tax share indicator, representing the brand that has the highest share in the market at the time of data collection. However, in very few cases of highly competitive markets, this brand represents a share as low as 15%. To try and correct for this, the WHO also collects and reports the price of a premium (expensive) brand and the cheapest brand in an effort to reflect the different price bands available in each national market (see price dispersion indicator referred to in Section 10.4).

Considerations are to be taken into account when interpreting tobacco tax share changes over time. Indeed, changes in the tobacco tax share indicator are not only dependent on tax changes but also on price changes. Particularly, in a given country, the most sold brand 20-cigarette pack can change over time. When this occurs, it can affect the comparability of the tax share indicator over time.

In most countries, estimates of retailer's and wholesaler's profit margins are rarely available. The zero retailer's and wholesaler's profit margins assumption – taken by WHO to calculate ad valorem excise taxes on locally produced cigarettes if no estimate is provided by national authorities – may lead to an overestimation of ad valorem excise taxes for countries with a tax base defined earlier in the value chain, such as the producer price.

Finally, in the case of imported products, changes in the CIF value over time, either reported by countries or collected from secondary sources, can influence the estimation of the tax share indicator.

Key lessons learned

While the tobacco tax share indicator has several limitations as described previously, it enables to measure existing levels of taxation in a way that can inform institutional opportunities or barriers to apply tobacco taxes, as recommended by the WHO Global Action Plan and the article 6 of the WHO Framework Convention on Tobacco Control. In addition, it allows for establishing a benchmark level for policy implementation and represents a powerful tool to advocate for excise tax increases, especially with ministries of finance.

The estimation of the tobacco tax share requires only tax design information and nominal price data for a 20-cigarette pack of the most sold brand, which are collected biennially from national authorities. Its relatively simple and standardised methodology enables comparisons of the level of taxation applied to tobacco products across more than 185 countries and over time since 2008. Finally, this very informative indicator is key for establishing best practices in tobacco tax design to reach the ultimate goal of reducing the consumption of tobacco products.

10.3.2. Adapting the tax share methodology to the unique characteristics of alcoholic beverages and SSBs

The tobacco tax share experience shows that it is a very informative indicator, and that in order to develop such indicator, different steps are required: (1) developing a methodology to calculate such standardised indicator; (2) collecting tax legislation and price data; (3) analyse data and calculate estimates.

Lessons learned from the experience of monitoring tobacco taxes with a quantitative tax share indicator can be applied to the monitoring of taxes on alcoholic beverages and SSBs. Nevertheless, one facilitating factor in developing the tobacco tax share indicator is that it is calculated only for cigarettes as they represent the main tobacco product consumed in the world (as indicated in Section 10.3.1, some efforts are made by the WHO to collect similar information for other tobacco products that are prevalent in specific countries or regions but it is less extensive). Alcoholic beverages and SSBs are much more diverse, not only in terms of product types consumed, but also volume sizes and content. Hence, the development of tax share indicators for these products would require adapting the methodology to their unique characteristics.

Data collection

Due to the high diversity of alcoholic beverages and SSBs consumed, criteria need to be established to determine for which product types (and categories or brands) tax share indicators would be calculated. Criteria may include the following: (1) regional or global patterns of consumption,

(2) representativeness of the categories or brands selected and (3) price dispersion. It is important to note that it is impossible to collect data on all desired alcoholic beverages and SSBs when such an endeavour is undertaken to collect data for a large number of countries, therefore, some decisions have to be made to limit the information collected while taking into account consumption and market share trends. For example, while data collection for the tobacco tax share has historically been focusing mostly on cigarettes – and some other nationally or regionally prevalent conventional tobacco products – the recent introduction and increase in the consumption of heated tobacco products and electronic nicotine delivery systems are leading to new challenges in terms of additional data requirements. In GTCR 2019, for the first time, the WHO reported price and tax share estimates for heated tobacco products for a limited number of countries. Additionally, for future editions, the WHO is now collecting such data for electronic nicotine delivery systems.

As described in Chapter 3 of this book, in response to variations in taxes and prices, there is a potential for substitution within types of the taxed products (e.g. to cheaper brands) or products taxed at relatively low rates and to non-taxed products (some of which may also be harmful to health).[22,23] Assessing potential substitutions is crucial to inform tax policy design. A tax share indicator would need to be at least calculated for the three major types of alcoholic beverages: beer, wine and spirits. Regarding SSBs, such indicator would ideally be calculated for most types such as carbonated SSBs,[m] fruit juices,[n] fruit drinks,[o] sugar-sweetened milk drinks,[p] energy

---

[m] Carbonated SSBs are beverages that contain carbonated water, free sugars added by the manufacturer, and natural or artificial flavouring. A carbonated SSB may also contain caffeine, colourings, preservatives, and/or other ingredients; e.g. sodas.

[n] Fruit juices are beverages that contain naturally present free sugars, but do not contain any added sugars or sweetening material; e.g. 100% pure orange juice with no added sugar or sweetening ingredients.

[o] Fruit drinks are processed sugar-sweetened juices/nectars (<100%). They are beverages that contain water, unpasteurised or pasteurised juice, free sugars (both naturally present in fruit juices and fruit juice concentrates and added by the manufacturer), and may also contain artificial or natural flavourings, preservatives and/or additives; e.g. processed orange juice with added sugar.

[p] Milk-based SSBs are beverages that contain dairy milk, yogurt or kefir, including plant-based milk substitutes, and added sugars. They are usually flavoured and may also contain thickeners; e.g. strawberry-flavoured milk sold in a container.

drinks[q] and isotonic drinks.[r] In addition to the information collected to build the tax share indicator, information should also be collected on healthy substitutes such as non-sweetened milk and water to measure taxation, price and affordability contrasts.

As in the case of tobacco products, an average national price may be difficult to collect for most countries. Therefore, for each beverage type, the tax share indicator could be calculated on the most sold brand, identified using secondary data or information from ministries of finance. The price of the cheapest brand and/or a premium brand could also be collected to assess price dispersion.

In order to allow cross-country comparisons, a tax share indicator for a given beverage type needs to be calculated for the same volume size across countries. However, alcoholic beverages and SSBs are sold in different container volume sizes across countries. The selected volume size to be requested for each beverage type should be selected based on regional or global consumption and container size patterns. When the data collected differ from the requested volume size, there will be a need for standardisation. A linear transformation of prices could be assumed. However, usually, as the container volume size of a beverage increases, the price per millilitre of this beverage decreases. Therefore, although the standardisation of volumes allows for comparisons, it might alter the calculation of the tax share or other price and affordability indicators.

Finally, the calculation of tax share indicators for alcoholic beverages and SSBs requires to collect sugar content and alcohol concentration information for each beverage. Indeed, some excise taxes are based on this information. In addition, in the case of alcoholic beverages, this information is key to calculate indicators of prices per litre of pure alcohol and taxes per litre of pure alcohol that would allow comparisons between alcoholic beverage types but also across countries.

---

[q] Energy drinks are beverages that contain large amounts of caffeine, added sugars, other additives, and legal stimulants such as guarana, taurine, and L-carnitine.

[r] Isotonic drinks are beverages that contain water, minerals, and added sugars; e.g. sports drinks.

Methodology

The methodology to calculate tax share indicators for alcoholic beverages and SSBs can be adapted from the well-established WHO tobacco tax share methodology. Calculating the share of VAT or sales tax would follow the same methodology. Although the methodology would be the same for amount-specific excise taxes, it would also need to allow for amount-specific excise taxes based on beverage volume, sugar content or alcohol concentration.

In the case of ad valorem excise taxes for locally produced beverages with a tax base set early in the value chain, such as the producer price, the assumption of zero margins for retailers and wholesalers – taken by the WHO in the tobacco tax share methodology – may not hold for alcoholic beverages and SSBs. Indeed, distribution margins – retailers' and wholesaler's margins – are expected to be higher for alcoholic beverages and SSBs than for tobacco products due to the smaller tax burden applied on these products. Assuming distribution margins to be zero would overestimate the base for ad valorem excise taxes and in turn the amount of ad valorem excise taxes and the share of ad valorem excise taxes in the final retail price. On the other hand, there is a risk of underestimating the tax base by assuming high distribution margins in countries where the distribution of alcoholic beverages and SSBs is very competitive. Consequently, assumptions on distribution margins have to be made carefully and, as much as possible, based on available information and evidence. Applying the same non-zero distribution margins to all countries using a tax base set early in the value chain, such as the producer price, would allow for comparisons of excise tax share estimates among them. In addition, it would allow for fairer comparisons with countries using tax bases fixed later in the value chain – closer to the retail price, such as the retail price excluding VAT – as it would estimate a relatively higher tax base for these countries.

For imported alcoholic beverages and SSBs, as it is the case for the tobacco tax share, the share of ad valorem excise taxes, import duties and other indirect taxes would be calculated either based on CIF value information provided by countries or using secondary sources such as the UN Comtrade database. In the case of SSBs, some harmonised tariff codes do not differentiate between beverages containing added sugar or other sweetening matter (e.g. HS code 2009), reducing the precision in the CIF value data. However, in the case of alcoholic beverages, the collection of CIF value data would be facilitated by the fact that their harmonised tariff codes differ from non-alcoholic beverages and are defined per beverage type.[24] Finally, secondary sources, such as the UN Comtrade database, can sometimes present beverage traded volume data in kilograms, requiring taking into account beverages density[s] to obtain the CIF value per litre.[25]

Environment levies are sometimes applied to some beverages based on their container type (e.g. on cans or plastic bottles). In some countries, they work as a deposit that is refunded when the container is returned. Even in this case, since such levies can have an impact on the final retail price that consumers face, it would be interesting to account for their value in the calculation of the tax share. However, this would require the collection of information on the type of container for each beverage.

Finally, in following an adapted methodology from the tobacco tax share, tax share indicators for alcoholic beverages and SSBs would have the same limitations, in terms of price representativeness and caution in interpreting changes over time, as discussed in Section 10.3.1. Nevertheless, these tax share indicators would provide a baseline assessment of the current taxes in place on alcoholic beverages and SSBs and would represent very useful tools to communicate the status of the implementation of such taxes, their evolution and how they vary across countries. They would also be instrumental in defining best practices in terms of tax design and informing institutional opportunities to improve the health impact of taxes on alcoholic beverages and SSBs.

---

[s] Defined as the ratio of mass per unit volume. See the following source to obtain an estimation for each beverage type: Food and Agriculture Organization. INFOODS Databases. Density Database Version 2.0. Rome: Food and Agriculture Organization; 2012.

10.4. Other important indicators for the monitoring of health taxes

While a tax share indicator is an important measure, complementary affordability and price indicators and information on the structure and administration of health taxes is needed to effectively monitor them. This section presents the supplementary tax information collected and reported in the GTCR for tobacco products. It discusses the relevance of collecting and reporting similar information for alcoholic beverages and SSBs. Additionally, this section proposes an approach to adapt the data collection and definition of certain indicators to the unique characteristics of alcoholic beverages and SSBs, and identify additional relevant information to be collected and reported for the monitoring of taxes on these products.

10.4.1. Affordability and price indicators

From a public health perspective, the goal behind the use of fiscal policy instruments is to reduce the consumption of health harming products by increasing their prices and decreasing their affordability. Therefore, it is key to monitor prices and measure the affordability of tobacco products, alcoholic beverages and SSBs.

Affordability

In the GTCR, following previous work in the literature,[26] the WHO measures the affordability of cigarettes by calculating the share of per capita GDP required in each WHO Member State to purchase 100 packs of 20 cigarettes (2,000 cigarette sticks) of the most sold brand (GTCR Table 9.6).[13] Across countries, a higher value indicates that cigarettes are relatively more expensive in relation to income.

In 2017, a study used a similar indicator to analyse global trends in the affordability of SSBs, defining the indicator as the share of per capita GDP required to purchase 100 L of carbonated SSBs.[27] For SSBs, one affordability indicator per type of beverage could be defined. By standardising the volume to the same value for each beverage type, such as 100 L, it would allow cross-country and cross-beverage type comparisons of affordability levels. For alcoholic beverages, additionally, alcohol concentration would need to be standardised. This could lead to the definition of an affordability indicator per litre of pure alcohol, for example. However, such standardisation of volumes for alcoholic beverages and SSBs would require an assumption on the transformation of prices, leading to some limitations as previously discussed in Section 10.3.2.

Changes in affordability over time

Decreasing the affordability of health harming products – that is, increasing prices more than income during a given period – tends to discourage their consumption. Therefore, assessing changes in affordability over time is key to reflect the effectiveness of tax policies in a more comprehensive way. An indicator of affordability trend was introduced in the last editions of the GTCR. In 2019, it assessed whether cigarettes had become more affordable (meaning the affordability indicator decreased), less affordable (meaning the affordability indicator increased) or did not change significantly (meaning that the least square rate of change in the affordability indicator was not different from zero at the 5% significance level) between 2008 and 2018 (GTCR Table 9.6).[28]

Figure 10.2 shows global affordability trends of cigarettes between 2008 and 2018 by income group. Between 2008 and 2018, less than 35% of low- and middle-income countries saw cigarettes become less affordable, compared to over 65% of high-income countries. In addition, it is concerning to notice that in more than 20% of middle-income countries, cigarettes have actually become more affordable in the last decade.

Measuring affordability trends in alcoholic beverages and SSBs would be instrumental. Studies have found that the affordability of these products is increasing in most countries.[27,29–31] The same approach as the GTCR could be applied in the case of alcoholic beverages and SSBs. This would require the periodic monitoring of prices for these products.

Fig. 10.2. Change in affordability of cigarettes by income group, 2008–2018.

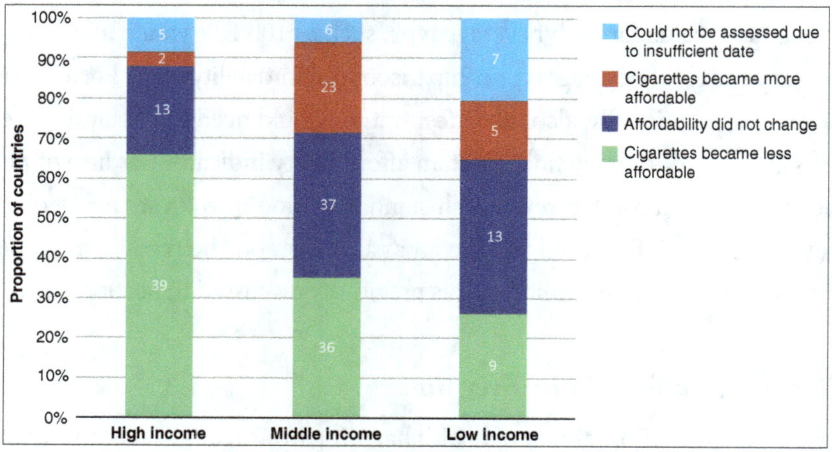

Source: World Health Organization. *WHO Report on the Global Tobacco Epidemic, 2019: Offer Help to Quit Tobacco Use*. Geneva: World Health Organization; 2019, p. 110.

Note: Changes in affordability are computed as the least squares rate of change in the per capita GDP required to purchase 2,000 cigarettes of the most sold brand in local currency in any given year. Please refer to Technical Note III of the GTCR for details of computation.

Nevertheless, measuring trends in affordability alone does not offer a complete assessment of the use of fiscal policy instruments to reduce affordability, as affordability of tobacco products, alcoholic beverages or SSBs can decrease due to reductions in income levels or increases in prices without any action taken by government authorities to increase taxes. Conversely, as the economic situation improves, as it is desired for any jurisdiction, the affordability of these products could increase, with its respective negative health consequences, highlighting the need for health taxes to be periodically increased. Therefore, it is key to analyse changes in affordability along with tax and price levels for a more comprehensive monitoring of tax policies.

Prices in international dollars at purchasing power parity and in US dollars

In order to compare prices of tobacco products across countries, the WHO converts them into international dollars adjusting for purchasing power parity. The international dollar is a hypothetical unit of currency that has the same purchasing power parity that the U.S. dollar had in the United States at a given point in time. Given that this currency is hypothetical, the GTCR also converts all prices from local currency unit to US dollars (GTCR Table 9.1).[13] However, prices in US dollars do not take into account differences in purchasing power between countries. Comparing both the affordability indicator and prices in international dollars or US dollars between countries is very useful when advocating before government authorities for increasing prices through the increase of excise taxes.

The same approach could be applied in the case of alcoholic beverages and SSBs. However, the comparison of alcoholic beverage and SSB prices across countries would require the standardisation of volumes. In addition, for alcoholic beverages, an indicator of prices per litre of pure alcohol and taxes per litre of pure alcohol, in international dollars adjusting for purchasing power parity, could be calculated to allow comparisons between alcoholic beverage types as well as across countries.

Price dispersion

Only analysing the price of the most sold brand or its affordability does not inform on the price and affordability of cheaper brands. In the GTCR, the WHO reports a price dispersion indicator, defined as the share of the final retail price of the cheapest brand in the final retail price of a premium brand (GTCR Table 9.2).[15] The smaller the gap between the two prices, the higher the value of the indicator.

The same approach could be applied to alcoholic beverages and SSBs defining one price dispersion indicator per type of beverage. This would require the collection of prices on at least two brands for each beverage type.

Price and tax share for other products

While cigarettes represent the main tobacco product consumed in the world, other tobacco products are prevalent in specific countries or regions. For this reason, the WHO collects prices and estimates the tax share for the most sold type of smoked tobacco product other than cigarettes (e.g. roll-your-own, cigars or bidis), smokeless tobacco product (e.g. chewing tobacco or dry snuff), and heated tobacco products. However, this information is only available for a small number of countries (GTCR Table 9.3).[13]

Alcoholic beverages and SSBs are more diverse in terms of product types. Given the high degree of possible substitutions, analysing differences in prices and taxes between beverage types is essential. Therefore, as indicated in Section 10.3.2, tax share indicators would need to be calculated for several types of alcoholic beverages and SSBs. However, it is important to note that decisions have to be made to limit the information collected and the burden on survey respondents and data collectors when such an endeavour is undertaken to collect data for a large number of countries. For the beverage types with low regional or global market shares, for which tax share indicators would not be calculated, only prices could be collected and reported to allow price and affordability comparisons, while reducing the data collection requirements. In addition, for non-alcoholic beverages, prices of healthy substitutes such as non-sweetened milk and water could also be collected, reported and their affordability compared to SSBs.

10.4.2. Tax structure indicators

In addition to the tax share, affordability and price indicators, many other aspects of health taxes need to be taken into account in order to effectively monitor them. In particular, as explained in Chapter 8, the structure of an excise tax has implications on its effectiveness in meeting the goal of reducing consumption. Monitoring tax structure information allows to assess health taxes design and the development of best practices.

Type of excise taxes applied

The GTCR reports the type of excise taxes applied on tobacco products in all WHO Member States. Excise taxes are either amount-specific, ad valorem, a mix of the two, or not applied to tobacco products (GTCR Table 9.5).[13]

Table 10.3 shows the diversity in the types of excise taxes applied on cigarettes across income groups and WHO regions. Tobacco taxation best practices recommend the use of amount-specific excise taxes.

In the case of alcoholic beverages and SSBs, in addition, some countries apply a combined excise tax structure, in which at least one beverage type is taxed by an ad valorem excise tax and at least one other beverage type is taxed by an amount-specific excise tax, but no beverage type is taxed by both. The WHO already collects information on the type of excise taxes applied on alcoholic beverages.[14] Similar information could also be collected

Table 10.3. The types of cigarette excise taxes applied by income group and WHO region, in 2018.

Excise tax systems on cigarettes					
By income group	Only amount-specific	Only ad valorem	Both amount-specific and ad valorem (mixed)	No excise	Total countries
High	16	6	29	4	55
Upper middle	21	10	19	6	56
Lower middle	19	10	13	2	44
Low	9	16	2	3	30
By WHO region					
AFR	13	23	7	1	44
AMR	17	8	7	1	33
EMR	3	5	6	7	21
EUR	10	2	39	0	51
SEAR	5	1	2	2	10
WPR	17	3	2	4	26
All countries*	**65**	**42**	**63**	**15**	**185**

*Countries for which data are available.

Source: Authors' calculations based on: World Health Organization. *WHO Report on the Global Tobacco Epidemic, 2019: Offer Help to Quit Tobacco Use*. Geneva: World Health Organization; 2019 (Appendix VII, Table 9.5). Updating: World Health Organization. Technical manual on tobacco tax administration. Geneva: World Health Organization; 2010 (Table 2, p. 35).

Note: AFR: African Region; AMR: Region of the Americas; EMR: Eastern Mediterranean Region; EUR: European Region; SEAR: South-East Asia Region; WPR: Western Pacific Region.

and reported for SSBs. Information for alcoholic beverages and SSBs could also further specify between volume-based and alcohol-content or sugar-content-based specific excise taxes.

Uniform versus tiered excise tax system

Excise taxes on tobacco products, alcoholic beverages and SSBs can either be applied using multiple tax rates – tiered design – as opposed to applying one single tax rate to all product types subject to the excise tax – uniform design. Tobacco taxation best practices recommend applying a uniform excise tax system to tobacco products.[20] The GTCR reports this information for excise taxes on tobacco products (GTCR Table 9.5).[13]

Similar information could also be collected and reported for alcoholic beverages and SSBs. For these products, tiered excise tax systems are most often defined by beverage type, harmonised tariff code or sugar content and alcohol concentration.

Minimum amount-specific excise tax policy

When ad valorem or mixed excise tax systems are applied, the use of a minimum amount-specific excise tax provides protection against products being undervalued. This type of policy is important to monitor as it forces unhealthy products prices up since they are not allowed to be lower than the amount-specific excise tax to be paid. The WHO monitors the use of minimum amount-specific excise taxes on tobacco products (GTCR Table 9.5).[13] This information could also be collected and reported for alcoholic beverages and SSBs.

Minimum price policy

While the introduction of a minimum price – or floor price – is pretty common to protect suppliers in agricultural product markets (e.g. in the

European Union), they can also be used to raise prices of unhealthy products to disincentivise their consumption. Therefore, it is important to track the implementation of such policy on tobacco products, alcoholic beverages and SSBs.

The WHO reports the countries that impose minimum prices on tobacco products (GTCR Table 9.5).[13] This information is also collected for alcoholic beverages.[14] While minimum price policies are not commonly applied on SSBs, there is ample literature on their effectiveness on alcoholic beverages prices and health outcomes.[32,33]

Retail price as base for ad valorem taxes on non-imported products

For ad valorem excise taxes, the tax base is defined as the value of the taxed product. A product's value may be assessed at different stages of the value chain. Tobacco and alcohol taxation best practices recommend fixing the tax base later in the value chain, closer to the final retail price. If the tax base for non-imported products is fixed earlier in the value chain, for example as the producer price, ad valorem tax rates are applied to a smaller base value, diminishing the impact of the excise tax on final retail prices.[20,23]

For countries applying ad valorem or mixed excise tax systems on tobacco products, the WHO reports if they apply ad valorem tax rates to the retail price or the retail price excluding the VAT for locally produced cigarettes (GTCR Table 9.5).[13] This information could also be collected and reported for locally produced alcoholic beverages and SSBs.

Automatic adjustment of amount-specific excise taxes

The real value of amount-specific excise taxes and their effectiveness in reducing consumption tend to diminish over time if they are not regularly adjusted to account for inflation and also, ideally, for income growth. For amount-specific and mixed excise tax systems applied on cigarettes, the

GTCR reports whether countries automatically adjust their amount-specific component for inflation or other economic indicators (GTCR Table 9.5).[13] This information is also collected and reported for excise taxes on alcoholic beverages.[15] It could also be collected and reported for SSBs.

10.4.3. Tax administration and other indicators

Information on tax administration, extracted from the legislation, can also provide complementary useful inputs to inform decision-making on taxation policies.

Tax stamps or fiscal marks and track and tracing systems

Tax stamps, fiscal marks, banderoles or other types of marking on tobacco products are recommended to ensure compliance with tax payment requirements. They are also useful to help administrators detect illicit tobacco products. It is recommended that countries implement such marking systems on tobacco products and use unique identifiers.[10] In the GTCR, the WHO reports whether countries have such systems in place. In addition, it reports countries using marking systems with additional features for tracking and tracing purposes (GTCR Table 9.5).[13]

This information is important to collect and report. Indeed, tax evasion offsets the impact of health taxes and is used as a common argument against the introduction or the increase of such taxes. However, the evidence shows that tax and price differentials are not the only factors explaining tax evasion. Corruption, lack of commitment to addressing illicit trade and ineffective customs and tax administration play an equal or greater role.[6] Finally, even in the presence of tax evasion, there are still significant public health and revenue benefits from health taxes.

The WHO collects and reports information on countries using duty-paid excise or tax stamps on alcoholic beverages.[15] Smuggling tobacco products or alcoholic beverages is more profitable than smuggling SSBs. Therefore, information on tax stamps and fiscal marks for SSBs is less important to collect as SSB tax avoidance and evasion is likely to be low.

Ban on sales of duty free

In most countries, tobacco products and alcoholic beverages are sold without taxes in duty-free shops in airports or other tax-free shops for travellers going out or entering a country. In addition to increasing the risk that these products end up in the illicit market, duty-free sales incentivise the purchase of health harming products while the associated foregone taxes represent tax revenue losses for governments.

In the GTCR, the WHO reports if countries ban the sales of duty (or excise) free cigarettes (GTCR Table 9.5).[13] This information could also be collected and reported for alcoholic beverages.

Tax revenue

Excise taxes on tobacco products, alcoholic beverages and SSBs generate tax revenue. In the GTCR, the WHO collects and reports data on tax revenues from taxes applied on tobacco products. The data are disaggregated by types of indirect taxes and are reported in local currency unit (GTCR Table 8.1).[13] This information could also be collected and reported for alcoholic beverages and SSBs.

While data are not comparable between countries due to differences in tax structure, tax administration and local currency, reporting this information is useful to give a sense of the magnitude of the tax revenue collected through health taxes. Tax revenue data can be compared to estimations of the direct health care costs, indirect productivity losses and other social costs associated with the consumption of such health harming products in order to advocate for excise tax increases.

Earmarking

Although their participation in total national fiscal revenue can be small, tax revenue from excise taxes on tobacco products, alcoholic beverages and SSBs can constitute a source of stable and readily available funds,[34] which could be used, for example, to attend emergencies such as health emergencies or natural disasters.[t]

---

[t] Among many examples, there is the case of Chile, which after a devastating earthquake in 2010, increased tobacco taxes with the explicit objective of raising revenue for the country

The UN Third International Conference on Financing for Development identified tobacco excise taxes as a revenue stream for financing the post-2015 Sustainable Development Goals.[35] In some cases, these taxes can represent substantial sources of revenues, such as in the Philippines where, following a major tax reform in 2012, earmarked excise taxes on tobacco products and alcoholic beverages contributed substantially to expand the country's Universal Health Care Programme coverage to millions of additional poor members.[36]

Some countries dedicate tax revenues from excise taxes on unhealthy products to the prevention of NCDs or other health programmes. This can serve as one way of partially correcting the negative economic and social externalities of the consumption of these products. In the GTCR, the WHO reports the countries that earmark tobacco taxes to fund specific tobacco control or health programmes (GTCR Table 9.4).[13] This information could also be collected and reported for alcoholic beverages and SSBs. Currently, the WHO NCD Country Capacity Survey collects information on whether countries earmark excise taxes on unhealthy products for health promotion or health service provision.[16] However, it gives no detail on whether excise taxes on all three groups of products are earmarked or if only excise taxes on one of these unhealthy products are earmarked.

10.4.4. Additional indicators to monitor taxes on alcoholic beverages and SSBs

Since alcoholic beverages and SSBs vary in products type, size and sugar content or alcohol concentration, additional indicators than the ones used to monitor tobacco taxation are needed to better monitor taxes applied to these products.

Excise tax systems based on alcohol concentration

According to the WHO, excise taxes calculated based on alcohol concentration – that is, volume of ethanol – can have a greater impact on

reconstruction (see: https://lta.reuters.com/articulo/latinoamerica-economia-chile-reconstrucc-idLTASIE63F17620100417).

alcohol consumption, particularly in high income countries where alcohol consumption and the prevalence of current drinker tend to be higher. Indeed, they encourage the production of low ethanol content beverages and increase beverage prices per litre of pure alcohol.[23] Therefore, it is important to monitor whether countries use an excise tax system taxing alcoholic beverages based on their alcohol concentration.

Excise tax systems based on sugar content

According to the WHO, excise taxes calculated based on sugar content can have a greater impact on SSB consumption. Indeed, they create a tax burden differential between options based on sugar content within a product category. This can incentivise consumers to substitute to beverages with lower sugar content while simultaneously encouraging producers to reformulate their beverages.[22] Therefore, it is important to monitor whether countries use an excise tax system taxing SSBs based on their sugar content.

List of product types on which excise taxes apply

In the GTCR, a country is reported as applying an excise tax on tobacco products as long as the excise tax is applied at least on cigarettes. Information on whether the excise tax applies on other tobacco products is only reported for countries for which price and tax data for another type of tobacco products is reported by survey respondents and the tax share for this product is calculated.

Nevertheless, it is important to collect and report information on the list of product types taxed by excise taxes for alcoholic beverages and SSBs. Indeed, there is a higher diversity of product types across alcoholic beverages and SSBs than across tobacco products. For SSBs, for example, in addition to carbonated SSBs, it is important to assess whether the definition of taxable products includes energy drinks, fruit juices, fruit drinks, sugar-sweetened milk drinks, isotonic drinks, or powders, concentrates or syrups used to make SSBs by adding water or carbonated water, among others, to evaluate whether an excise tax is applied to a broad scope of SSBs or includes loopholes, incentivising undesirable substitutions and tax evasion. In addition, it is also important to identify if countries apply excise taxes on plain water bottles as this undermines the ability of excise taxes to incentivise consumers to switch from consuming SSBs to a healthier alternative.

Box 10.1. List of indicators and information that could be monitored for taxes on alcoholic beverages and SSBs based on the experience of tobacco tax monitoring

Tax share indicators

- Total tax share
- Excise tax share
- Total and excise tax share for other products than the most common product type (e.g. fruit juices, energy drinks)

Affordability and price indicators

- Affordability and affordability trend over time
- Prices in international dollars at purchasing power parity and US dollars
- Price dispersion
- Price of other products than the most sold brand of the most common product type (e.g. fruit juices, energy drinks) but also healthy substitutes (e.g. water bottles)

Tax structure indicators

- Type of excise tax system (e.g. amount-specific, ad valorem)
- Uniform versus tiered excise tax system
- Minimum amount-specific excise tax policy
- Minimum price policy

- Retail price as base for ad valorem taxes on non-imported products
- Automatic adjustment of amount-specific excise taxes

Tax administration and other indicators

- Tax stamps or fiscal marks and track and tracing systems
- Ban on sales of duty free
- Tax revenue
- Earmarking

Additional indicators to monitor taxes on alcoholic beverages and SSBs

- Excise tax systems based on alcohol concentration
- Excise tax systems based on sugar content
- List of product types on which excise taxes apply

Box 10.2. Developing tax share, price, affordability and tax structure and tax administration indicators to monitor SSB taxation in Latin America and the Caribbean

Since 2016, the Pan American Health Organization (PAHO), WHO Regional Office for the Americas, has been engaged in improving the understanding of the panorama of taxes applied on SSBs and developing tax share, price, affordability and tax structure and tax administration indicators in Latin America and the Caribbean. As part of this effort, PAHO developed a pilot methodology, which was discussed and validated with researchers and ministries of finance in 2018.[11] The methodology benefitted from their valuable inputs on how to adequately capture the intricacies, unique characteristics and regional consumption patterns of SSBs.

Following the validation of the methodology, PAHO conducted a comprehensive search and review of the tax legislation in place – collected through existing PAHO/WHO monitoring tools, secondary sources and surveying ministries of finance – to characterise the current excise taxes on SSBs in Latin America and the Caribbean. Out of the 33 PAHO/WHO Latin American and Caribbean Member States, the analysis found that 21 applied excise taxes on SSBs as of March 2019 (no information was available for Haiti). While this is promising, there is heterogeneity between subregions as most Caribbean countries do not impose such taxes. In addition, there is a high diversity in excise tax design in terms of tax structure, tax base or beverages taxed. Existing excise taxes could be further leveraged to improve their impact on population health and countries would benefit from additional guidance. Table 10.4 presents some of the results of this analysis.[37]

Simultaneously, PAHO implemented a survey using a questionnaire – modelled after the WHO GTCR Excel-based tax and price questionnaire for monitoring tobacco taxation – filled out by Ministry of Finance officials in charge of excise taxes in all PAHO/WHO Latin American and Caribbean Member States to collect price, volume, sugar content, and tax data on an internationally comparable brand of carbonated SSB, the cheapest brand of carbonated SSB and the most sold brand of fruit drink, fruit juice, sugar-sweetened milk drink, energy drink, isotonic drink, plain milk and plain water bottle.

Standardised tax share and price dispersion indicators were then calculated. Tax design and tax administration information was also analysed. Estimates have been calculated and validated by national authorities. PAHO expects to publish the results of this analysis in 2022.

Finally, in late 2020, PAHO launched a survey questionnaire in the Region of the Americas to collect price, volume, alcohol concentration and tax data on beer, wine and spirits – based on the WHO GTCR Excel-based tax and price questionnaire and building on its experience collecting such data for SSBs. PAHO has calculated preliminary tax share estimates, as well as other price indicators and tax design information, which have been sent for validation to national authorities.

10.5. Institutional considerations

The tax share and other tax, affordability and price indicators and the information on tax structure and tax administration reported in the GTCR contribute to tracking aspects of the implementation of tobacco taxes for all WHO Member States. Having similar indicators for alcoholic beverages and SSBs, for all WHO Member States, would allow the WHO to monitor the level of implementation of all three tax policies recommended by the WHO Global Action Plan. However, as it is the case for tobacco products, the collection of tax and price data for alcoholic beverages and SSBs needs to be part of a routine global monitoring system. Indeed, the added value of the tax share and all the other indicators previously described is not only to characterise the taxation of these products at a particular point in time but also to identify changes when comparing their value over time.

The routine global monitoring system used by the WHO for the biennial GTCR consists in tax and price data collection through contacts with ministries of finance and regional data collectors. The information is collected using an Excel-based questionnaire sent to national authorities. Once the tax share and other price and tax indicators are estimated and the other components of the MPOWER policy package are evaluated, every data point for which legislation was the source is assessed and validated independently by WHO Headquarters and the respective WHO Regional

Table 10.4. Summary of excise taxes on SSBs in Latin America and the Caribbean (based on legislation as of 31 March 2019).

	Countries	Tax structure	Applies on bottled water	Ad valorem tax base for locally produced beverages	Automatic adjustment of amount-specific tax for inflation or another economic indicator
Latin America	Argentina	Ad valorem	Yes	Retail price excluding VAT	–
	Bolivia (Plurinational State of)	Amount-specific	No	–	Yes
	Brazil	Ad valorem	No[d]	Producer price	–
	Chile	Ad valorem	No	Retail price excluding VAT	–
	Costa Rica	Amount-specific	Yes	–	Yes
	Ecuador	Combined[b]	No	Retail price excluding VAT and excise	Yes
	El Salvador	Ad valorem (Energy drinks mixed)[c]	No	Retail price excluding VAT and excise	No[f]
	Guatemala	Amount-specific	Yes	–	No
	Honduras	Amount-specific	No	–	Yes
	Mexico	Amount-specific (Energy drinks mixed)[c]	No	Producer price[e]	Yes
	Nicaragua	Ad valorem	Yes	Retail price	–
	Panama	Ad valorem	No	Retail price	–
	Paraguay	Ad valorem	No	Producer price	–
	Peru	Ad valorem	No	Retail price excluding VAT and excise	–
	Uruguay[a]	Amount-specific	Yes	Fixed tax base “precios fictos”	No[g]

Table 10.4. *(Continued)*

	Countries	Tax structure	Applies on bottled water	Ad valorem tax base for locally produced beverages	Automatic adjustment of amount-specific tax for inflation or another economic indicator
Caribbean	Barbados	Ad valorem	No	Producer price	_
	Belize	Amount-specific	Yes	_	No
	Dominica	Combined[b]	No	Producer price	No
	Saint Kitts and Nevis	Ad valorem	No	Retail price excluding VAT	_
	Saint Vincent and the Grenadines	Ad valorem	No	Retail price excluding VAT	_
	Suriname	Amount-specific	Yes	_	No

[a] Uruguay: The excise tax on SSBs is structured as an ad valorem tax applied on fixed tax base amounts – 'precios fictos' – per volume varying per beverage type, effectively operating as an amount-specific tax and classified as such in this analysis.

[b] Combined: At least one type of non-alcoholic beverage is taxed by an ad valorem excise tax and at least one other type is taxed by an amount-specific excise tax. No beverage type is taxed by both.

[c] Mixed: At least one type of non-alcoholic beverage is taxed by both an ad valorem excise tax and an amount-specific excise tax. In El Salvador and Mexico, only energy drinks are subject to a mixed excise tax structure.

[d] Brazil: Only non-aerated waters are exempted from excise taxes.

[e] Mexico: The ad valorem component applies only to energy drinks.

[f] El Salvador: The amount-specific component applies only to energy drinks.

[g] Uruguay: The fixed tax base amounts – 'precios fictos' – are usually adjusted annually, however, it is not mandated by law.

Source: Sandoval RC, Roche M, Belausteguigoitia I, Alvarado M, Galicia L, Gomes FS, Paraje G. Excise taxes on sugar-sweetened beverages in Latin America and the Caribbean. Revista Panamericana de Salud Pública. 2021 Apr 30; 45: e21.

Note: The following Latin American PAHO/WHO Member States do not apply excise taxes on SSBs: Colombia, Cuba, Dominican Republic and Venezuela (Bolivarian Republic of). The following Caribbean PAHO/WHO Member States do not apply excise taxes on SSBs: Antigua and Barbuda, Bahamas, Grenada, Guyana, Jamaica, Saint Lucia and Trinidad and Tobago. No information available for Haiti.

_ : Not applicable

Office. Finally, validated data for each country are sent to the respective national authorities for review and sign-off.[38] The process requires a close communication between ministries of finance which validate the information and estimations for tobacco taxes and prices – "R" component of the MPOWER policy package to be reported in the GTCR – and the ministries of health. While this demands cooperation from already significantly busy ministry of finance personnel, in general their response has been very positive and has motivated some to study further tobacco taxes and other excise taxes in their respective country or internationally.

Despite recent regional efforts in the European Region and the Region of the Americas,[11,39] as seen in Section 10.2, the routine global monitoring systems for taxes on alcoholic beverages and SSBs are yet to be expanded. The WHO GTCR Excel-based tax and price questionnaire could be adapted to collect similar tax and price data for alcoholic beverages and SSBs. Indeed, national authorities are used to the format of this questionnaire and have experience in responding to it since 2008. Building on the tobacco experience, the collection of tax and price data for alcoholic beverages and SSBs could follow similar processes and build on potential synergies from data collection, to the estimation of indicators, validation and sign-off by national authorities.

However, an institutional decision would be needed as to determine if two other similar questionnaires should be developed – adapting the GTCR Excel-based tax and price questionnaire for alcoholic beverages and SSBs – and incorporated along with the already existing global monitoring tools for alcoholic beverages and SSBs, or if only one comprehensive questionnaire should be sent to national authorities biennially to collect the data for all three products.

Finally, the tax share and other tax, affordability and price indicators and the information on tax structure and tax administration need to be analysed vis-à-vis consumption and prevalence information. The WHO collects and reports prevalence data for tobacco use and prevalence and consumption data for alcohol use.[13–15] While some studies have analysed the consumption of SSBs at country or global level, the WHO does not report on the consumption or prevalence of the use of SSBs.[40–42] Given that, from a public health perspective, the objective of the use of excise taxes on unhealthy products is to reduce their consumption, it would be crucial to better monitor it. However, considerations about consumption and prevalence go beyond the scope of this chapter.

10.6. Conclusion

Health taxes are cost-effective evidence-based NCD prevention policies that require consistent and standardised monitoring as to assess progress in their application at country level, establishing best practices and help countries achieve both the WHO Global Action Plan and the UN Sustainable Development Goals targets.

Since 2008, the WHO biennially monitors tobacco taxes through the calculation of quantitative standardised tax share, price and affordability indicators which are comparable across countries and over time for all WHO Member States, as well as reports tax structure and tax administration information. However, comparable measures are not available for taxes on alcoholic beverages and SSBs at the global level. Existing WHO global monitoring tools do not allow for tracking progress on tax policies in a comparable manner across these groups of products.

As described in this chapter, lessons learned from the experience in measuring and monitoring taxes on tobacco products stand out as applicable to alcoholic beverages and SSBs, particularly in regard to the benefits of developing standardised indicators measuring taxation levels, affordability and prices for alcoholic beverages. Developing such indicators would require the development of new global monitoring tools or the adaptation of existing ones in order to collect country-level information on tax structure, tax rates and bases, nominal retail prices, beverage volume sizes and sugar content and alcohol concentration. As it is the case for the monitoring of tobacco taxes, such monitoring should be systematic, periodic and expanded to all regions, and should involve national authorities – particularly ministries of finance.

Nevertheless, a balance is to be reached in applying the tobacco tax share relatively simple and consistent methodology to taxes on alcoholic beverages and SSBs between comparability among countries, clarity in an indicator and the precision of this indicator. Indeed, alcoholic beverages and SSBs have a wider product type and price variance, as well as more differences in product sizes and composition – in terms of sugar content or alcohol concentration. Consequently, there is a need for selecting the beverage types and standardised volume sizes of alcoholic beverages and SSBs for which such tax share indicator would be estimated, in light of the diversity of global or regional consumption patterns and as to inform on the possible substitution between beverage types or brands.

Other indicators on affordability and prices, and other information regarding the tax structure and tax administration – such as whether countries automatically adjust their amount-specific excise taxes periodically or whether they earmark excise tax revenues – would also need to be monitored in order to assess the multiple dimensions of taxation policies. For this additional information, it is also possible to build on and adapt the experience monitoring tobacco taxes to the unique characteristics of alcoholic beverages and SSBs.

It is essential to ensure that policymaking is informed by sound data to achieve key long-term objectives. While the proposed approach based on the experience of monitoring tobacco taxes has its own limitations – mostly due to data availability constraints and the need for standardisation to allow comparability between countries – it would allow to characterise prices, affordability, tax structure and tax administration and existing levels of taxation on alcoholic beverages and SSBs in a way that can inform institutional opportunities or barriers to apply excise taxes with a health rationale. It would allow the better identification of best practices in tax design and tax administration and facilitate WHO's technical support to governments on health taxes. Finally, by enabling comparisons across countries and time through standardised indicators, the routine monitoring of taxes applied on alcoholic beverages and SSBs would provide a powerful tool for advocacy, especially with ministries of finance to promote fiscal and health policy coherence.

Key messages

- Monitoring health taxes is essential in fostering the effective design and implementation of this cost-effective NCD prevention tool and to ensure that policymaking is informed.
- Since 2008, the WHO has been monitoring taxes applied on tobacco products via quantitative standardized tax share, prices, and affordability indicators, as well as other qualitative indicators on tax structure and tax administration.
- No comparable measures and information are currently monitored by the WHO for taxes applied on alcoholic beverages and sugar-sweetened beverages (SSBs).
- The experience of measuring and monitoring tobacco taxes, particularly the tobacco tax share indicator, has proven very useful in the communication of the status of the implementation of tobacco taxes, their evolution and how they vary across countries. It has also been instrumental in substantially increasing the knowledge about global tobacco tax designs and determining best practices, as well as establishing a benchmark level for policy implementation. It represents a powerful tool to advocate for excise tax increases, especially with ministries of finance.
- Learning from the experience of measuring and monitoring tobacco taxes, we propose a similar approach with an adapted methodology and additional indicators for monitoring taxes on alcoholic beverages and SSBs.
- Due to the higher diversity of alcoholic beverages and SSBs, institutional decisions are needed for the selection of product types and the frequency and tools for that monitoring.

References

1. World Health Organization. *Global Health Estimates 2016: Deaths by Cause, Age, Sex, by Country and by Region, 2000–2016*. Geneva: World Health Organization; 2017. https://www.who.int/healthinfo/global_burden_disease/estimates/en/index1.html (accessed 10 August 2019).
2. Bloom DE, Cafiero E, Jané-Llopis E, Abrahams-Gessel S, Bloom LR, Fathima S, Feigl AB, Gaziano T, Hamandi A, Mowafi M, O'Farrell D. *The Global Economic Burden of Noncommunicable Diseases*. Geneva: World Economic Forum; 2011. http://www3.weforum.org/docs/WEF_Harvard_HE_GlobalEconomicBurdenNonCommunicableDiseases_2011.pdf (accessed 10 August 2019).
3. World Health Organization. *Global Action Plan for the Prevention and Control of Noncommunicable Diseases 2013–2020*. Geneva: World Health Organization; 2013. https://www.who.int/publications/i/item/9789241506236 (accessed 10 August 2019).
4. World Health Organization. *Tackling NCDs: "Best Buys" and Other Recommended Interventions for the Prevention and Control of Noncommunicable Diseases*. Geneva: World Health Organization; 2017. http://apps.who.int/iris/bitstream/10665/259232/1/WHO-NMH-NVI-17.9-eng.pdf?ua=1 (accessed 10 August 2019).
5. World Health Organization. *Health Taxes: A Primer*. Geneva: World Health Organization; 2019. https://www.who.int/publications-detail/health-taxes-a-primer (accessed 20 December 2019).
6. U.S. National Cancer Institute and World Health Organization. *The Economics of Tobacco and Tobacco Control. National Cancer Institute Tobacco Control Monograph 21*. NIH Publication No. 16-CA-8029A. Bethesda, MD: National Cancer Institute; and Geneva: World Health Organization; 2016. https://cancercontrol.cancer.gov/brp/tcrb/monographs/21/ (accessed 10 August 2019).
7. Marquez PV, Moreno-Dodson B. *Tobacco Tax Reform at the Crossroads of Health and Development: A Multisectoral Perspective*. Technical report of the World Bank Group global tobacco control program. Washington DC: World Bank Group; 2017. https://elibrary.worldbank.org/doi/abs/10.1596/28494 (accessed 10 August 2019).
8. Wagenaar AC, Salois MJ, Komro KA. Effects of alcohol beverage price and tax levels on drinking: a meta-analysis of 1003 estimates from 112 studies. *Addiction*. 2009; 104(2): 179–190.
9. Task Force on Fiscal Policy for Health. Health Taxes to Save Lives: Employing Effective Excise Taxes on Tobacco, Alcohol, and Sugary Beverages. Chairs: Michael R. Bloomberg and Lawrence H. Summers. New York: Bloomberg Philanthropies; 2019. https://www.bbhub.io/dotorg/sites/2/2019/04/Health-Taxes-to-Save-Lives.pdf (accessed 20 October 2019).
10. World Health Organization. *WHO Report on the Global Tobacco Epidemic, 2008: The MPOWER Package*. Geneva: World Health Organization; 2008. https://apps.who.int/iris/handle/10665/43818 (accessed 12 August 2019).
11. Pan American Health Organization. Meeting report: "Meeting to Develop a Standardized Tax Share Indicator for Alcoholic and Sugar-Sweetened Beverages," 24–25 July 2018,

Washington D.C. Pan American Health Organization; 2019. http://iris.paho.org/xmlui/handle/123456789/51715 (accessed 20 November 2019).

12. World Health Organization. *Noncommunicable Diseases Progress Monitor 2020.* Geneva: World Health Organization; 2020. https://www.who.int/publications-detail/ncd-progress-monitor-2020 (accessed 12 February 2020).
13. World Health Organization. *WHO Report on the Global Tobacco Epidemic, 2019: Offer Help to Quit Tobacco Use.* Geneva: World Health Organization; 2019. https://apps.who.int/iris/bitstream/handle/10665/326043/9789241516204-eng.pdf?ua=1 (accessed 20 October 2019).
14. World Health Organization. *Global Survey on Progress on SDG Health Target 3.5.* Geneva: World Health Organization; 2019. https://www.who.int/health-topics/alcohol#tab=tab_1 (accessed 14 February 2020).
15. World Health Organization. *Global Status Report on Alcohol and Health.* Geneva: World Health Organization; 2018. http://apps.who.int/iris/bitstream/handle/10665/274603/9789241565639-eng.pdf?ua=1 (accessed 26 October 2019).
16. World Health Organization. *Assessing National Capacity for the Prevention and Control of Noncommunicable Diseases: Report of the 2019 Global Survey.* Geneva: World Health Organization; 2020. https://www.who.int/publications-detail/ncd-ccs-2019 (accessed 6 May 2020).
17. World Health Organization. *Global Nutrition Policy Review 2016–2017.* Geneva: World Health Organization; 2018. https://www.who.int/nutrition/publications/policies/global_nut_policyreview_2016-2017/en/ (accessed 21 November 2019).
18. Jawad M, Leet JT, Glantz S, Millett C. Price elasticity of demand for non-cigarette tobacco products: a systematic review and meta-analysis. *Tobacco Control.* 2018; 27(6): 689–695. http://dx.doi.org/10.1136/tobaccocontrol-2017-054056 (accessed 14 May 2020).
19. World Health Organization. *WHO Report on the Global Tobacco Epidemic, 2017: Monitoring Tobacco Use and Prevention Policies.* Geneva: World Health Organization; 2017. Technical Note III: Tobacco taxes in WHO Member States. http://apps.who.int/iris/bitstream/10665/255874/1/9789241512824-eng.pdf?ua=1&ua=1 (accessed 12 August 2019).
20. World Health Organization. WHO technical manual on tobacco tax policy and administration. Geneva: World Health Organization; 2021. https://www.who.int/publications/i/item/9789240019188 (accessed 14 May 2021).
21. Rodríguez AY, Araque A, Calderón LV, Franco C, Góngora P, Iunes R. Impuestos al tabaco. Bogota: Ministerio de Salud y Protección Social; 2016 June 30. https://ideas.repec.org/p/col/000504/014825.html (accessed 12 January 2020).
22. World Health Organization. *Fiscal Policies for Diet and the Prevention of Noncommunicable Diseases.* Technical meeting report, 5–6 May 2015. Geneva: World Health Organization; 2016. http://apps.who.int/iris/bitstream/10665/250131/1/9789241511247-eng.pdf?ua=1 (accessed 26 October 2019).

23. Sornpaisarn B, Shield KD, Österberg E, Rehm J. *Resource Tool on Alcohol Taxation and Pricing Policies.* Geneva: World Health Organization; 2017. https://www.who.int/publications/i/item/resource-tool-on-alcohol-taxation-and-pricing-policies (accessed 24 January 2020).
24. World Customs Organization. *HS Nomenclature 2017 edition.* Brussels: World Customs Organization; 2017. http://www.wcoomd.org/en/topics/nomenclature/instrument-and-tools/hs-nomenclature-2017-edition/hs-nomenclature-2017-edition.aspx (accessed 21 May 2020).
25. Food and Agriculture Organization. *INFOODS Databases. Density Database Version 2.0.* Rome: Food and Agriculture Organization; 2012. http://www.fao.org/3/ap815e/ap815e.pdf (accessed 18 May 2020).
26. Blecher EH, Van Walbeek CP. An international analysis of cigarette affordability. *Tobacco Control.* 2004; 13(4): 339–346.
27. Blecher E, Liber AC, Drope JM, Nguyen B, Stoklosa M. Global trends in the affordability of sugar-sweetened beverages, 1990–2016. *Preventing Chronic Disease.* 2017; 14.
28. World Health Organization. *WHO Report on the Global Tobacco Epidemic, 2019: Offer Help to Quit Tobacco Use.* Geneva: WHO; 2019. Technical Note III: Tobacco taxes in WHO Member States; 136–141. https://www.who.int/publications/i/item/9789241516204 (accessed 20 December 2019).
29. Rabinovich L, Brutscher PB, de Vries H, Tiessen J, Clift J, Reding A. *The Affordability of Alcoholic Beverages in the European Union.* UK: European Commission; RAND Corporation; 2009. http://citeseerx.ist.psu.edu/viewdoc/download?doi=10.1.1.183.3387&rep=rep1&type=pdf (accessed 15 May 2020).
30. Kan MY, Lau M. Comparing alcohol affordability in 65 cities worldwide. *Drug and Alcohol Review.* 2013; 32(1): 19–26.
31. Paraje G, Pincheira P. Affordability of beer and sugar-sweetened beverages in 15 Latin American countries. *Pan American Journal of Public Health.* 2018; 42: e49. https://pdfs.semanticscholar.org/ea4c/49e3ea15718061e5789888ec098c53a2e14d.pdf (accessed 15 May 2020).
32. Sheron N, Chilcott F, Matthews L, Challoner B, Thomas M. Impact of minimum price per unit of alcohol on patients with liver disease in the UK. *Clinical Medicine.* 2014; 14(4): 396. https://dx.doi.org/10.7861%2Fclinmedicine.14-4-396 (accessed 13 May 2020).
33. Stockwell T, Zhao J, Martin G, Macdonald S, Vallance K, Treno A, Ponicki W, Tu A, Buxton J. Minimum alcohol prices and outlet densities in British Columbia, Canada: estimated impacts on alcohol-attributable hospital admissions. *American Journal of Public Health.* 2013; 103(11): 2014–2020.
34. Cashin C, Sparkes S, Bloom D. *Earmarking for Health: From Theory to Practice.* Geneva: World Health Organization; 2017. https://www.who.int/publications-detail/earmarking-for-health (accessed 14 May 2020).

35. United Nations. *Addis Ababa Action Agenda of the Third International Conference on Financing for Development.* New York: United Nations; 2015. https://www.un.org/esa/ffd/wp-content/uploads/2015/08/AAAA_Outcome.pdf (accessed 14 May 2020).
36. World Health Organization. *WHO Report on the Global Tobacco Epidemic, 2015: Raising Taxes on Tobacco.* Geneva: World Health Organization; 2015. Higher tobacco taxes in the Philippines are a win-win for both health and revenues (p. 87). https://apps.who.int/iris/handle/10665/178574 (accessed 14 May 2020).
37. Sandoval RC, Roche M, Belausteguigoitia I, Alvarado M, Galicia L, Gomes FS, Paraje, G. Excise taxes on sugar-sweetened beverages in Latin America and the Caribbean. Revista Panamericana de Salud Pública. 2021 Apr 30;45:e21.
38. World Health Organization. *WHO Report on the Global Tobacco Epidemic, 2019: Offer Help to Quit Tobacco Use.* Geneva: WHO; 2019. Technical Note I: Evaluation of existing policies and compliance. https://apps.who.int/iris/bitstream/handle/10665/326043/9789241516204-eng.pdf?ua=1 (accessed 26 October 2019).
39. World Health Organization. Regional Office for Europe. Alcohol pricing in the WHO European Region. Update report on the evidence and recommended policy actions. Copenhagen: World Health Organization Regional Office for Europe; 2020. https://apps.who.int/iris/bitstream/handle/10665/336159/WHO-EURO-2020-1239-40989-55614-eng.pdf?sequence=1&isAllowed=y (accessed 14 May 2021).
40. Singh GM, Micha R, Khatibzadeh S, Shi P, Lim S, Andrews KG, Engell RE, Ezzati M, Mozaffarian D. Global Burden of Diseases Nutrition and Chronic Diseases Expert Group (NutriCoDE). Global, regional, and national consumption of sugar-sweetened beverages, fruit juices, and milk: a systematic assessment of beverage intake in 187 countries. *PLoS One.* 2015; 10(8): e0124845.
41. Barquera S, Hernandez-Barrera L, Tolentino ML, Espinosa J, Ng SW, Rivera JA, Popkin BM. Energy intake from beverages is increasing among Mexican adolescents and adults. *The Journal of Nutrition.* 2008; 138(12): 2454–2461.
42. Duffey KJ, Popkin BM. Shifts in patterns and consumption of beverages between 1965 and 2002. *Obesity.* 2007; 15(11): 2739–2747.

https://doi.org/10.1142/9781800612396_0014

Chapter 11

Health Taxes and Trade Law

Benn McGrady* **and Kritika Khanijo***

Multilateral, regional and bilateral agreements establish the rules governing international trade. This chapter examines the interplay between trade obligations and the rights states retain to impose domestic taxes for health purposes. Customs and monetary unions can establish very specific rules governing domestic taxation, such as through harmonised excise or sales taxes, or harmonised approaches to tax administration. These agreements set out the most detailed international obligations concerning health taxes, but are not described or compared in detail in this chapter as they are particularistic. This chapter focuses on World Trade Organization (WTO) law, which places relatively clear limits on the use of customs duties (whether used for health or other purposes) and establishes principles of non-discrimination. Disputes can arise where it is alleged that the effect of a tax measure discriminates against imported products as compared to domestic products. The case law as a whole suggests that even where a health tax has the effect of favouring domestic products, it may still be lawful under trade agreements, so long as that effect is justifiable in health terms. This will be the case, for example, where any differential treatment of product categories is justified by reference to differences in the risks they pose to health. This requires care in establishing the tax base and in setting tax rates to ensure

* World Health Organization, Switzerland.

that these are related to a health objective and justifiable by reference to that objective. Overall, international trade rules protect freedom to adopt and implement domestic tax measures for health purposes.

11.1. Introduction

The political economy of taxation is shaped by political incentives to seek political rewards for reducing taxes and to avoid political costs associated with increasing taxes. The policy problems created by this dynamic are sometimes also amplified by domestic legal structures as they allocate responsibility for taxation between the executive and legislative branches of government. A knock-on effect is that when introducing new taxes, governments sometimes attempt to guard against public backlash or shield special interests, including domestic firms. This can not only undermine achievement of any health objectives underpinning a fiscal policy, but depending on tax structure and design, raise questions of compliance with international trade agreements.

With tax policymakers (not trade lawyers) in mind, this chapter describes the relevance of international trade agreements to health taxes. Although states retain the right to regulate and tax for health purposes under trade agreements, and there have been relatively few trade disputes concerning health taxes, trade agreements do place limits on domestic fiscal policies, including taxes. These limits can play a negative role in the political economy of taxation, such as when industry invokes trade rules in attempting to discourage taxation. But, they can also play a positive role, such as if governments use trade agreements to shield themselves from special interests, or if agreements require minimum levels of health taxes to be implemented.

As the discussion below in the chapter illustrates, there are a number of things to know about the impacts of trade agreements on tax policy design.

First, international agreements governing customs harmonisation often underpin health taxes because they define customs codes that are then often used for purposes of defining categories of products subject to taxation.

Second, agreements governing customs and monetary unions sometimes establish minimum or maximum levels of excise or sales taxes on specific product categories and may also harmonise rules governing tax administration. These rules are specific to each agreement and a comparative analysis is beyond the scope of this chapter.

Third, trade agreements place upper limits on the imposition of customs duties (tariffs). So-called 'progressive liberalisation' (the making of new commitments under trade agreements) also means that those upper limits will generally be further reduced under future trade agreements. These factors, combined with the fact that customs duties are not well tailored to achieving health objectives (discussed below), creates a preference for taxes where health objectives are pursued.

Fourth, trade agreements discipline the use of subsidies on agricultural and non-agricultural goods either by prohibiting them, limiting them or by authorising trading partners to respond, such as through use of countervailing duties on imports. But subsidies are not the focus of this book and how trade agreements govern them is not therefore discussed in this chapter.

Fifth, trade agreements govern discriminatory taxes, such as taxes that favour domestic production. Article III:2 of the World Trade Organization's (WTO) General Agreement on Tariffs and Trade 1994 (hereinafter simply GATT) provides a good example. As a general rule, taxes that discriminate on their face (such as by applying only to imported goods) and taxes that discriminate through their effect (such as by falling heaviest on imports) are prohibited. Principles of non-discrimination are relevant to:

- Setting the tax base (whether 'like' imported and domestic products are taxed);
- Setting tax rates (whether graduated rates afford protection to domestic production);
- Policies seeking substitution (whether imported products are substituted with domestic products).

But, a tax with discriminatory effects might be justified under a health exception if:

- it pursues a health objective;
- there is sufficient evidence of the tax contributing to that health objective;
- distinctions drawn between imported and domestic products are legitimate (in terms of the health objective).

Principles of non-discrimination can also be relevant to tax administration, such as where administrative requirements differ in ways that favour domestic as compared to imported products. These differences can also be justified, however, where among other things necessary to secure compliance with tax laws.

These points, and the rules and disputes substantiating them are described in further detail below.

11.2. Domestic tax laws

Before describing trade law in further detail, it is worthwhile to describe what a health tax is and how that is reflected in domestic law. In the truest sense, a health tax is a tax that pursues a health objective. In a broader sense, taxes on health harming products such as tobacco, alcoholic beverages and sugary drinks might be considered health taxes even if not explicitly pursuing a health objective. For a detailed discussion on the role of health taxes and their revenue raising capacity, please refer to Chapter 2 of this book.

The elements of health tax will be similar even if there are differences in design or purpose. For example, a typical excise tax law (the combination of legislation and any regulation), will set out:

- The grant of powers to the executive branch of government
- Detailed provisions defining liability for a tax, including at a minimum:
    - Territorial scope
    - Excisable goods
    - Tax rates
    - Methods of calculation

    - Definitions of taxable events (such as upon sale or transfer of goods)
    - Tax suspension arrangements
    - Specific rules governing products for export
    - Reporting
    - Indexation
    - Stamps
    - Earmarking
- Tax collection and administration, including at a minimum:
    - Movement of excise goods
    - Procedural rules for free zones and duty-free shops
    - Licencing and/or registration for importation, production, holding goods (such as tax warehousing) and tax suspension
    - Refunds
    - Control and inspection
    - Evasion and penalties
    - Disputes

In legal terms, this illustrates that health taxes have many elements. The design of elements of a domestic tax might be influenced by specific rules governing customs valuation under WTO law, or tax administration under regional commitments. But as foreshadowed above, they might also be shaped by principles of non-discrimination, such as when determining the tax base, tax rates or when designing taxes with substitution in mind. In this context, it is important to understand how excisable goods (what falls within and outside the scope of a tax) are typically defined.

First, an excise tax law may define excisable goods by reference to harmonised product nomenclature developed by the World Customs Organization (WCO), often referred to as the Harmonized System Code or HS Code. In line with the International Convention on the Harmonized Commodity Description and Coding System, customs authorities use the HS Code for purposes of developing national customs codes that categorise products based on their characteristics. These national customs codes facilitate customs declarations, the levying of customs duties and, by extension, commitments with respect to upper limits on customs duties under trade agreements. Most importantly, customs codes distinguish between product categories based on characteristics other than the risks posed to health. Where health goals are pursued, this can limit the usefulness of customs codes for purposes of defining excisable goods or for establishing tiered excise taxes within a product category.

Some excise tax laws may define excisable goods without reference to the HS Code. This may be necessary where the HS Code does not distinguish between different product categories in a way that would facilitate achievement of the objectives of an excise tax. For example, if two product categories fall within a single customs heading and a government seeks to discourage consumption of one category, but not the other, one means of addressing this is to create a statutory definition of excisable goods separate from a national customs code. Another approach is to create more detailed sub-headings that separate the goods in question under the national customs code, but this option may not always be available, such as if a country has harmonised its customs code with others through a customs union.

The need for statutory definitions of excisable goods may also arise as a consequence of the emergence of new categories of products into a market. For example, in May 2019, the UK introduced an amendment to the Tobacco Products Duty Act 1979 to include a separate category of 'Tobacco products for heating' to maintain the effectiveness of the tobacco duty regime.[1] This pre-empted amendments to the HS Code to create sub-headings that will explicitly cover heated-tobacco-products, which will come into force in 2022.

Although the mechanics of defining excisable goods may seem banal, there are a few observations, including that:

- the HS Code, as well as any customs codes agreed as part of a customs union, can affect how excisable goods are defined if used in a tax law to define what is subject to taxation.
- these instruments need to be used cautiously in this context because they distinguish between product categories based on characteristics other than the risks posed to health.

For a detailed discussion about tax design considerations to maximise effectiveness of heath taxes, please refer to Chapter 8 of the book.

11.3. A brief word on customs and monetary unions

As is observable below, for the most-part, WTO law establishes a system of what is often referred to as 'negative integration'. By prohibiting and disciplining certain conduct WTO law creates a minimum level of economic integration. Many customs unions go beyond this to create a system of positive integration whereby national laws are harmonised to deepen economic integration. This can include some degree of harmonisation on excise and other taxes, which can have a substantial impact on the form that health taxes may take.

For example, under EU law, EU Member States must apply excise duties to products, including tobacco, alcohol and energy.[2] EU law also sets out common rules regarding the product, storage and movement of excise goods. The latter rules ensure some elements of a common approach to tax administration within the EU, whereas the requirement that Member States impose minimum levels of excise tax is intended to 'ensure the smooth functioning of the internal market'. In essence, a common minimum excise reduces the incentives associated (for consumers to engage in cross-border shopping) and the incentives for Member States to compete through a 'race to the bottom' style approach of lowering excise taxes.

Other rules within EU law, such as those governing 'state aid' can also affect taxes. For example, the Finnish government introduced a tax on confectionery, chocolate, ice cream and soft drinks to curb sugar consumption.[3] After complaints[4] were received concerning the tax, the European Commission informally indicated to Finland that the tax was incompatible with state aid rules because the tax was not based on the sugar content of different foods, but instead applied to designated categories while exempting other competing products. For example, chocolates were taxed whereas chocolate and other biscuits were not. The Finnish Cabinet Committee therefore decided to remove the tax.

Other customs unions have taken different approaches. For example, until recently the Economic Community of West African States (ECOWAS) placed an upper limit on excise taxes that could be levied on tobacco products. Rather than empowering Member States to impose excise taxes, or supporting functioning of the market where they are in place, this approach limited their potential. Accordingly, the Council of Ministers reversed this approach in 2017 through Directive on the Harmonization of Excise Duties on Tobacco Products in ECOWAS Member States.[5] This Directive obliges ECOSWAS Member States to impose a minimum *ad valorem* duty of 50% or more.[5] Similarly, the Western African Economic and Monetary Union (WAEMU) stipulated minimum and maximum rates for alcoholic (15%–50%) and tobacco products (15%–45%).[6]

Another example can be found in the Gulf Cooperation Council's (GCC) Excise Treaty, which forms the common framework for the introduction of excise tax across all six Member States, with the aim to reduce consumption of goods deemed most harmful to the social and economic fabric of the region.[7,8] Under the common framework, tobacco and tobacco derivatives are taxed: 100%, energy drinks: 100%, carbonated drinks: 50%, and 'special purpose goods' (including alcohol and pork products): 100%. Saudi Arabia, United Arab Emirates, Bahrain, Qatar and Oman have implemented the framework, joined by Kuwait in April 2020. In effect, this framework led to imposition of excise taxes covering these products for the first time in GCC countries.

Describing how a particular customs union governs health taxes is beyond the scope of this chapter. These examples merely illustrate the potential role of regional integration organisations as either stumbling blocks or enablers for health taxes. The legal agreements governing taxation within a customs union, or practical considerations like cross-border shopping, can constitute obstacles to the use of health taxes. Conversely, however, when mobilised these bodies can scale up the use of health taxes widely.

11.4. The World Trade Organization and internal taxation

The World Trade Organization (WTO) Agreement[9] is the central multilateral treaty governing international trade. The Agreement is an umbrella agreement that encompasses a number of WTO 'covered agreements', which discipline the ways in which WTO Members may restrict or regulate trade in goods and services. This includes disciplines governing the imposition of customs duties, internal taxes, and non-tariff measures such as regulations. Agreements also govern agricultural and non-agricultural subsidies, although these fiscal policies are beyond the scope of this chapter, as are WTO rules relating to other issues such as intellectual property rights.

These disciplines are backed by a binding system of dispute settlement, whereby one WTO Member can bring a claim against another alleging the violation of an obligation under the covered agreements (non-compliance).[10] In the event of a violation, a Member failing to bring its trade measure (normally a law or regulation) into compliance may face authorised retaliation in the form of temporary suspension of trade concessions in proportion to the violation (until compliance is eventually attained).

A number of WTO disputes relevant to health taxes are discussed below. A handful of alcoholic beverage taxes have been challenged on grounds that they discriminate in favour of domestic products and administration of a handful of tobacco taxes has been challenged on the same grounds. None of these cases has been decided on health grounds, but they do illustrate the relevance of WTO rules prohibiting discrimination to health taxes.

The GATT applies to trade in goods and a number of its provisions are relevant to health taxes.

First, GATT Article II prohibits WTO Members from levying customs duties above and beyond what they have each agreed in their Schedules of Concessions.[a] In this respect, the GATT does not prohibit the imposition

[a] For an overview, see: https://www.wto.org/english/tratop_e/schedules_e/goods_schedules_e.htm.

of customs duties by a WTO Member, but does impose ceilings on them based on that Member's negotiated commitments.

Second, upper limits on customs duties are complemented by a provision on most-favoured nation (MFN) treatment in GATT Article I:1. This provision prohibits a WTO Member from treating the imports of one country more favourably than those of any other WTO Member. In essence, the general rule is that where a WTO Member applies a customs duty on a given product that Member must impose the same duty to all products within that category from other WTO Members.

As with many general rules, exemptions and exceptions exist, including with respect to GATT MFN obligations. In this case, subject to certain conditions, GATT allows a WTO Member to treat imports from one Member more favourably than those of another Member where this is pursuant to a free trade agreement (FTA) or customs union. For example, where goods are traded free of customs duties pursuant to such an agreement, a WTO Member is not obliged to extend that 'treatment' (i.e. duty-free) to goods from all other WTO Members not part of that agreement. The effect of this system is that while, as a general rule, WTO Members have upper limits on customs duties under the GATT, exceptionally they may also be allowed to commit to and apply lower limits only for imports from their trading partners in FTAs or customs unions.

At this point, it is worth noting that the upper limits on customs duties (referred to as 'bound tariffs' in WTO parlance) negotiated under Article I of the GATT reduce the usefulness of customs duties, for health purposes. This limited usefulness is further compounded by a dynamic of so-called 'progressive liberalisation', whereby new FTAs and customs unions drive down customs duties or lead to their elimination altogether. But, from a health perspective this is not necessarily a bad outcome because customs duties are not well tailored to achievement of health goals. They apply only to imported products and are thereby limited in their design even where a product category is typically imported. Put simply, they distinguish between products based on their origin rather than their risk profile.

Third, GATT Article III prohibits a Member to discriminate against imported goods from WTO Members in favour of its own domestic goods through either taxation or regulation. GATT Article III:2 prohibits discriminatory taxes, whereas Article III:4 prohibits other discriminatory non-fiscal measures, such as regulations. As mentioned above, these 'national treatment' provisions have been invoked in a number of WTO disputes concerning taxation, including of products such as alcoholic and non-alcoholic (soft drinks) beverages and tobacco.

Fourth, where a tax or other fiscal measure does violate GATT Article III, it might nonetheless be lawful if one of the 'general exceptions' GATT itself provides can be successfully invoked. For example, it might be possible to argue that a health tax is, among other things, not more trade restrictive than necessary to protect human life or health. As the discussion below illustrates, much will turn on whether any discriminatory effect of a measure (be it in terms of MFN or national treatment) can be justified in health terms.

Recognising the inherent limits of customs duties, this section focuses on how principles of non-discrimination have been applied in the context of internal taxes and tax administration.

11.4.1. Internal taxes under GATT Article III:2: Principles of non-discrimination

As a general rule, WTO Members retain the right to impose domestic taxes and to set them at levels they deem appropriate. As mentioned above, this is subject to GATT Article III:2. This provision prohibits tax discrimination both in form or effect. Taxes that discriminate through their *form* are those that formally (i.e. they state so explicitly) apply higher taxes to imported products ('de jure' discrimination, in WTO parlance). These are relatively easy to identify. This may not be the case of facially neutral taxes (i.e. they state that all products, domestic and imported, are subject to the same tax rate). Such facially neutral taxes may sometimes nonetheless discriminate through their relative *effects* on imported products when seen as applied in practice ('*de facto*' discrimination, in WTO parlance). These latter types of discrimination can be more difficult to determine (and in fact most of the WTO disputes on tax discrimination involve allegations of '*de facto*' discrimination).

Before briefly describing these rules it is worth noting that many health taxes may be structured with either the aim or prospect of product substitution in mind. For example, alcoholic beverage taxes may impose a heavier tax burden on beverages with higher amounts of alcohol by volume. Similarly, sugary drink taxes might use thresholds on sugar content to impose a higher burden on products higher in sugar. This approach can both encourage consumer substitution and product reformulation in order to reduce total consumption or heavy episodic consumption. But this approach also favours one product category over another, giving rise to the question of whether one product category is discriminated against. GATT Article III is concerned with whether a WTO Member discriminates in favour of domestic products, not one product category over another *per se*. Nonetheless, Article III may be relevant, such as if the effect of the measure falls heaviest on imported products.

To some extent, this limits the importance of discussing Article III from a health policy standpoint. Inadvertent violations are conceivable and in such a situation the key question will be whether the tax structure is justifiable in terms of the general exceptions discussed below.

Article III:2 establishes two separate rules. The first sentence of Article III:2 imposes a strict rule prohibiting any excess taxation of imported products where they are highly competitive with domestic products (so-called 'like products'). Where imported products are in a less competitive relationship with domestic products ('directly competitive or substitutable'), the second sentence prohibits dissimilar taxation that acts to afford protection to domestic production.

Article III:2 first sentence	Article III:2 second sentence
Prohibits internal taxes or charges: • in excess of those applied to • like domestic products	Prohibits internal taxes or charges where: • directly competitive or substitutable products • are not similarly taxed and • this acts so as to afford protection to domestic production

On its face, this provision is arcane to say the least. But, the two rules are underpinned by common concepts, albeit with different thresholds for violation.

Under each rule, for a violation to occur, at least two product categories must have a different tax burden ('excess' taxation in the first sentence and 'dissimilar' taxation under the second sentence). The concept of *excess taxation* in the first sentence is strict in the sense that any excess taxation of imported products satisfies the test. The concept of *dissimilar taxation* in the second sentence is not as strict, but there is no quantitative or pre-defined threshold other than to say that it must be more than *de minimis*, which is to be assessed on a case-by-case basis.[11] The concept has been interpreted to mean that a greater tax burden is levied on imported products than on domestic 'directly competitive or substitutable products'.[b]

There must also be a relationship of competition between the imported and domestic products in question ('like products' under the first sentence and 'directly competitive or substitutable' products under the second sentence). For products to be considered 'like' under the first sentence they must be in a highly competitive relationship. By contrast, it is easier to establish that products are 'directly competitive or substitutable because they need not be so highly competitive and can be established if they offer alternative ways of satisfying a particular need or taste.[12] The nature and extent of a competitive relationship is evaluated by reference to factors

[b] Appellate Body Reports,[11] p. 26.

including product characteristics, consumer tastes and habits, end uses and tariff classification.

In the case of the second sentence, there is an additional requirement that the dissimilar taxation acts so as to afford protection to domestic production.

A number of WTO disputes have illustrated how GATT Article III:2 applies to excise taxes.

Philippines – Distilled Spirits provides the clearest example of how the rules in the first and second sentences of Article III:2 differ. The Philippines taxed spirits differently depending on the primary ingredient used in their production. Spirits using sugar-cane, coconut and other ingredients ('designated raw materials') were subject to lower flat tax rates than spirits using other ingredients such as wheat and potato ('non-designated raw materials').

On its face, this tax appeared to be origin-neutral (and thus, at least formally, non-discriminatory) because any distilled spirit, imported or domestic, made from 'designated raw materials' would be always taxed at the lower rate. In practice ('*de facto*') however, the effect of this tax measure on imported spirits was found to be markedly different from that on domestic spirits. As the Panel observed, because in practice *all* 'designated raw materials' were grown in the Philippines and *all* domestic distilled spirits were produced from such materials, all Philippine spirits (e.g. domestic sugar-based whisky) would be always taxed at the lower tax rate. By contrast, since the vast majority of imported distilled spirits were *not* made from 'designated raw materials' (e.g. imported wheat-based whisky), they were therefore subject to the higher tax rates. For the Panel, this meant that '*de facto*' the measure resulted in all domestic distilled spirits enjoying the favourable low tax, while the vast majority of the imported spirits were subject to taxes between 10 and 40 times higher.[c] Ultimately, therefore, the

[c] Appellate Body Reports,[12] paras 245 and 255 (referring to the Panel Reports, paras 7.182 and 7.183).

effect of this tax regime was found to be discriminatory contrary to the first and second sentences of Article III:2.[d]

Philippines' excise tax was found to be inconsistent with the *first* sentence of Article III:2 because the distinction between raw materials resulted in each *type* of imported distilled spirits (e.g. Scotch whiskies) having to pay excise taxes that were higher than (and thus 'in excess of') those levied on 'like' domestic distilled spirits of that same *type* (e.g. Philippine whiskies).

An important point in *Philippines – Distilled Spirits* concerned how to assess if products are 'like' for the purpose of the first sentence of Article III:2; which, as explained above, is relatively harder than establishing that products are 'directly competitive or substitutable' for the purpose of the second sentence. In this case, the Appellate Body also provided further guidance on the boundaries between 'like(ness)' and 'directly competitive or substitutable'.

The Appellate Body in that case agreed with the Panel's conclusion that, in the Philippine market, *all* imported and domestic products of the *same type* were in more than significant degree of competition with each other (e.g. imported gins in relation to domestic gins; imported brandies in relation to domestic brandies and imported whiskies in relation to domestic whiskies). These group types were thus considered as 'like' within the meaning of the first sentence of Article III:2.[e]

However, the Appellate Body disagreed with the Panel's broader factual conclusion that, in the Philippine market, *absolutely all* distilled spirits were 'like' irrespective of their types. For the Appellate Body, distilled spirits of *different* types could not be considered 'like products' with respect to each other (e.g. imported 'wheat-based' whiskies with respect to domestic 'sugar-based' brandies) within the meaning of Article III:2, first sentence.[f] The Appellate Body found that these groups of products were not 'like' because: there was not a more than a *significant* degree of competition or

[d] Appellate Body Reports,[12] paras 174 and 258, respectively.

[e] Appellate Body Reports,[12] paras 172 and 174.

[f] Appellate Body Reports,[12] paras 175–183.

substitutability[g] among them; that not all distilled spirits have the same organoleptic properties and that the fact that the products fall within the same customs code is not decisive because of the breadth of the tariff heading.[h]

As indicated above, 'like' products under the first sentence of Article III:2 are a narrow subset of the broader category of 'directly competitive or substitutable products' found in the second sentence of Article III:2.[13] But in *Philippines – Distilled Spirits*, the Appellate Body further clarified that this does not mean that *only* products that are *perfectly* substitutable can fall within the scope the first sentence.[14] Rather, it said, under the first sentence, products that are 'close to being perfectly substitutable' can also be 'like', whereas products that 'compete to a lesser degree' would instead fall within the scope of the second sentence (Figure 11.1).[i]

The Philippines' excise tax was also found inconsistent with the second sentence of Article III:2 in respect of certain types of imported and domestic distilled spirits that were in a lesser degree of competitive relationship. For example, even though they were not 'like products' under the first sentence, domestic *rums* produced with 'designated raw materials' (attracting lower tax rates) were still considered to be 'directly competitive or substitutable' with imported *vodkas* produced from 'non-designated raw materials' (attracting much higher tax rates). In this context, such dissimilar taxation violated the second sentence because it was applied 'so as to afford protection to domestic production'.[15]

Earlier WTO disputes on alcohol taxes also illustrate how the 'so as to afford protection' element of the second sentence has been applied. In the early WTO dispute *Japan-Alcoholic Beverages II*, a liquor tax law based on

---

[g] Appellate Body Reports,[12] para. 181 (stating that a finding of 'likeness' under the first sentence requires a degree of competition that is 'higher than merely *significant*') (emphasis original).
[h] Appellate Body Reports,[12] paras 180–183.
[i] Appellate Body Reports,[14] paras 149 and 181. The Appellate Body made these pronouncements to clarify the meaning of a statement it had made in earlier disputes (*Canada – Periodicals* and *Korea – Alcoholic Beverages*) that 'perfectly substitutable products' fall within the first sentence of Article III:2, while 'imperfectly substitutable products' are covered by the second. Appellate Body Reports,[14] paras 148–149.

Fig. 11.1. Like products and directly competitive or substitutable products under GATT Article III:2.

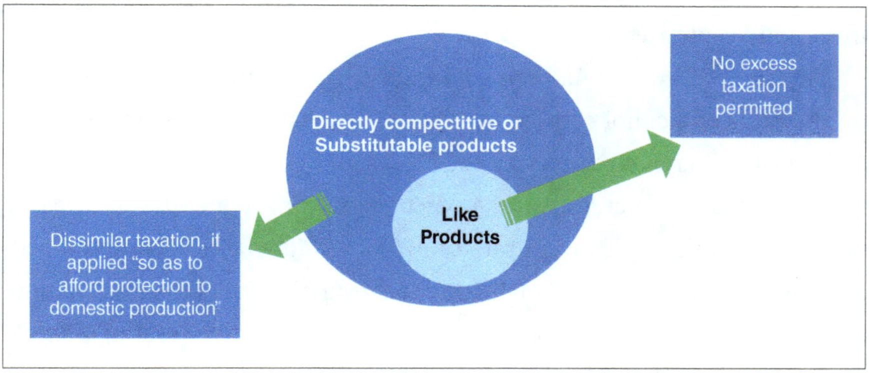

the strength of the alcohol was held to violate Article III:2. Japan's Liquor Tax Law (Shuzeiho) laid down a system of internal taxes for domestically produced and imported beverages and classified the various types of alcoholic beverages into ten categories.[16] Different tax rates were applicable to each of the categories:

Alcoholic beverage (both domestic and imported)	Tax rate
Shochu (25 degrees alcohol strength)	¥155,700 per litre plus ¥9,450 for each degree above 25
Vodka (37 degrees alcohol strength)	¥367,300 per litre plus ¥9,930 for each degree above 37
Whisky (40 degrees alcohol strength)	¥982,300 per litre plus ¥24,560 for each degree above 40

The dispute concerned application of the second sentence and, specifically, whether the measure was designed so as to afford protection to domestic production (domestically produced shochu). Japan contended that the Liquor Tax intended to ensure neutrality and equity and did not aim to protect domestic production. The Appellate Body looked to what it referred to as the 'design, architecture and the revealing structure' of the measure, rather than Japan's stated intent, in order to discern whether the tax was 'so as to afford protection to domestic production'.[17] It was held that the design of the differentiated internal tax was such that it managed to isolate domestically produced shochu from foreign competition, violating the second sentence of Article III:2.[j]

In *Chile – Taxes on Alcoholic Beverages*,[18] a Chilean law taxed all spirits on the basis of alcohol content by volume. Spirits with an alcohol content of 35° or less were taxed at a rate of 27% *ad valorem*. The tax rate increased from this figure in increments of 4 percentage points per additional degree of alcohol, until a maximum rate of 47% *ad valorem* was reached for all spirits over 39°. The WTO Panel found that roughly 75% of the total volume of domestically produced spirts were taxed at the lower level of 27% *ad valorem* while over 95% of the total volume of imported spirts were taxed at the rate of 47% *ad valorem*. Chile argued that its tax was not 'so as to afford protection' because several of its domestic products such as Chilean whisky, brandy, rum, gin, vodka fell in the highest tax bracket. The Appellate Body rejected this argument. After evaluating the impact on imported products as compared to domestic products as a whole, the Appellate Body stressed that the tax burden on imported products was heavier than on domestic products (Figure 11.2).[k]

To illustrate the analysis outlined in the flowchart above, it is possible to examine a hypothetical situation. Country X levied an excise tax of 67% (*ad valorem*) on all e-cigarette products without any exception. The tax on e-cigarettes is higher than the excise tax of 30% (*ad valorem)* levied on smokeless tobacco products. A WTO Member (Country Y) that exports e-cigarettes to Country X alleges that the tax is protectionist and prohibited under WTO rules.

The first step in this analysis is to examine, whether imported e-cigarettes and domestically produced smokeless tobacco products are 'like products' under the first sentence. This is based on the nature and extent of a competitive relationship between the products. Analysis may examine

---

[j] Appellate Body Report,[17] p. 31.

[k] Appellate Body Report,[18] para 53.

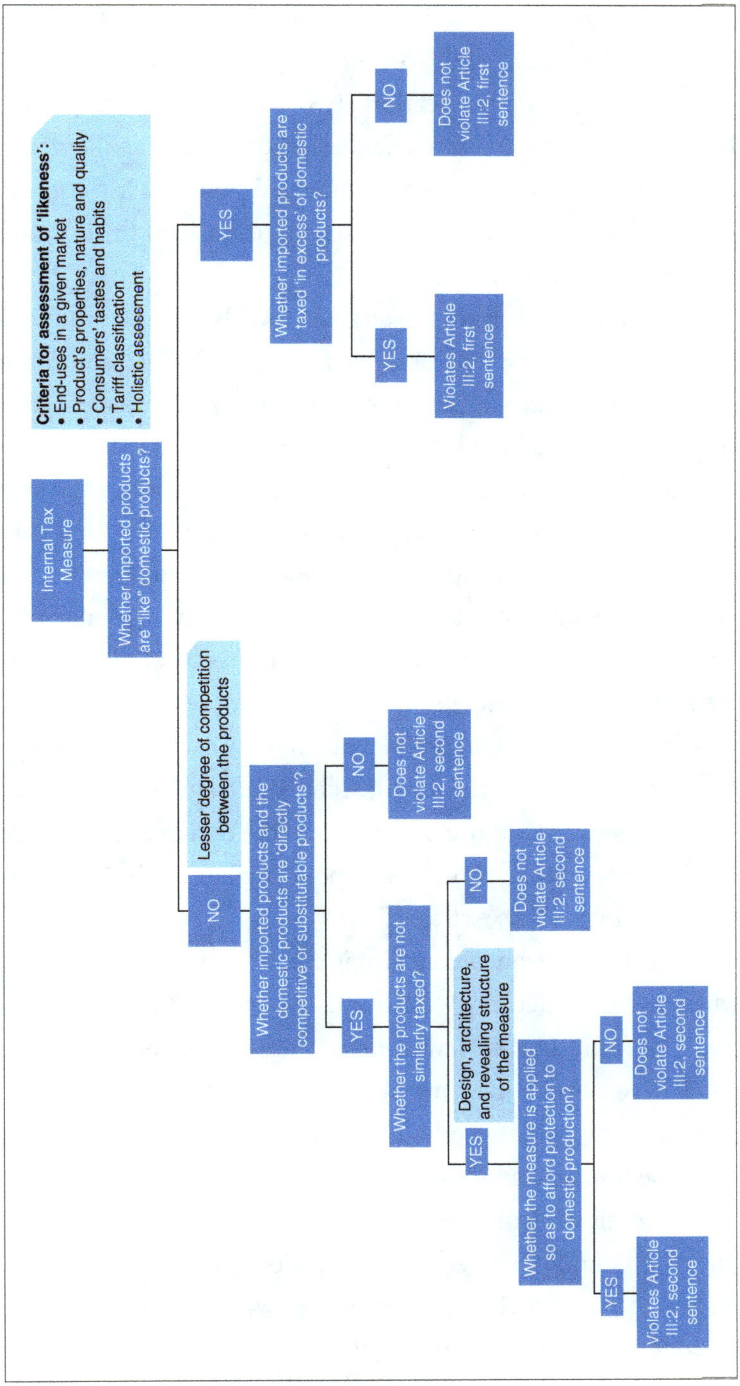

Fig. 11.2. Analysis under GATT Article III:2.

factors including a product's end-uses in a given market, consumers' tastes and preferences (specific to the country), a product's properties, nature and quality, and the tariff classification (HS Code). In the event the analysis establishes e-cigarettes and smokeless tobacco products as 'like', the question turns to whether excess taxation of imported products has arisen. On this issue a Panel might consider factors such as the size of the tax differential, both in relative and absolute terms.

By contrast, in the event the analysis reveals that the products are not 'like', the tax measure will be assessed under Article III:2, second sentence. Under the second sentence, the first step is whether imported e-cigarettes and domestically produced smokeless tobacco products are 'directly competitive or substitutable products'. Using factors outlined above for the assessment of 'likeness', the second sentence establishes a lower threshold concerning the competitive relationship of the products in the marketplace. A panel might also consider factors such as price elasticity, evidence of price or other competition, whether distribution channels overlap in evaluating the nature and extent of competition.[19] Thereafter, the second question to be answered is whether the two products are not similarly taxed. If they are not, the final step is whether the design, architecture and revealing structure of the measure is so as to afford protection to the domestic production.

This step-wise analysis will assist policymakers in deciding whether or not the measure violates Article III:2.

To date, WTO disputes concerning alcoholic beverages have not turned on whether tax structures were in place to protect health, or protected health.[20] As such, the case law under Article III:2 does not illustrate how Article III:2 would be interpreted if the effect of a tax treated a category of (primarily imported) products less favourably on health grounds. For example, the case law has not addressed a situation where alcoholic beverages with lower levels of alcohol by volume were subjected to lower tax rates for health reasons, and it happens that the majority of high alcohol by volume beverages are imported. Nonetheless, we know from case law on Article III:4, which concerns discriminatory regulation, that the focus of analysis under

Article III is on whether a tax or regulation discriminates, not on whether that tax is justifiable on health grounds.

11.4.2. Justifying discriminatory taxation under GATT general exceptions

Although the cases above were not defended on health grounds, where a tax or regulation is implemented to protect human life or health, but violates Article III, the WTO Member implementing the measure may nevertheless argue that the tax is justified by the general exceptions. In particular, GATT Article XX(b) states:

> Subject to the requirement that such measures are not applied in a manner which would constitute a means of arbitrary or unjustifiable discrimination between countries where the same conditions prevail, or a disguised restriction on international trade, nothing in this Agreement shall be construed to prevent the adoption or enforcement by any Member of measures:
>
> . . .
>
> (b) necessary to protect human, animal or plant life or health;

When applying Article XX(b) a panel will first determine whether the measure in question is a measure for the protection of human life or health.[21] To do so, a panel will examine whether there is a risk to health, and if so, whether the measure is designed to address that risk.[22] This is a fairly low threshold test, meaning that a tax pursued for health purposes should ordinarily be considered a measure for the protection of human health.

To evaluate necessity, a panel will then weigh and balance the trade restrictiveness of the tax measure against its contribution to the objective pursued, in light of the importance of that objective. For example, the extent to which a tax restricts international trade would be weighed against the contribution that the tax makes to the government's health objectives, in light of the importance of those objectives. This functions somewhat like a proportionality test whereby the proportionality of the discriminatory effect is evaluated by reference to contribution to the health goal. In this vein, the greater the contribution of the measure to the health objective pursued, the easier it may be to justify any unintended and incidental discrimination through the effect of a measure.

A panel may also consider whether there are reasonably available alternative measures that are less trade restrictive but capable of achieving the objective pursued. Depending on what is argued by a complainant, a panel might examine whether an entirely separate measure such as a regulatory measure is available, or it might examine whether tax structure could be altered to reduce or eliminate discrimination while achieving the health objective.

In the absence of reasonably available alternatives, the panel then examines whether the measure complies with the introductory paragraph (chapeau) of Article XX. This requires assessing whether a measure is applied in a way that results in arbitrary or unjustifiable discrimination or a disguised restriction on trade. In doing so, a panel will commonly examine whether there is a rational connection between the policy goal and how the measure is applied.[l]

With risk of over-simplifying the rule, in practice, whether a WTO Member can rely on the health exception will generally turn on whether any differential tax treatment is justifiable by reference to a health goal. This might turn on what is included and excluded from the definition of excisable goods, or on differences in the rates applied to different product categories. The prospect of a tax being discriminatory in effect is also most apparent where the goal or likely effect is substitution. In such a situation, much will turn on which categories of goods are domestically produced or imported.

[l] Appellate Body Report,[22] p. 1527, paras 226–227.

Analysis of the exception under GATT Article XX (b)[23]

Step 1. Does the measure fall within the range of policies considered to protect human health?

1. Does a risk to human health exist?
2. If so, is the policy goal underlying the measure to reduce that risk?

Step 2. The panel will weigh and balance relevant factors in light of the importance of the regulatory goal in order to reach a preliminary determination on necessity.

1. How important is the regulatory goal?
   The case-law suggests that protection of human health is important to the highest degree (*European Communities-Asbestos; Brazil-Retreaded tyres)*.
2. To what extent does the measure contribute to achievement of the regulatory goal?
3. How trade-restrictive is the measure i.e. to what extent does it limit international trade?

Step 3. Are less trade restrictive measure reasonably available?

1. Are the purported alternatives less trade-restrictive?
2. Do the purported alternative achieve the respondent's risk tolerance or chosen level of protection?
3. Are the purported alternative true alternatives, or are they actually complementary measures?
4. Are the purported alternatives reasonably available to the Member in question?

Step 4. Is the measure applied in a manner which would constitute a means of arbitrary or unjustifiable discrimination between countries where the same conditions prevail, or a disguised restriction upon trade?

1. Do reasons given for discrimination in application of the measure bear a rational connection to the policy goal or go against that goal?
2. Does a lack of connection between application of the measure and its objective suggest that the measure is applied as a disguised restriction on trade?

11.4.3. Tax administration cases

There have also been a number of tax administration cases under Article III of the GATT, including cases in which arrangements for administration of tobacco taxes have been found to be discriminatory. In addition to Article III:2 of the GATT, these disputes have concerned Article III:4, which prohibits measures that treat imported products less favourably than like domestic products. Essentially, Article III:4 prohibits discriminatory regulation, whereas Article III:2 prohibits discriminatory taxation. Two disputes illustrate how tax administration measures can fall afoul of Article III:4.

Dominican Republic – Importation and Sale of Cigarettes concerned measures implemented to address illicit trade in tobacco products. In this dispute, Honduras brought a claim against the Dominican Republic concerning a requirement that tax stamps be affixed to cigarettes at the point of importation in the Dominican Republic. This requirement meant that imported products had to be unpacked and stamped on importation, which increased the cost of production and undermined the capacity of foreign manufacturers to control how their products were presented. In contrast, domestic manufacturers could comply with the stamping requirement at the point of manufacture. It was found that this measure resulted in less favourable treatment for imported cigarettes under Article III:4 of the GATT.[24]

However, another Honduran claim was rejected under Article III:4. Honduras argued that an import-bonding requirement (designed to secure payment of taxes) was less favourable to imported products because the greater market share of imported goods meant that higher bonds had to be paid by importers than by domestic producers who had a smaller market share (and lower tax liability). In this context, the WTO Panel found that the fact that an importer held the majority market share of an adversely affected good did not mean that a measure was necessarily less favourable to imported goods. As such, this second claim under Article III:4 failed.[m]

In its defence, the Dominican Republic also invoked Article XX(d) of the GATT, which permits measures necessary to secure compliance with laws or regulations (such as tax laws) provided those laws are themselves not inconsistent with the GATT. Honduras argued that less restrictive means existed, such as providing secure stamps for exporters so that the stamps could be affixed under supervision of an agent of the Dominican Republic at the point of production. The Dominican Republic failed to rebut the showing that this would be a reasonably available alternative measure.[n] As such, the Dominican Republican did not succeed in justifying its measure under Article XX(d).

Although not argued in this dispute, it is also worth noting that labelling measures such as tax stamp requirements may constitute technical regulations under the Agreement on Technical Barriers to Trade (TBT Agreement). This creates additional obligations, such as an obligation to ensure that the regulations are not more trade restrictive than necessary to protect human health.

In *Thailand – Customs and Fiscal Measures on Cigarettes from the Philippines*, the Philippines brought claims against Thailand concerning Thailand's treatment of Philip Morris cigarettes imported from the Philippines.[25]

Some of the claims related to the process of customs valuation, which occurs when a good is imported. If tariffs and other taxes are based on the value of a good (i.e. *ad valorem* taxes), the customs valuation forms the basis for determining the taxes due. The Philippines alleged that Thailand was overvaluing cigarettes imported from its territory, resulting in the payment

[m] Panel Report,[24] paras 7.281–7.311.

[n] Panel Report,[24] para. 7.228.

of tariffs and taxes at a higher rate than was due. Thai customs rejected the transaction value of the cigarettes (the price at which the imported cigarettes were purchased) as the basis for valuation. Thailand argued that the exporter and importer, both of which are Philip Morris companies, are related parties and that the transaction value was lower than the true value of the imported cigarettes. The Panel agreed with the Philippines, finding that Thailand's Customs authorities had violated a number of procedural obligations governing how imported goods should be valued.

Other claims related to the administration of the Thai tobacco tax system. One claim related to the calculation of the tax base for purposes of Thailand's value-added tax. It was found that Thailand had departed from its general methodology for the calculation of the tax base in respect of imported cigarettes on a number of occasions. The Panel found that the effect of these departures was to increase the amount of tax due on imported cigarettes, but not on domestic cigarettes, resulting in a violation of Article III:2 of the GATT.[o]

The Philippines also took issue with Thai laws imposing value-added tax on resellers for the sale of imported cigarettes, but not for domestic cigarettes. Whereas domestic cigarettes qualified for an automatic exemption, resellers were forced to apply for a rebate of the tax in respect of sales of imported cigarettes. The Philippines argued that this violated Article III:2 of the GATT because imported cigarettes were taxed more heavily than domestic cigarettes. The Panel agreed, finding that the procedural obligation to apply for a rebate created a risk of discrimination that was sufficient to violate Article III:2 of the GATT.[p] In this respect, there was a risk that a reseller might not be granted the rebate if adequate documentation could not be provided. The Panel also found that the additional procedural burden of having to apply for a rebate resulted in violation of Article III:4 of the GATT. In this respect, the Panel found that the less favourable treatment of imported products was based on their foreign origin.[q]

[o] Panel Report,[25] para. 7.567.

[p] Panel Report,[25] para. 7.637.

[q] Panel Report,[25] paras 7.744–7.748.

Thailand argued that these measures were necessary to secure compliance with tax laws under Article XX(d). However, the Panel ruled that the administrative requirements in question were not compliant with Article III:2 and, therefore, Article XX(d) could not be invoked. This aspect of the Panel's decision was reversed by the Appellate Body, although the Appellate Body ultimately held that Thailand had not substantiated its defence under Article XX(d).[26]

On the whole, these disputes illustrate a variety of ways in which principles of non-discrimination may be relevant to excise and other taxes. For example, they may be relevant to which products are taxed, or not taxed, and the rates applied to different product categories. Wherever substitution of one product category for another is an intended or anticipated outcome, product categories will compete with one another to some extent. Whether discrimination will arise will then depend ultimately on the relative effect of tax structures on competition between imported and domestic products.

Although the tax measures in those disputes were not defended on health grounds, discussion of Article XX(b) also illustrates the importance of establishing health objectives during the policy process. Provided that health objectives are reflected in tax design, those objectives can open an avenue to defending a tax that discriminates through its effect. This avenue is available provided that the differential tax treatment in question is justifiable by reference to the relative risks posed by the product groups in question.

Finally, the tax administration disputes reflect the variety of ways in which tax administration arrangements may be discriminatory through their effect. Although this does not impact the right to regulate for health purposes *per se*, it highlights the need for care in tax administration arrangements.

11.5. Conclusion

This chapter has set out four key observations concerning how trade agreements affect tax design.

First, harmonisation of customs codes, such as through the HS Code, affects domestic customs codes, which are often used for purposes of defining the categories of products subject to taxation. However, caution should be used both in use of customs codes in this way because customs codes do not distinguish between product categories based on health risk, but instead based on other characteristics.

Second, customs and monetary unions often establish rules governing imposition of taxes, including health taxes. Other rules may also affect health taxes or tax administration.

Third, trade agreements (both WTO law and other agreements) place upper limits on customs duties. This embeds a preference for domestic taxes, which in any case are more suited to achieve health objectives.

Fourth, trade agreements establish general rules that prohibit discriminatory taxes and discriminatory tax administration unless the discrimination is *inter alia* necessary to protect human health. Application of these rules is complex and they are less definitive than other aspects of trade agreements relevant to taxation. In this context, the simplest approach to ensure compliance is to ensure that distinctions drawn between different product categories or products within a category are legitimate in health terms. That means ensuring that relative risk to population health should guide distinctions drawn between products for tax purposes.

Key messages

- Agreements governing customs and monetary unions may establish rules governing health taxes, including minimum or maximum levels of excise or sales taxes on specific product categories or harmonised rules governing tax administration.
- Trade agreements place upper limits on the imposition of customs duties (tariffs), creating a preference for taxes where health objectives are pursued.
- Trade agreements prohibit taxes that discriminate against imported products, meaning that care must be taken not to favour domestic products in setting the tax base, tax rates and particularly where product substitution is anticipated.

- But, taxes with discriminatory effects might be justified if they pursue a health objective, there is sufficient evidence of a contribution to that objective and any distinctions drawn between imported and domestic products are legitimate.
- Approaches to tax administration that have discriminatory effects may also be justified provided they are necessary to secure compliance with tax laws.

References

1. HMRC, *Tax Information and Impact Note – The Tobacco Products (Descriptions of Products) (Amendment) Order*, 2019. https://www.gov.uk/government/consultations/draft-legislation-tobacco-for-heating/tax-information-and-impact-note-the-tobacco-products-descriptions-of-products-amendment-order-2019 (accessed 10 February 2020).
2. Official Journal of the European Union, Concerning the general arrangements for excise duty and repealing Directive 92/12/EEC, 2008, OJ 2 9/2. https://eur-lex.europa.eu/legal-content/EN/TXT/PDF/?uri=CELEX:02008L0118-20200101&from=EN (accessed 14 October 2020).
3. European Commission, *Food Taxes and Their Impact on Competitiveness in the Agri-Food Sector: A Study*, 2014, 27. https://ec.europa.eu/docsroom/documents/5827/attachments/1/translations/en/renditions/native#:~:text=Overall%2C%20this%20study%20on%20the,fat%20levels%20of%20the%20product (accessed 15 October 2020).
4. ETL Complaint, 2013. http://www.etl.fi/media/aineistot/lausunnot/kannanotot/state_aid_complaint_excise_duty_in_finland.pdf (accessed 15 October 2020).
5. Economic Community of West African States (ECOWAS), *Directive C/DIR.1/12/17 on the Harmonization of Excise Duties on Tobacco Products in ECOWAS Member States*, December 2017. https://untobaccocontrol.org/impldb/wp-content/uploads/sierra_leone_2018_annex-5_ECOWAS_directive_tobacco_2017.pdf (accessed 22 July 2020).
6. Western African Economic and Monetary Union (WAEMU), *Directive 03/1998/CM/UEMOA and Directive 03/2009/CM/UEMOA*. http://www.uemoa.int/sites/default/files/bibliotheque/directive_03_2009_cm_uemoa.pdf (accessed 22 July 2020).
7. Gulf Cooperation Council, *Excise Treaty*. https://www2.deloitte.com/content/dam/Deloitte/xe/Documents/tax/GCC-EXCISE-tax-treaty-English-July-2017.pdf (accessed 23 July 2020).
8. Kingdom of Saudi Arabia, *Excise Tax Guidelines, General Authority of Zakat and Tax*. https://extranet.who.int/ncdccs/Data/SAU_NCD_SAU_Excise%20Tax%20Guidelines%20form%20Tax%20Authority.pdf.
9. *Marrakesh Agreement Establishing the World Trade Organization*, 1867, U.N.T.S. 154.
10. World Trade Organization (WTO), *Dispute Settlement Rules: Understanding on Rules and Procedures Governing the Settlement of Disputes, Marrakesh Agreement*

Establishing the World Trade Organization, Annex 2, 1869 U.N.T.S. 401, 33 I.L.M. 1226, 1994. https://www.wto.org/english/docs_e/legal_e/28-dsu.pdf (accessed 13 October 2020).

11. Appellate Body Reports, *Philippines – Taxes on Distilled Spirits*, WT/DS396/AB/R / WT/DS403/AB/R, adopted 20 January 2012, DSR 2012:VIII, paras 181, 250.
12. Appellate Body Reports, *Philippines – Taxes on Distilled Spirits*, WT/DS396/AB/R / WT/DS403/AB/R, adopted 20 January 2012, DSR 2012:VIII, paras 181, 205.
13. Appellate Body Report, *Korea – Taxes on Alcoholic Beverages*, WT/DS75/AB/R, WT/DS84/AB/R, adopted 17 February 1999, para. 118.
14. Appellate Body Reports, *Philippines – Taxes on Distilled Spirits*, WT/DS396/AB/R / WT/DS403/AB/R, adopted 20 January 2012, DSR 2012:VIII, para. 149 (reasoning that such a view 'would be too narrow an interpretation and would reduce the scope of the first sentence essentially to identical products').
15. Appellate Body Reports, *Philippines – Taxes on Distilled Spirits*, WT/DS396/AB/R / WT/DS403/AB/R, adopted 20 January 2012, DSR 2012:VIII, paras 244–57.
16. Panel Report, *Japan – Taxes on Alcoholic Beverages*, WT/DS8/R, WT/DS10/R, WT/DS11/R, adopted 1 November 1996, paras 2.1–2.4.
17. Appellate Body Report, *Japan – Taxes on Alcoholic Beverages*, WT/DS8/AB/R, WT/DS10/AB/R, WT/DS11/AB/R, adopted 1 November 1996, DSR 1996:I, p. 29.
18. Appellate Body Report, *Chile – Taxes on Alcoholic Beverages*, WT/DS87/AB/R, AT/DS110/AB/R, adopted 12 January 2000.
19. Appellate Body Reports, *Philippines – Taxes on Distilled Spirits*, WT/DS396/AB/R / WT/DS403/AB/R, adopted 20 January 2012, DSR 2012:VIII, para. 242.
20. Appellate Body Report, *Japan – Taxes on Alcoholic Beverages*, WT/DS8/AB/R, WT/DS10/AB/R, WT/DS11/AB/R, adopted 1 November 1996, DSR 1996:I, p. 97; Appellate Body Report, *Korea – Taxes on Alcoholic Beverages*, WT/DS75/AB/R, WT/DS84/AB/R, adopted 17 February 1999, DSR 1999:I, p. 3; Appellate Body Report, *Chile – Taxes on Alcoholic Beverages*, WT/DS87/AB/R, WT/DS110/AB/R, adopted 12 January 2000, DSR 2000:I, p. 281.
21. Appellate Body Report, *EC – Asbestos*, paras 156–63.
22. Appellate Body Report, *Brazil – Measures Affecting Imports of Retreaded Tyres*, WT/DS332/AB/R, adopted 17 December 2007, DSR 2007:IV, paras 133–82.
23. World Health Organization, *Confronting the Tobacco Epidemic in a New Era of Trade and Investment Liberalization*, 2012, 32. https://apps.who.int/iris/bitstream/handle/10665/70918/9789241503723_eng.pdf;jsessionid=7BCF80DC2B083184EB24FAF873E80A1C?sequence=1 (accessed 28 July 2020).
24. Panel Report, *Dominican Republic – Measures Affecting the Importation and Internal Sale of Cigarettes*, WT/DS302/R, adopted 19 May 2005, paras 7.184–7.202. This finding was upheld by the Appellate Body (AB Rep, para. 128(a)).
25. Panel Report, *Thailand – Customs and Fiscal Measures on Cigarettes from the Philippines*, WT/DS371/R, adopted 15 July 2011.
26. Appellate Body Report, *Thailand – Customs and Fiscal Measures on Cigarettes from the Philippines*, WT/DS371/AB/R, adopted 15 July 2011, paras 162–80.

https://doi.org/10.1142/9781800612396_0015

Chapter 12

A Political Economy Analysis of Health Taxes

Thomas F Babor[*], Jeff Collin[†], and Maristela G Monteiro[‡]

Industry sectors involved in the production, distribution, sales and promotion of tobacco, alcohol, unhealthy foods, and sugar-sweetened beverages (SSBs) tend to oppose health taxes because they can decrease the demand for their products and thus reduce shareholder profits. This creates an inherent conflict of interest between the commercial goals of these industries and the public health responsibilities of governments. These industries have become increasingly concentrated into a small number of global corporations that account for a large proportion of the market for these products, especially in low- and middle-income countries (LMIC). There are similarities in the way these products are marketed and purchased, explaining the historical and emerging linkages across industries in how they conduct political activities that influence the policy environment for their products. To illustrate this development, we conducted a broad search for examples of the tactics used by these industries in their treatment of health taxes and pricing policies. Sixty-four documented examples were identified that illustrate how five general corporate political strategies are implemented in a wide variety

[*] University of Connecticut, USA.

[†] University of Edinburgh, UK.

[‡] Pan American Health Organization, USA.

of countries: (1) using information to gain access to political decision-makers; (2) constituency-building with influential political decision-makers; (3) promoting alternative policies or voluntary measures as substitutes for statutory regulation; (4) using financial incentives to influence government policymakers to act in ways favourable to industry interests; and (5) legal measures employing trade agreements as well as pre-emption, litigation, and circumvention.

Framing health taxes in terms of their economic, social, and public health benefits rather than allowing industry to define them as a liability can be a persuasive argument that could increase the chances of implementing effective NCD prevention. To achieve this aim, there is a need to build coalitions at the local, national, and international levels capable of working collaboratively in the interests of public health.

12.1. Introduction

> "*Sugar*, *rum*, and *tobacco*, are commodities which are no where necessaries of life, which have become objects of almost universal consumption, and which are therefore extremely proper subjects of taxation."
>
> Adam Smith, *An Inquiry into the Nature and Causes of the Wealth of Nations*, 1776

No less of an authority than Adam Smith in his 1776 essay on the Wealth of Nations made an excellent case for the taxation of commodities like sugar, rum and tobacco because they are not considered as 'necessaries of life…' As documented in previous chapters of this book, health taxes provide governments with a clear and effective opportunity to save lives, generate revenues and at the same time reduce the health and social costs of non-communicable diseases (NCDs).

Health taxes aim at reducing the affordability of tobacco, alcohol, foods with high salt, sugar and fat content and sugar-sweetened beverages (SSB), with the objective that these products will be consumed less and thus improve population health. A second aim of health taxes is to compensate society for the enormous social, economic and healthcare costs of such products, which are borne primarily by society rather than by the producers or the consumers.[1]

Despite these benefits, the sectors involved in the production, distribution, sales and promotion of tobacco, alcohol, unhealthy foods and SSBs tend to oppose health taxes given that taxes decrease sales and thus may reduce profits for shareholders. As a result, an inherent conflict exists between the commercial goals of these industries and the public health and economic equity goals of governments.

In this chapter, we consider the following questions: What is the political economy of health tax policy? Who are the major players in this policy arena? How do their political and economic activities have an impact on public health? The answers to these questions are not simple. They may vary across countries and between different levels of government within countries and potentially across product sub-categories. The first part of this chapter focuses on how the affected industries interfere with the policymaking process. The second part goes one step further by analysing how different stakeholders, who often have competing priorities, can build lasting coalitions or otherwise work to promote public benefit through health taxes. The chapter addresses a gap in the existing literature by providing a political economy analysis of the roles of influential stakeholders (especially the producer industries and government agencies) and how governance mechanisms can be used to promote public health.

Implicit in our review is a model of the policymaking process that comprises the institutions, stakeholders and the environment within which policy decisions are made. One highly stylised model of the policy process forms a cycle, beginning with an assessment of NCD-related health problems, followed by implementation of evidence-based interventions and concluding with systematic evaluation and corrective action if necessary. But the reality of the policymaking process is rarely that simple or straightforward.

In this chapter, policy formation in the area of health taxes is understood as a more complicated political and economic process influenced by a combination of state and non-state actors. State-centric accounts of policymaking emphasise the roles of government institutions at the local and national levels, as well as international agencies, such as the World Health Organization. Relevant non-state actors include civil society organisations, particularly non-governmental organisations and commercial interests like the tobacco, SSB, food and alcoholic beverage industries, which variously attempt to influence the policymaking process directly through political lobbying or indirectly by changing public opinion. Other relevant actors include the mass media, health scientists, medical practitioners and public health advocates. As this chapter will show, the extent to which any interest group can influence NCD-related tax policy depends on both the political power of a particular group and the governing images of the various NCD problems to which the policymakers subscribe.

12.2. Political economy analysis, policy coherence and the whole of society approach

The commitment to work across sectors in a 'whole of society' approach to achieving the NCD targets agreed upon for the Sustainable Development Goals promoted by the United Nations includes increased emphasis on engagement with the private sector and other non-state actors (NSA). Within SDG17, this commitment to advancing multi-sectoral collaboration is intended to ensure *policy coherence* for sustainable development, implying that health and development policies across different sectors and policy spheres should be synergistic, reinforcing and coordinated.[2] While the influence of unhealthy commodity producers on policymaking has emerged as a major barrier to the promotion of such coherence,[3] this can also be impeded by other, often neglected factors that shape the policy process. Economic sectors of governments, including those in low- and middle-income countries (LMIC), are often heavily influenced by international norms of economic development. Such norms focus on economic growth, employment and revenue generation as a primary policy objective and they are realised in part through trade agreements and development plans established by international agencies and national governments. In such contexts, policymakers often pursue the singular mandate of economic growth to the neglect of other goals such as health promotion and disease prevention, not simply because of industry pressure, but because this pressure coincides with economic development norms and international commitments. In this way, economic norms can condition an openness to industry practices and products that may harm the health of populations. A common barrier to health sector pursuit of health goals across sectors is that these sectors operate within distinct policy communities with different ideas or paradigms of the 'public good'.

Addressing NCDs and their risk factors is a high priority for investments and multi-sectoral health and development efforts globally. It is also a compelling example of the challenges of mobilising an all of society response. Engagement with the private sector, which includes industries that produce, distribute, market and sell the products that are the leading risk factors for NCDs on one side, and a wide range of industries that can contribute to reducing the burden of NCDs on the other, pose a significant challenge to efforts to promote and protect health and sustainable development.

Although historically labelled 'behavioural risk factors', alcohol, tobacco, unhealthy foods and SSBs are intimately tied to global political economic conditions, which structure product environments and create environments of risk. A political economy analysis positions the consumption of these products within environments where behaviours and health outcomes are shaped by social, political and economic structures, suggesting that a better understanding of these factors could help to overcome impediments to public health.[4,5]

Political economy analysis can be a powerful tool for bridging the traditional concerns of politics, economics and public health in order to bring stakeholders together in a whole-of-society approach. It helps to identify political, economic, social and cultural factors that drive or impede reforms and to design better policies. In this chapter, we use the term 'political economy' to refer to the political and economic dimensions of policy adoption, implementation and enforcement, as well as an analytical approach to explaining important challenges to the use of health taxes as a way not only to control the consequences of these NCD risk factors but also the healthcare costs of managing the conditions resulting from them. One key aspect of political economy analysis is focused on the political strategies of key stakeholders in the policymaking process.[5] In the area of NCDs, these stakeholders include international organisations, government legislative bodies, academic institutions, public health professionals as well as a variety of organisations linked to unhealthy commodity industries manufacturing products that drive NCD epidemics.

Political economy analysis covers a variety of tools, ranging from in-depth theory-based analyses to rapid assessment studies that provide a survey of the main stakeholders, their power relations and their implications for policy. In this chapter, we focus on the latter approach, beginning with a specific policy question that is likely to influence the successful implementation of NCD risk factor mitigation measures. Our analysis is focused on the extent to which industries engaged in the manufacture, sale and marketing of tobacco, alcohol, unhealthy foods and sugar-sweetened beverages can be considered partners in the development, implementation and enforcement of effective policies, or should be kept at arms length so that other stakeholders can work more effectively with government agencies and policymakers. To address this issue, we critically evaluate the strategies and tactics of four industries that are strategically threatened by the use of taxation and pricing policies to promote public health.

We begin this chapter with a brief overview of the tobacco, alcohol and SSB industries and their global relevance. We then describe how these industries have sought to influence decision-making in the area of health taxes at the global, national and local levels, across high-income and LMIC contexts. After considering the arguments used to challenge taxation policies as well as the counterarguments that can be used to promote them, we close with a discussion of how civil society, governments and the public health community can work together to implement health taxes in order to prevent NCDs and other health conditions.

12.3. The global tobacco, alcohol, food and SSB industries

The tobacco, alcohol, food and SSB industries have become increasingly concentrated into a small number of global corporations that account for a large proportion of the market for these products. The network of consumer corporations, financial institutions, advertising agencies, law firms and lobbying groups as well as the politicians, lobbyists and others they support constitute what has been called a 'corporate consumption complex',[6] which is considered to be a fundamental part of a culture of hyper-consumption of unhealthy products associated with premature mortality and chronic disease. In addition, such corporations are connected to and often support each other and have been expanding their reach globally, nationally and locally, making it difficult for governments to regulate them and keep health at the centre of policymaking.

The corporate consumption ideology is summarised in Box 12.1 as it applies to tobacco, alcohol and SSBs.

This ideology has been widely disseminated through significant investments in marketing and political activity, supported by an economic model of development based on consumption as a driver of growth.[7] However, it is the position of this book that the global epidemic of NCDs is one of the predictable if unintentional consequences of such a paradigm.

Box 12.1. Main propositions of the corporate consumption ideology

1. Lifestyle, not the products themselves, is the main influence on health
2. Companies produce what customers want

3. Advertising helps consumers choose wisely
4. Government should not tell people or companies what to do
5. Free trade is good for everyone
6. Criticising big business is unwise
7. Promoting consumption is essential for economic growth and prosperity

Source: Freudenberg (2014).[6]

12.3.1. The alcohol industry

The term 'alcohol industry' here refers to producers of beer, wine and distilled spirits and their network of distributors and retailers. Trade associations and social aspects/public relations organisations (SAPROs), which are funded to promote industry interests, are also included in this definition. In recent years, the global alcohol market has become highly concentrated in terms of beer and spirits production, though wine remains more fragmented. Table 12.1 describes the changes over a 37-year period in shares of the global market volume among the 10 leading multinational producers of beer, distilled beverages and wine.

In the malt beverage sector, multinational corporations have been purchasing local companies and regional breweries, and establishing local partnerships, especially in the global South. AB InBev's portfolio of over 500 beers includes seven of the top 10 global beer brands and 18 other brands that together generate more than USD 1 billion in retail sales.[8] Anheuser-Busch InBev (AB InBev), a Belgian company, took over the largest American beer producer in 2008 and purchased the second largest brewer in the US market, MillerCoors, as part of its takeover of SABMiller in 2016.[8] This single company now produces and markets more than a quarter of the world's commercial beer. According to Jernigan and Ross,[8] what is significant in the beer sector is the rapid pace of consolidation in the global industry.

Table 12.1. Share of global market volume of the 10 leading multinational producers of alcoholic beverages, by category.

Global market share			
Corporation	Headquarters	1979–1980	2017
Beer[8,10]			
AB Inbev	Belgium	6.5% (AB)[a]	26.8%
Heineken	Netherlands	2.8%	10.9%
China Resources Holdings Ltd.	China	[b]	6.1%
Carlsberg Breweries A/S	Denmark	[b]	6.0%
Molson Coors Brewing Co.	United States	0.8% (Molson), 1.9% (Coors)	4.8%
Tsingtao Brewery Co. Ltd.	China	[b]	4.1%
Asahi Group Holdings Ltd.	Japan	[b]	3.2%
Beijing Yanjing Beer Group Corp.	China	[b]	2.4%
Kirin Holdings Co. Ltd.	Japan	3.1%	1.4%
Diageo	United Kingdom	0.9% (Grand Metropolitan)	1.3%
Total market share of top 10		**27.99%**	**67.0%**
	Headquarters	2006	2016
Distilled spirits			
Diageo	United Kingdom	10.8%	20.0%
Pernod Ricard	France	8.3%	9.7%
Beam Suntory	Japan	3.7% (Beam only)	4.9%
Bacardi Ltd.	Bermuda	3.7%	2.9%
Allied Blenders and Distillers	India	[b]	2.8%
Gruppo Campari	Italy	1.7%	2.2%
Sazerac Co. Inc.	United States	[b]	2.2%

(Continued)

Table 12.1. *(Continued)*

Global market share			
Corporation	Headquarters	1979–1980	2017
Brown-Forman Beverages Worldwide	United States	1.8%	2.0%
Roust	Russia	[b]	2.0%
Group La Martiniquaise	France	[b]	1.9%
Total market share of top 10		**42.3%**	**50.5%**
	Headquarters	2006	2016
Wine[10]			
E&J Gallo Winery	United States	2.5%	3.10%
Constellation Brands	United States	2.0%	1.50%
Treasury Wine Estates	Australia	1.4%	1.40%
The Wine Group	United States	1.5%	1.30%
Group Castel	France	1.1%	1.20%
Vina Concha y Toro	Chile	0.9%	1.10%
Accolade Wines Ltd.	Australia	1.2%	1.10%
Pernod Ricard Groupe	France	1.0%	0.90%
Grupo Penaflor SA	Argentina	0.9%	0.90%
FeCoVItA Coop Ltda	Argentina	1.0%	0.80%
Total market share of top 10		**13.50%**	**13.30%**

[a] Parentheses indicate rank of predecessor companies when applicable.
[b] Indicates the company was not listed among the leading producers in that category in that year.
Source: Jernigan and Ross.[8]

The top-10 companies sold 68% of the world's beer in 2017, compared with 28% in 1980.[9,10]

Although distilled spirits production is not as heavily concentrated, the growing role of Diageo, the world's largest distilled spirits producer, in both the beer and distilled spirits indicates how that company's size reflects a related trend toward cross-sector concentration.

Wine production, on the other hand, remains decentralised in many countries, especially in Argentina, Chile, South Africa, Australia and New Zealand. Traditionally a family business, big corporations such as Kendall-Jackson in California, Moet & Chandon and Lafite-Rothschild in France and Freixenet in Spain have nevertheless been purchasing wine-growing land and buying into existing vineyards.[11]

In addition to mergers and acquisitions, alcohol beverage companies also achieve growth through vertical integration, which occurs when a company controls different stages of production, such as distribution or supply functions. These trends suggest that the alcohol industry is an important part of the environment in which drinking patterns are learned and practiced – especially with the growth of modern industrial production, the proliferation of new products (e.g. caffeinated alcohol 'energy drinks' and alcopops) and the development of sophisticated marketing and promotional techniques. Latin America, Africa and Asia have been identified by the industry as having high growth potential because of increasingly stable economies, growing income levels, a relatively high proportion of abstainers and a large youth population.[3,12]

12.3.2. Tobacco

Over the past 20 years, the tobacco industry has grown by means of a large number of privatisations, mergers and acquisitions that have strengthened the position of the four largest transnational tobacco companies (TTCs) in the world market (Philip Morris International (PMI), British American Tobacco (BAT), Japan Tobacco and Imperial Tobacco). Using a commonly accepted measure of market concentration, Hawkins et al.[13] have shown that the tobacco industry in almost all countries is often the most concentrated sector in an economy. Other significant changes in the global market include those designed to decrease the exposure of PMI and BAT assets in the United States to litigation against the tobacco companies.

In 2003, RJ Reynolds Tobacco Holdings and BAT's Brown & Williamson Tobacco Corporation combined their assets to create Reynolds American Inc, with BAT holding 42% of the shares of the new company. In 2008 Altria, until then the parent company of Philip Morris USA and PMI, spun off PMI, as a separate legal entity. Following China's 2001 entry into the World Trade Organization, China National Tobacco Corporation, the national state tobacco monopoly, increased its ambitions for global expansion and is the largest tobacco company in the world by volume, accounting for around 40% of global cigarette production.[14] Despite progress with implementation of the WHO Framework Convention on Tobacco Control (WHO FCTC), tobacco industry expansion continues globally, with greater functional integration of domestic, regional and global business strategies, which results in greater political and economic power.[15]

12.3.3. Unhealthy food and sugar-sweetened beverage industries

Ten food companies now control the majority of the world's leading food and beverage brands (i.e. Nestlé, PepsiCo, Coca-Cola, Unilever, Danone, General Mills, Kellogg's, Mars, Associated British Foods and Mondelez). Collectively, they generate over a billion dollars of revenue a day in an industry valued at over $7 trillion dollars in 2013.[16] SSBs are also manufactured by large corporations including Coca Cola, PepsiCo, Nestlé and Dr Pepper. Their products include soft drinks, fruit drinks, sports drinks, vitamin waters, flavoured waters, sweetened teas and caffeinated energy drinks. Of particular concern from a public health perspective is the dominance of highly processed food products. The global market in soft drinks has the strongest growth prospects of any consumer packaged goods.[17] The Asia Pacific region is projected to account for almost half (47%) of global volume growth with India the most rapidly expanding market.[10]

12.3.4. Structural links across industries and their political, economic and public health implications

In addition to the concentration of these industries into a small number of Transnational Corporations (TNCs), and their expansion across markets in the LMIC, there are similarities in the way that unhealthy food products, SSBs, alcohol and tobacco are marketed and purchased, which are potentially significant to understanding challenges confronting fiscal policy for health. Three of the top 10 soft drinks companies (Suntory, Asahi Group and Kirin) are also significant manufacturers of alcohol products in the Asia Pacific region. Broader links are reflected in integrated bottling operations and distribution chains.[13] There are also historical links between the tobacco, food and alcohol industries[19] that remain significant in some national and regional contexts. Altria Group, Inc. ('Altria') owns Ste. Michelle Wine Estates, and as of 2010, retained 27.1% economic and voting interests in SABMiller plc ('SABMiller'), the world's second largest beer company[20] before it merged with AB InBev in 2014.

The growing concentration of large industries producing products that are hazardous to health and the structural links among them have important public health implications. First, the economies of scale that come with concentration have allowed these TNCs to use sophisticated marketing techniques to create new or expanded markets in areas of the world where consumption has been traditionally low (e.g. Africa, Asia, Latin America) and where economies are expanding. Second, with increased consumption of these products comes greater risk of NCDs and other health hazards. Indeed, TNCs representing unhealthy commodity industries have been identified as major drivers of NCD epidemics.[21] Third, with increased concentration and global coordination across sectors, the alcohol, tobacco, food and beverage TNCs can conduct political activities that influence the policy environment for their products (see, e.g. Refs.[13,22]). As a result, they are able to prevent new players from competing with the existing ones (in economics, this is known as creating 'barriers to entry' in the marketplace).

12.4. Strategies and tactics employed by four industries to oppose health taxes

Strategies and tactics to advance political objectives, or corporate political activity (CPA), have been documented and analysed in many areas of business.[23] As shown in Table 12.2, core political strategies used across a variety of industries, including those involved in the production of NCD risk factors, are (1) using information to gain access to political decision-makers; (2) constituency-building with political decision-makers; (3) promoting alternative policies or ineffective voluntary measures; (4) using financial incentives to influence government policymakers to act in ways favourable to industry interests and (5) legal measures employing trade agreements as well as pre-emption, litigation and circumvention. Each long-term strategy includes a variety of tactics or short-term activities. Such taxonomies[24–26] have been used to evaluate how these industries promote their commercial and political interests, but the tactics have rarely been compared across all four industries in relation to taxation issues to examine whether the industries act in similar ways when their interests are threatened by public health measures. To the extent that these strategies and tactics are found to be similar, this information could be used to inform tax policy implementation across leading NCD risk factors.

In the preparation of this chapter, we conducted a broad search for examples of the tactics used by these industries in their treatment of health taxes and pricing policies. Search procedures were similar across the four industries. We combined two domains of keywords: the title of the tactic and the name of the industry. We searched for published research studies, journal review articles, books, book chapters, open data websites, newspaper articles and reports that addressed strategies and tactics used by these industries to prevent (or promote) tax or regulation policy related to public health. For the food industry, health taxes included varying names such as 'fat tax', 'sugar tax', 'grocery tax' depending on which types (fast foods, Food Corporation, restaurants) of food the article was talking about. Therefore, we used multiple combinations of keywords including 'food industry' and 'strategies' or 'food industry' and 'tax' or 'food industry' and 'the name of the tactic'.

Table 12.2. Categorisation and description of strategies.

Strategy	Tactics
Access/information	Political and other campaign contributions Direct and indirect lobbying (meetings and correspondence with policymakers) Use of misinformation; measures to shape the evidence base (funding and dissemination of research, use of paid consultants, position papers, technical reports) Partnerships/collaboration (working/advisory groups, technical support, advice)
Constituency-building	Forming alliances with trade associations, other industry sectors Forming alliances with or mobilizing civil society organisations, consumers, employees and/or the public Creation of SAPROs and fake grass-roots ('astroturf') consumer advocacy organisations Corporate-image advertising[a] Advocacy advertising[b] (press releases, mass media campaigns)
Policy substitution	Develop/promote self-regulation Develop/promote alternative regulatory policy Develop/promote voluntary activities
Financial incentives	Contributions to political parties Hiring or offering future employment to people with political connections Other financial enticement (gifts, travel)
Legal actions	Pre-emption Litigation (or threat of litigation) Circumvention

Source: Adapted from Hillman and Hitts[24] and Savell et al.[25]

[a] Corporate-image advertising seeks to build a favourable image and keep the company's name in the public eye.

[b] Advocacy advertising is defined as an advertisement or public communication that attempts to influence public opinion on a specific issue.

Major search engines such as Google, Google Scholar, PubMed (from early 2000 to 2019) were used. Although we tried to include sources from multiple languages, English-language sources predominated because of the nature of the primary search engines. In addition to the major search engines, other articles were found by tracing sources found in reference lists. Five different sources of information were included in the analysis: newspaper articles, original studies and reviews published in scientific or biomedical journals, books or book chapters, open data websites and reports. The largest proportion was derived from qualitative and quantitative studies published in peer reviewed scientific journals, followed by news reports.

Although Denmark started taxing soft drinks and juices in the 1930s, and the tobacco and alcohol industries were active in health policy issues since the 1970s, we limited the search primarily to examples identified since the year 2000 in order to make the search more relevant to contemporary health policy issues. Nevertheless, due to the Master Settlement Agreement (MSA) in 1998 in the United States, a vast quantity of internal tobacco industry documents became available, exposing strategies and tactics the industry utilised prior to 2000. We therefore included some earlier tobacco industry examples where relevant.

Articles that discussed industry activities in areas other than taxes were excluded, unless the more general tactic could be applied to tax policies, such as policy substitution. For example, we included some instances of food labelling and marketing regulation if the industry was likely to use these strategies to prevent health taxes. Editorials, letters and commentaries were excluded.

Table 12.3 summarises 64 documented examples related to the five general strategies and specific tactics used to implement these strategies. Evidence for almost every tactic was found for each of the four industries. Although the United States accounts for 45% of the examples, 25% were classified as international in scope and the remainder were found in Europe, Latin America, some Sub-Saharan African countries and several large metropolitan Asian cities such as Hong Kong and Bangkok. Many of the articles documenting these strategies and tactics were published around the time of major tax initiatives associated with national health policies. For

Table 12.3. Examples of strategies and tactics employed by four industries to oppose health taxes.*

Strategies	Tactics	Sugar-sweetened beverage industry	Tobacco industry	Alcohol industry	Food industry
Access and information	**Political and other campaign contributions**	Nine sugar farm or refinery groups made more than 900 separate contributions totaling nearly $1.5 million to candidates, parties and political funds[27] (1, USA).	A study of the US elections in five states during the mid-1990s demonstrated that tobacco industry campaign contributions influenced tobacco control policymaking. As tobacco industry contributions increased, a legislator's tobacco policy score became more pro-tobacco[28] (2, USA).	Alcohol distributors actively influenced state alcohol policies by donating $14.6 million to state candidates, and federal alcohol policies by giving approximately $5.9 million to congressional contests[29] (2, USA).	14 leading US restaurant chain Political Action Committees including unhealthy food companies contributed nearly $6 million to political groups between 2011 and 2014[30] (1, USA).
	Direct and indirect lobbying (meetings and correspondence with policymakers)	Sugar represents just 2% of the total value of US crop production, but the industry accounts for 33% of total campaign donations and 40% of total lobbying expenditures to protect US sugar producers[31] (5, USA).	A systematic review of 17 studies reported evidence of traditional lobbying techniques, with industry targeting key decision-makers both directly and indirectly[32] (2, INT). Two of the largest U.S. tobacco companies spent a combined $147,000 lobbying lawmakers and successfully defeated a Montana tobacco tax bill, which would have raised the state tax on cigarettes by $1.50 a pack and set a 74% tax on the wholesale price of vaping products[33] (1, USA).	A major alcohol producer was found to be secretly producing National Alcohol Policy drafts for four Sub-Saharan countries undermining public health approaches, including taxes, despite claiming to be an impartial observer at national conferences[34] (2, INT). An analysis of 35 policy debates on the United Kingdom's alcohol pricing found UK industry actors at every stage of the policy process by accessing and lobbying political members involved in policy-making[35] (2).	Food and beverage industries collectively spent $29,121,465 in their lobbying efforts[36] (4, USA). An Australian study documented 148 lobbying occurrences by the five key food and beverage industry actors between 2012 and 2015[37] (2, INT). The global food industry doubled their lobbying expenditures to $175 million during 2008–2011[38] (5, INT).
	Partnership/ collaboration (working/ advisory groups, technical support, advice)	From 2011 to 2015, two major beverage companies sponsored 95 national health organisations and lobbied against 29 public health bills intended to reduce soda consumption or improve nutrition[39] (2).	Between 1988 and 1998, the tobacco industry developed coalitions with African, American and Latinx trade unionists to influence excise taxes and smoke-free worksite policies[40] (2, USA). The tobacco industry established a political relationship with the Coalition of Labour Union Women to oppose smoke free worksite policies and increased tobacco taxes[41] (2, USA).	A major alcohol producer collaborated with think tank Demos and London Economics, a consultancy firm, to produce reports to influence the evidential content of UK's minimum unit pricing (MUP) alcohol policy debate[42] (2, UK).	At least 2 of the 15 advisors from the WHO Nutrition Guidance Expert Advisory group drafting new guidelines for sugar, salt and fat in the diet had direct financial ties to the food industry[38] (5, INT).

(Continued)

Table 12.3. *(Continued)*

Strategies	Tactics	Sugar-sweetened beverage industry	Tobacco industry	Alcohol industry	Food industry
Constituency-building	**Forming alliances with trade associations, other industry sectors**	A powerful Washington, D.C., trade organisation that represents major beverage companies funded a group to oppose a ballot measure to raise taxes on soda and other sweetened beverages[43] (1, USA). The soda industry pushed statewide measures to strip cities and towns of their ability to tax soda[44] (1, USA). Trade Associations formed a coalition called 'Americans Against Food Taxes' at the URL 'nofoodtaxes.com' to prevent taxation on sugar sweetened beverages using social media[45] (1, USA).	The tobacco industry built a coalition with alcohol and other industries to oppose cigarette excise taxes, clean indoor air policies and tobacco advertising constraints[20] (2, USA).	Hong Kong beer and wine formed the Hong Kong Wine & Spirits Industry Coalition along with catering and trade industries to lobby government officials on alcohol duties and strengthen its position on alcohol tax reduction. Hong Kong eliminated all duties on alcohol except for spirits in 2008[46] (2, China). The drinks industry in Ireland collaborated with civil society partners and governmental agencies to produce a report that created controversy about a public health approach to alcohol taxes and supported the industry's positions on reducing alcohol taxes[47] (2, Ireland).	
	Forming alliances with or mobilising civil society organisations, consumers, employees and/or the public	Dozens of Hispanic and African-American civil rights groups, health advocacy organisations and business associations joined the SSB industry in opposing soda regulation, arguing that such measures are discriminatory, paternalistic or ineffective[48] (2, USA).	Smoke shop owner/operators in the US state of Oklahoma formed a coalition that spearheaded a statewide campaign to end the continuing taxation of tobacco products[49] (1, USA). Tobacco industry financed the Consumer Tax Alliance, an interest group in 1989 that used media outreach to build public opposition to excise tax increases in US federal budget deficit negotiations[50] (2, USA).	The industry created front groups and used fake citizen groups (called 'astrotuf' organisations) to influence alcohol policy on behalf of the alcohol industry[35] (2, UK).	The food industry created front groups such as The Center for Consumer Freedom that criticised public health science that threatened corporate interests[51] (2, INT).

Table 12.3. *(Continued)*

Strategies	Tactics	Sugar-sweetened beverage industry	Tobacco industry	Alcohol industry	Food industry
	Creation of social aspects/ public relations organisations (SAPROs) and CSR campaigns	All leading US SSB firms launched corporate social responsibility (CSR) initiatives with elaborate, multinational cause marketing campaigns.[52] (2, INT).	A major tobacco company developed CSR programs to represent themselves as socially responsible, enable access to policymakers and increase the company's chances of influencing policy decisions[53] (2, UK).	The alcohol industry created social aspects organisations (SAOs) such as the Portman Group, Drinkaware and Challenge 25 to portray themselves as socially responsible partners in the policy process[35] (2, UK). An analysis of the alcohol industry's SAPROs such as the Foundation for Advancing Alcohol Responsibility in the USA, DrinkAware (UK) and DrinkWise (Australia) found they serve as fronts for the industry to lobby for ineffective approaches and against effective countermeasures[54] (2, INT).	The food industry created front groups to manipulate media, policymakers and general public into trusting industry-produced information such as reports, panels, and professional conferences[55] (1, USA).
	Corporate-image advertising	SSB corporations use CSR initiatives to align themselves with good causes to burnish their public image and improve their standing among consumers, the press, legislators, and regulators who make policy decisions[52] (2). Internal emails detailed the overarching strategy of a major beverage producer to defeat local, national and international policy efforts, including soda taxes, by building political power, positioning itself as a public health partner, and appearing to the public as socially responsible[56] (1, INT).	Companies build their corporate reputations by marketing their ethical sincerity to the public by admitting nicotine is addictive and by supporting the Youth Smoking Prevention Department with an annual budget of $100 million[57] (2).	The alcohol industry used media sources to portray themselves as socially responsible economic actors that generate tax revenue and employment during the excise tax debate in Poland[58] (2, Poland).	The food industries in Thailand associated with charitable foundations to improve their public image by promoting health, sports and research[59] (2, Thailand).

(Continued)

Table 12.3. *(Continued)*

Strategies	Tactics	Sugar-sweetened beverage industry	Tobacco industry	Alcohol industry	Food industry
	Advocacy advertising (press releases, publicity campaigns)	A leaked email from the American Beverage Association showed that a major beverage company was actively trying to 'shape' media coverage including print, digital, radio and television in coordination with 'off record conversations' with the *Wall Street Journal* reporter before Philadelphia's soda tax vote[56] (1, USA).		The Drinks Industry Group of Ireland held a press conference to express concerns about increased taxation in 2004 after the publication of a report incorporating WHO strategies to alcohol policy[60] (2, Ireland).	
Policy substitution	**Develop/ promote self-regulation**	Public health lawmaking and litigation triggered self-regulation initiatives such as the 2006 Beverage Industry Voluntary Guidelines to curtail sales of SSBs in schools[61] (2).	The tobacco industry's 'We Card' youth tobacco access prevention program was created in 1995 to improve the industry's image through publicity and to reduce regulation and law enforcement activity focused on tobacco control[62] (2, USA).		When the Mexican government was advised to raise taxes on products high in sugar, fat and salt, the bakery giant Grupo Bimbo cut sodium in its leading bread and rolls in response[38] (5, Mexico).
	Develop/ promote alternative regulatory policy or voluntary activities	In 2016, Latin American beverage companies responded to the regulatory initiatives to reduce SSBs, pledging to sell only water, drinks with over 12% fruit juice and cereal-based drinks in primary schools in Colombia and only water, fruit juice, coconut water and dairy products in schools for children under 12 years in Brazil[22] (2, INT).	Between 1999 and 2001, three major tobacco producers executed Project Cerberus to develop a global voluntary regulatory regime as an alternative to the WHO FCTC and FDA regulation on the USA tobacco industry[63] (2, INT).	When the Scottish Parliament and United Kingdom considered measures to increase the minimum price of alcohol, the industry promoted non-price interventions, especially education and proposed targeted approaches instead[64] (2, UK). Diageo's Responsible Drinking Fund supported more than 130 programs lacking evidence of effectiveness in more than 40 countries, covering education, public awareness and responsible retail practices in 2009[65] (2, INT).	When the industry was threatened by the government's obesity-related public health measures, they launched self-regulation efforts as an alternative[66] (2, USA).

Table 12.3. *(Continued)*

Strategies	Tactics	Sugar-sweetened beverage industry	Tobacco industry	Alcohol industry	Food industry
Financial measures	**Contribution to political parties**	The soft-drink industry gave a total of $95,300 to Council candidates in 2010–2011 to stop efforts to revive soda tax in Philadelphia, a nearly 800% increase from 2006 to 2007, when the industry contributed just $10,600[67] (1, USA).	The tobacco industry donated $2.4 million to members of Congress between 1991 and 1992. The more tobacco money a member received, the less likely the member was to support tobacco control legislation[68] (2, USA).	Due to the alcohol industry's heavy contributions to political parties, it is difficult to amend alcohol policies[69] (2, USA).	The number of registered lobbyists increased from 15,000 to 20,000 between 1997 and 1999, spending an estimated $1.42 billion on behalf of food industry clients to influence the US Congress in 1998[70] (3, USA).
	Hiring or offering future employment to people with political connections	In its efforts to oppose taxes on sugary drinks in California, the soda industry engaged a research firm that had previously worked for Michelle Obama's *Let's Move!* Initiative and the Robert Wood Johnson Foundation, the nation's largest public health philanthropy organisation[71] (1, USA).		When 10 of the world's largest distilled spirits and beer marketers created the International Centre for Alcohol Policies, they hired a former employee of WHO to create programs that focused on countering the influence of the WHO and leading alcohol researchers[72] (2, INT).	The European Food Information Council, an industry sponsored think tank, hired former EU lobbyist-in-chief for snack company Mars to conduct its scientific operations[73] (5, INT).
Legal actions	**Pre-emption**	The food and beverage industry successfully pushed for a state law that prevents or nullifies the government's power to tax sugary drinks in Santa Fe, New Mexico[74] (1, USA).	In 1995, the tobacco industry promoted legislation that pre-empted local tobacco regulation in 29 states and introduced 26 bills regarding pre-emption in 1996 state legislation session[75] (2, USA).	A study reported that 31 states had pre-empted local alcohol tax authority[76] (USA, 2).	State pre-emption was used to impede local food and nutrition policies and government-initiated litigation. Between 2008 and 2018, 12 states enacted 13 pre-emptive laws on food-related policies and taxes[77] (2, USA).
	Litigation (or threat of litigation) and circumvention	In Mexico's 'Taxes on Soft Drinks' (2005) case, the United States challenged Mexico's 20% excise tax measures on soft drinks, syrups and other beverages that used any sweetener including high-fructose corn syrup and beet sugars other than cane sugar. The World Trade Association found the tax discriminatory and Mexico had to withdraw the measures[78] (1, Mexico).	The tobacco industry used federal equal protection claims under the 14th Amendment and claims of state pre-emption of local ordinance violations in litigation to overturn local tobacco control ordinances[79] (2, USA).	The Scottish Whiskey Association delayed the implementation of Minimum Unit Pricing by litigating the issue in the European Court[64] (2, UK).	Denmark's fat tax was repealed as a result of the food industry's lobbying, threatened lawsuits and juridical actions at the EU level[80] (2, Denmark). In France, the food industries promoted deregulation or promised to make their products healthy when threatened with taxes or regulation by the government[81] (2, France).

*At the end of each entry, in parentheses, is a number and either a country name or INT. The numbers refer to the following sources: (1) newspaper article, (2) journal article or case study (3) book, (4) Open Data Website, (5) report. INT refers to 'international' indicating that the tactic was used in multiple countries.

example, Finland reinstated a soft drink tax in 2011 and France introduced a targeted tax on sugary drinks at a national level in 2012.

It should be noted that these examples are provided for illustrative purposes only. They represent neither a complete nor a representative inventory of industry activities. Many come from the United States, in part because of the availability of internal industry documents obtained through litigation cases against the tobacco industry, in part because of the concentration of many TNCs in the United States.

Almost all of the examples describe the activities of TNCs and their social aspects organisations and trade associations. This suggests that opposition to health taxes may be a primary concern of the largest producers, which often own a large portfolio of products and services. The table also suggests that individual tactics tend to be part of long-term strategies that are conducted to achieve broad industry goals such as reduced regulation, lower taxation and un-regulated marketing. Some articles[72,73] identified direct coordination or common interests across industries, such as tobacco and alcohol, especially during a period when a large TNC owned both alcohol and tobacco brands. This suggests the likelihood of cross-fertilisation through TNC ownership of food, beverage, alcohol and tobacco companies. Marion Nestle's (2015) book, *Soda Politics: Taking on Big Soda (and Winning)*,[70] describes the soda industry's adoption of the business tactics developed by the tobacco industry, which built a coalition with the alcohol producers and other industries to oppose cigarette excise taxes, clean indoor air policies and tobacco advertising constraints.[20] Financial ties between the tobacco and pharmaceutical companies have weakened smoking cessation efforts as well by sharing technology to develop nicotine products that are profitable to both industries.[82]

The tobacco industry pioneered the use of strategies to frame the issues and create controversy about tobacco policy by manipulating research at multiple stages. For instance, through its funding mechanisms, the industry attempted to control the research agenda and types of questions asked about tobacco, and the industry's lawyers and executives were involved in the sponsorship of research as well as the suppression of research findings that were unfavourable to the industry.[83] While tobacco companies' involvement in the political process has been well documented, there has also been an increase in their efforts to promote themselves as responsible corporate citizens as well as important partners in the development of legislation and regulation, particularly in markets where there is less political support for tobacco control.[63] As new threats to industry profits emerge, new industry strategies develop, such as the exploitation of bilateral trade agreements to oppose national tobacco control measures and to undermine implementation of the WHO Framework Convention on Tobacco Control (WHO FCTC).[68]

Some industry tactics cut across several strategies. Box 12.2 shows the typical arguments used by these industries in advocacy campaigns against health taxes, illustrating tactics such as information dissemination, advocacy advertising, constituency building and promoting alternative regulatory policy. Several policy reviews have concluded that these arguments are not consistent with the scientific evidence.[17,32,84–86] For example, the claim that raising tobacco taxes will serve to increase smuggling is a misleading but longstanding and often influential argument. It has persisted despite evidence that tobacco companies have been actively complicit in cigarette smuggling in order to maintain their market share in jurisdictions with high excise taxes.[32,86]

Box 12.2. Main arguments against health taxes

- Raising taxes leads to economic losses to the government and massive job losses in the retail sector
- Raising taxes will lead to illicit trade and consumption, as well as tax evasion and tax avoidance
- Raising taxes are against the rule of the WTO and free trade agreements
- Consumers will switch to cheaper and more dangerous products

- The poor and working class consumers are adversely targeted by taxation policies
- Consumers have the right to consume what they want and it is not the job of governments to interfere
- Countries with high taxes also have high consumption
- People who consume in moderation should not pay the price for the few who consume excessively and substitution of other products which would be more harmful

In the area of constituency-building, these industries have numerous allies who act as collaborators at country and local levels. Many such allies are groups that profit from the sale of alcohol, tobacco and SSBs, such as convenience stores, restaurants, bars, grocers, gas stations, pharmacies, tourism groups, hotels and advertising groups. Such industries also create front groups or third-party organisations to lobby on their behalf, forming alliances with NGOs and other civil society organisations. This generally occurs when these industries are facing a significant regulatory threat.[25]

Within each industry, companies act both individually and at times in collaboration to oppose tax increases, including by forming alliances with trade and business associations and with other sectors to oppose tax increases. For example, in 2014, Chile began tax reforms to finance free, quality public education. Proposed reforms included 'corrective taxes' on SSBs and alcohol. The proposed tax on alcohol would increase from 15% for beer and wine and 27% for spirits, to an ad valorem base tax of 18%, with 0.5% extra per each degree of alcohol content and 0.03 monthly tax unit per litre of pure alcohol. Shortly after the announcement, the country's largest brewer, along with several large food and beverage companies, announced the creation of an association, AB Chile, to represent the interests of the industry and fight the tax increase. Instead of supporting public health advocates, the government agreed to eliminate the per unit tax, resulting in a 50% drop in the proposed tax increase.[87]

Promoting alternative regulatory policy is a common tactic used by all four industries. Sometimes their interests converge around a particular policy proposal. In March 2016, government officials in Ecuador announced plans to increase taxes on cigarettes, alcohol and soda. Concerned by these proposed tax reforms, which would raise taxes on beer from USD 7.24 to USD 12 per litre of pure alcohol, executives from the national brewery presented their own proposal to the Economic Regime Commission instead suggesting a gradual increase in taxes whereby the company would maintain product prices under such reforms,[88] effectively neutralising the likely health impact of the taxes.

Another industry strategy that directly targets policymakers is the use of financial inducements or financial leverage, which occurs when a business uses its economic power to influence government. In response to proposed tax increases in El Salvador, the brewing and spirits industries threatened mass firings of their employees and reduced earnings, which would translate into lower revenue from taxes. Transcripts from an AmBev Earnings Conference Call[88–89] provide some insight into this process. Speaking to investors regarding a potential tax increase, the CEO of AmBev explained that:

> 'the federal tax is a discussion between the industry and the government. It has usually been like that in the past ... We are sitting with the government. The industry is sitting with the government as we speak to find out where this will end.' He goes on to say, 'I think one thing we can say is it's a different moment. When we sat down with the government last year, it was a moment where growth and jobs and everything were more important. They are always important, but they were more important. So the government sought the proposal that was sort of put together with the whole industry and the government about not moving federal tax at all.'

Research has also documented multiple instances of industry tactics over an extended period of time. McCambridge et al.[90] analysed 20 reports from 15 peer-reviewed journals between 1980 and 2016 that revealed the alcohol industry's strategies in influencing policymaking, especially tax laws.

The empirical and qualitative studies suggest that the industries' policy positions in engaging with taxation are focused on industry-related commercial issues rather than public health, even as public health is often advanced as the ostensible reason for their policy involvement. These findings suggest that a political economy analysis of health taxes needs to consider the corporate political activities in these industries and how that affects the ability of key stakeholders to create health policy networks capable of reversing global trends in NCDs.

12.5. Toward a public health approach based on a political economy analysis

The previous assessment of NCD risk factors has demonstrated that TNCs involved in the manufacture, marketing and sale of health damaging products engage in corporate political tactics that make it difficult to implement effective public health policies, notably including health taxes. Our analysis shows that many other stakeholders are involved in the development and implementation of health taxes and these should be considered in any political economy analysis. NGOs, government agencies, civil society groups, public health professionals and the scientific community can all play a role as part of a global health policy network.[91]

Bump and Reich[92] contend that one reason why tobacco has been so difficult to control is that the political economy of these products has not been adequately understood and addressed. That observation seems likely to be equally relevant to other NCD risk factors. Political economy analysis differs from the traditional public health approaches that dominate the health policy literature because it deals with the interactions between politics and economics, and it requires that attention be devoted in particular to transnational corporations (TNCs) that increasingly influence the framing, the discourse, the political processes and the economic policies that are likely to affect the future of health taxes nationally and internationally. The information presented in Table 12.3 provides a compelling case not only for studying and monitoring the activities of these industries, but also for seeking to exclude them from the public health policy process, as is provided for, in relation to the tobacco industry, by the WHO FCTC.

Bump and Reich[92] identified five policy areas where political economy analysis could make a positive contribution to the advancement of tobacco control policies: information problems concerning citizen knowledge; the roles of domestic producers; multinational corporations and trade disputes in consumption; smuggling; incentive conflicts between government branches and barriers to raising taxes. Based on the information summarised in Table 12.3, these areas can be broadly applied to other NCD risk factors to design and implement more effective NCD controls.

12.5.1. Information problems concerning citizen knowledge of the dangers of NCD risk factors

If the true costs of the products defined as NCD risk factors were universally known and accepted, it is unlikely that completely rational people would choose to smoke, drink alcohol excessively and consume SSBs and processed foods to the extent they do. But ignorance of these health consequences is common among both individual consumers and government policymakers. Many of the health interventions designed to inform consumers about NCD risk factors are based on the implicit assumption that providing accurate information about the public health benefits of regulation is sufficient to persuade consumers to quit smoking and reduce or eliminate their use of other harmful products. It is also assumed that such information is sufficient to empower control advocates and regulators.

Rather than let scientific and medical findings drive popular opinions, these industries, particularly through the influence of TNCs, have defined and promoted a positive culture of using these products that proved more persuasive for many individuals, particularly youth. Political economy analysis can be helpful for understanding the forces that shape opinions regarding these products because it focuses on information asymmetries. It can also move beyond description to suggest strategies for addressing public perceptions, including counter-marketing.

12.5.2. Domestic producers, TTCs and trade disputes

TTCs and the countries that support them have used trade liberalisation, agreements and disputes to open new markets for their products. By exercising their power in the context of international trade agreements, TNCs can undermine the authority of national governments even in their own domestic affairs. An important if partial exception to this pattern has been Thailand, whose success in establishing high taxes on tobacco and alcohol was due largely to the influence of non-government organisations and activists. Political economy analysis can help control advocates understand how TTCs gain access to closed or restricted markets and can identify relevant stakeholders to form more powerful coalitions.

12.5.3. The use of smuggling and unrecorded alcohol to undermine regulation

Cigarette smuggling and the illicit production of unregistered alcohol are large and profitable activities in which TTCs have been both 'complicit' and instrumental in misinterpreting as a policy lever.[93,94] Cigarette smuggling and illicit production of alcohol limit tax revenues by impacting on the legal trade and contribute to increased consumption because of lower prices. Political economy analysis could help explore the challenges of using international action to prevent diversion and smuggling and hold TTCs responsible for their products through improved tracking and tax enforcement, and by helping to identify stakeholders, build coalitions and prepare for TTC responses. A landmark development in this regard is the entry into force in 2018 of the Protocol to Eliminate Illicit Trade in Tobacco Products,[95] building on Article 15 of the WHO FCTC. The Protocol provides for multi-sectoral action and international cooperation to eliminate all forms of illicit trade in tobacco products and reaffirms the obligation for Parties to protect their policies from commercial and other vested interests of the tobacco industry.

12.5.4. Intra-governmental incentive conflicts

Political economy analysis can help explain conflicts among government agencies and how these conflicts can favour the profit-making agendas of powerful industries. Some ministries, such as finance, typically support such industries because of the tax revenues they generate. Other ministries, such as health, are likely to oppose NCD risk factor industries because of the death, disability and related illness costs that they cause. Further complexity comes from the asymmetric power of ministries of finance and health, which often favours the former in policymaking. Intragovernmental conflicts are often based on misinformation, which is frequently supplied by these industries as a means of promoting and protecting their interests. Such misinformation exacerbates the policy differences between tax authorities and health authorities, which need not be in conflict.

12.5.5. Barriers to implementing health taxes

Political economy analysis can be used to meet the challenges in adopting and implementing health taxes. As suggested by Table 12.3, the primary opposition to taxation is TTCs and their economically interested allies. A common strategy for opposing taxes is misinformation based on the argument that taxes will cause economic harm to affected businesses.[22] Attempts to raise taxes have also been countered by TTC lobbying efforts suggesting that increased taxes cause economic harm, and through the use of biased research, litigation, constituency-building, policy substitution and financial contributions to political parties.[22] Political economy considerations can also guide the work of public health activists to deal with opposition from TNCs by identifying the relevant stakeholders and assessing different political strategies. Potential allies include health NGOs, physicians, scientists and national health authorities.

12.6. Next steps: Methods and countermeasures

Documenting industry strategies and tactics in relation to the activities of these other stakeholders is just the first step in a political economy analysis. The next step is using this information and other research to develop countermeasures that enable decision-makers to act in the public interest. In this section we describe methods and countermeasures that can be used to build coalitions at the local, national in international levels capable of working with or without the cooperation of these industries in the interests of public health. Many of these strategies have been found to be instrumental in the design and implementation of health taxes in LMICs.[22,96] We begin with a review of stakeholder contributions that have been tried, tested or considered as potentially effective ways to promote, implement and enforce health taxes and related measures. We conclude with a description of how these stakeholder interests can be combined to work synergistically as health policy networks at the national and global levels.

12.6.1. World Health Organization and its regional offices

The World Health Organization[97] has developed an active program to provide its own staff and those of its Member States with the information and skills needed to promote health taxes by: (1) framing health taxes as health measures that can result in significant gains in population health; (2) understanding that health taxes generate stable, predictable revenues and (3) knowing the practical aspects of tax design and implementation such as the different types of excise taxes (e.g. specific duty versus ad valorem, earmarking) as well as issues of tax governance and administration. WHO's current guidance[98] for Member States emphasises the importance of collaboration between health and financial sectors, updating the evidence on fiscal policies in health and preventing or eliminating artificial financial incentives to consume products that are harmful to health.

WHO developed a series of information packages and policy briefs in collaboration with UN Development Program that describe the evidence base needed by decision-makers inside and out of government to make informed decisions about the reduction of NCDs, taking into account implications for agriculture, employment, revenue generation, illicit trade and social inequality. These efforts toward information dissemination and strategic support need to be supplemented with greater amounts of funding for technical assistance, monitoring and implementation support.

The 2018 report of the Independent High-Level Commission on NCDs[99] calls on governments to appropriately engage with the private sector while considering commercial and other vested interests, including the food and non-alcoholic beverage companies (though with the notable exception of tobacco). It called on WHO to support governments' efforts to engage with the private sector taking into consideration the rationale, principles, benefits and risks, as well as the management of conflicts of interest in such engagement. WHO should build on such efforts by continuing to examine terms of engagement with major industries whose products are responsible for NCD risk and by advising governments about the hazards of partnerships with industry organisations and groups. Such approaches can draw lessons from the guidelines for implementation of Article 5.3 of the WHO FCTC on the protection of public health policies with respect to tobacco control from commercial and other vested interests of the tobacco, and from WHO's development of a tool to support member states in the management of conflict of interest in nutrition policy.[98,100,101]

12.6.2. Governments

The UN interagency Task Force on the Prevention and Control of Non-communicable diseases[102] recommends that an acceptable national response requires greater policy coherence across government to deliver effective NCD action plans. In the area of health taxes, policy coherence can be achieved in the following ways:

- Design health taxes to be easy to administer, hard to manipulate and difficult to circumvent.
- Increase taxes, design better taxes, adjust taxes, enforce taxes.
- Develop national frameworks to achieve greater policy coherence, partnerships and stronger systems for surveillance.
- Use WHO information packages.

Governments can also improve their capacity to counter the strategies used by industry by setting rules about their ability to interfere with the political process, undertaking due diligence and having transparent processes in decision-making. This can be advanced by:

- Expanding people's right to know and corporations' duty to disclose health consequences of corporate practices and products.
- Requiring corporations to pay for health and environmental consequences of products and practices.
- Establishing local and national health standards for product design and marketing.
- Protecting science and universities from corporate intrusion.
- Restoring the 'visible hand' of government in public health protection.
- Preventing corporations from using money and power to manipulate democratic processes.

National and local governments are often the targets for much of the information dissemination undertaken by commercial and vested interests. It is important to correct the imbalance in resources to advocate for effective policies and at the same time conduct a critical appraisal of the industry's strategies. National and local governments can best fulfil their public health responsibilities by:

- Avoiding direct partnerships with commercial or vested interest groups, or their representatives, in the development or implementation of policy. Commercial conflicts of interest should be made explicit, and input from industry-financed groups on policy implementation must be critically evaluated in light of their vested interests. Public health must be placed above commercial interests.
- Establishing an independent governmental agency to address product-related issues and advise on policy options. Such an agency should be protected from influence of commercial and vested interests.
- Using tax revenues to establish funding sources independent of commercial and other vested interests to carry out research, public health advocacy work, prevention and treatment.
- Banning price promotions and other marketing strategies that encourage overconsumption.

12.6.3. Public health professionals

The public health community consists of a loose coalition of public health practitioners, academics and government officials who maintain and study the public health infrastructure at the local, national and international levels. The public health community can provide critical support for governments to implement health taxes by engaging in the following activities:

- Avoid funding from industry sources for prevention, research and information dissemination activities. Refrain from any form of association with industry education programs.
- Improve dissemination of information for advocacy and policy development to combat the extensive lobbying power of the alcohol industry.

- Make research published in peer-reviewed journals available and interpretable for non-technical audiences.
- Insist on industry support for evidence-based policies and cessation of anti-scientific lobbying activities.
- Insist on rigorous adherence to conflict-of-interest principles.
- Support independent research in developing countries on the public health impact of taxes on unhealthy commodities.
- Make all information and details relating to funding and/or partnership work transparent and available for public scrutiny.

12.6.4. Scientific community

Concerns have been raised about the involvement of food, beverage and alcohol companies in scientific organisations and their influence on scientists. Similarities of these tactics with the activities of the tobacco industry have been noted.[103] Tactics include the provision of research funding designed to raise methodological or substantive questions about the existing literature, controlling the research agenda to focus on alternatives to health taxes (e.g. education programs), and recruitment of reputable scientists to serve in industry-funded advisory committees and organisations. The response of the scientific community, including journal editors, has typically been to require funding disclosures and conflict of interest statements to be published along with industry-funded studies, but these measures can be easily circumvented and have little impact on public health except to demonstrate consistent evidence of biased findings and industry agenda-setting.[104] Nevertheless, in isolated incidents, health journalists, journal editors and public health advocates have been influential in exposing industry tactics and at the same time inadvertently promoting health taxes because of the counter-marketing effect of negative publicity on industry stakeholder marketing. Freedom of Information (FOI) requests, interviews with key informants and depositions gathered through legal challenges have been employed to draw public attention to industry tactics.

Bakke and Endal[34] published a paper exposing alcohol industry involvement in writing national policy documents in four African countries, including recommendations against alcohol tax increases. The effect of their article led to employer sanctions against an Australian academic who served as a consultant to the industry and had other repercussions in the countries where the industry interference occurred.[103]

To the extent that industry activities can serve as risk factors or inducers of NCDs, there is a need to include relevant industry indicators in public health surveillance systems that are used routinely to monitor health-related harms at the international and national levels. Public health surveillance of the activities of the alcohol, tobacco, unhealthy food and SSB industries can be conducted in several ways.[90,105] First, national governments can be encouraged to fund data collection centres to monitor industry activities and performance. An international NCD clearinghouse or monitoring centre could also be established to provide ongoing guidance, assemble existing research findings and develop protocols and instruments to monitor industry activities and facilitate cross-national research. Other mechanisms and tools for monitoring industry activities include:

- The use of FOI requests to investigate corporate political activity that occurs behind closed doors.
- Interviews with key informants who have been involved in or who have directly observed industry activities.
- Protection for whistle blowers who disclose unethical activity.
- Monitoring corporate progress towards the UN SDGs, which are reported in annual sustainable development reports.
- Pool resources to purchase, monitor and track market research data.
- Use industry financial data to monitor changes in patterns of consumption and sales.
- Analyse industry communications and documentation of any discrepancies between public statements and actual industry practices.
- Track spending for lobbying and campaign contributions.

12.6.5. Civil society groups and nongovernmental organisations

NGOs can be critical watchdogs and advocates for health-related issues.[106] They can facilitate the health literacy of parliamentarians and work with public health professionals and health scientists to bring pressure to act in the public interest. For example, a group of public health professionals in Chile created the *Frente por una Reforma Tributaria Saludable* ('Front for a Healthy Tax Reform')[107] to advocate for tax reform that would effectively reduce consumption of alcohol, tobacco and SSBs. The Front consists of 13 organisations, including academic institutions, NGOs, trade unions, medical associations and scientific societies. Its advocacy work is divided into three areas: media, parliament and civil society. The group has organised massive Twitter events, written articles in national newspapers and blogs, drafted an open letter to the Minister of Finance and met with the Minister of Health and several members of Parliament. Such efforts are consistent with effective policy advocacy in other areas of public health. Studies[108,109] suggest the reform of Corporate Political Activity is contingent upon the ability of rivals to pursue strategies comparable to those of industry.

'Grass roots' initiatives that bring together various segments of civil society can have a significant effect on public opinion when industry tactics are designed to capture the public discourse around tax initiatives. Lessons learned from US cities where sugary drink taxes were being debated (https://nyti.ms/2zbEw9B) suggest that community coalitions that build public awareness at the early stages of a policy debate are better able to withstand industry attacks that include lobbying, targeting key journalists and the formation of faux grass-roots organisations by Big Soda companies like Coca-Cola and their trade associations. In the case of health taxes, coalitions include teachers' unions, local ethnic and religious groups, civic leaders and health NGOs.

12.6.6. The food, beverage, alcohol and tobacco industries

In recent years several attempts have been made to better define an appropriate role for the private sector and its industries in matters that relate to public health. Wiist[110] developed illustrative examples of actions that could be taken by food and beverage corporations to be truly responsive to the needs of civil society and democratic governments. In relation to the tobacco industry, WHO has acknowledged that 'the tobacco industry has operated for years with the express intention of subverting the role of governments and of WHO in implementing public health policies to combat the tobacco epidemic' (WHA54.18). Article 5.3 of the WHO FCTC, adopted in 2003 under the auspices of WHO, requires that Parties to the Convention protect their public health policies from commercial and other vested interests of the tobacco industry. Further, WHO's Framework of engagement with non-State actors, adopted in 2016, commits WHO not to engage with the tobacco industry or non-State actors that work to further the interests of the tobacco industry.

In 2011 the United Nations General Assembly adopted the Political Declaration of the High-level Meeting of the General Assembly on the Prevention and Control of Non-communicable Diseases (resolution A/RES/66/2). The Declaration acknowledged that governments are primarily responsible for NCD prevention and control, but they also need the cooperation of private sector entities, including the alcohol, food and beverage industries. The Declaration cited the need to protect policies for the prevention and control of NCDs from undue influence from real, perceived or potential conflicts of interest. The issue of conflict of interest and its management was identified as the most important and critical aspect of WHO work on a framework of engagement with non-State actors (FENSA) which was adopted at the World Health Assembly in 2016.[111]

Similarly, a WHO Global Coordination Mechanism for the prevention and control of non-communicable diseases (GCM/NCD) included a working group on how to realise governments' commitments to engage with the private sector for the prevention and control of NCDs. The Working Group concluded:

> that governments (including government agencies) will need to engage or consult with the private sector in preventing and controlling NCDs, and may indeed be obliged to do so in the development of policies and legislation, even if this is solely related to implementation issues.

In 2017, the WHO Global Conference on NCDs held in Montevideo, Uruguay, led to the Montevideo Roadmap 2018–2030s on NCDs as a sustainable development priority. The document recognised the need to increase opportunities for participation of non-State actors, including the private sector, to address NCDs as a development priority. At the same time, it recognised that public health objectives and private sector interests can conflict and suggested conditions to engage constructively with private sector actors in ways that maximise public health benefits. This may include promoting verifiable commitments of non-State actors, as well as their reporting on the implementation of those commitments. In addition, the 2018 report of the Independent High-Level Commission on NCDs asked governments to collaborate and appropriately engage with the private sector while considering commercial and other vested interests, including the food and non-alcoholic beverage companies. In all these political declarations, the tobacco industry is excluded because of its past behaviour and the global governance provisions set forth in the WHO FCTC. To the extent that other industries have adopted the strategies and tactics of the tobacco industry, they have a corporate responsibility to respect human rights.[112] However, when it comes to tobacco: (1) it is recognised that the tobacco industry is like no other given that the core of its business is incompatible with the right to health (WHA39.14 'Tobacco or Health') and (2) the tobacco industry has used 'human rights' arguments in legal challenges against tobacco control measures.

Inappropriate commitments by these industries to prevent and reduce NCD-related problems can be defined as activities that have no scientific evidence of effectiveness, those that have evidence of potential harm and those that include implicit or explicit marketing messages that are associated with a particular brand and therefore may contribute to increased sales and consumption. This includes a variety of industry Corporate Social Responsibility (CSR) initiatives that appear to be designed to minimise health problems, but have little impact on reducing harmful use of these products and may actually serve as marketing activities themselves.[26] In the case of tobacco, Implementation Guidelines for Article 13 of the WHO FCTC explicitly call on Parties to ban contributions from tobacco companies to any other entity for 'socially responsible causes', as this is a form of sponsorship, as well as publicity given to 'socially responsible' business practices of the tobacco industry, as it constitutes advertising and promotion.

Another type of inappropriate activity that these industries should refrain from is lobbying against evidence-based taxation policies,[85] especially policies recommended by WHO as cost effective measures to reduce NCDs.

12.7. Conclusions and the way forward

According to some analysts[106,113] several frameworks or conceptual trends have characterised the public health field in the area of NCDs in the 21st century. Initially, attention was devoted to the social determinants of health and the impact of social and economic inequality. A second trend has been the growing interest in studying the commercial determinants of health, as suggested by much of the research reviewed in this chapter. A third trend is the study of political determinants of health, which overlaps with the first two trends).[105] Within the context of these conceptual developments, especially in relation to health taxes, there is a need for discourse on commercial determinants of health to include a specific focus on health taxes as an instrument of increased government revenues, reduced health care costs, as well as improved quality of life and increased longevity. Framing health taxes in terms of their economic, social and public health benefits rather than allowing industry to define them as a liability can be a persuasive argument that could increase the chances of implementing effective NCD prevention.

Nevertheless, there remain significant conflicts between commercial and public health goals. There are also significant regulatory challenges in most countries, including insufficient regulatory capacity; overlap of functions; lack of clarity of functions; regulatory processes which are not systematic, and sectors (e.g. finance, agriculture, health) that are working in opposite directions. As described in other chapters in this book (see, e.g. Chapters 9 and 10), several mechanisms should be in place to ensure independent decision-making in setting up taxation policies, including: technical consultations, social participation, protection of the right to health, transparency, risk assessment, management of conflicts of interest, enforcement of laws, monitoring implementation and evaluating results.

To effectively take advantage of these mechanisms, there is a need to expand the influence of health policy networks dedicated to the reduction of NCD risk factors at the national and international levels. In contrast to the fragmented activities that are conducted by independent groups of public health professionals, health NGOs, academics and government agencies, health policy networks can play a synergistic role in policies like health taxes by framing issues, assembling resources, mobilising support groups, setting up coordination structures and getting policies adopted and implemented.[91] Networks have historically been used to successfully address global health problems like tuberculosis, tobacco use, polio and neonatal mortality. What is needed are effective leaders, appropriate governance structures to pursue collective goals, communication channels that link scientists, advocates, policymakers and others from both high- and low-income countries and framing strategies that allow network actors to publicly position an issue. Box 12.3 describes the role of health policy networks in the progress made by tobacco control advocates, compared with those engaged in the prevention of other NCD risk factors. Because these diverse coalitions work independently, there may be value in encouraging greater collaboration among these networks, particularly around the common idea of health taxes.

Box 12.3. Why has tobacco control made greater strides than efforts to address other NCD risk factors?

Smoking, drinking and the consumption of unhealthy food and beverages contribute significantly to the burden of non-communicable diseases, especially in low- and middle-income countries. According to Gneiting and Schmitz,[91] tobacco control has made more sustained progress than alcohol control in terms of international and domestic policy commitments, resources dedicated to reducing harm and reduction of tobacco use in many high-income countries. Research suggests that one reason for the progress in tobacco control, compared with alcohol, SSBs and unhealthy food products, is the emergence of a global health network composed of individuals and organisations dedicated to tobacco control.[91,114] Networks that link scientists, advocates, policymakers and others may achieve better outcomes because diversity improves collective understanding and problem solving, especially in LMIC.[115]

Whereas the tobacco control network evolved from a group of dedicated individuals to a global coalition of membership-based organisations, the effectiveness of the alcohol control network has been limited by mixed messages about the harmfulness of alcohol, competing problem definitions, the segmentation of the treatment, harm reduction (e.g. alcohol-impaired driving) and policy groups and the influence of industry partnerships with civil society organisations.

The tobacco control network has been more effective in creating and maintaining wide-spread consensus about effective policies to harm reduction and has been successful in combining research with effective advocacy at the highest levels of the World Health Organisation. The WHO FCTC is both an example of and a key catalyst for the achievements of tobacco control. Although the tobacco industry has been relegated to the status of a pariah in public opinion and policy deliberations, the alcohol industry, as well as the producers of SSBs and harmful food products, are still viewed as legitimate stakeholders in shaping domestic and international policies aimed at the reduction of harm connected with their products. Among network and actor features, the existence of effective leaders, the quality of governance and the ability to mobilise external philanthropic and government funding may account for network effectiveness of tobacco control advocates, compared with similar networks dedicated to the reduction of other NCD risk factors.

As our political economy analysis suggests, defining roles and responsibilities of different stakeholders and collaborative advocacy for health taxes among health policy networks dealing with tobacco, alcohol, SSBs and unhealthy foods may be a way to directly address industry interference with public health policy, and at the same time reduce the burden of disease and disability associated with NCD risk factors. Indeed, a scoping review of the world literature[22] found the following factors instrumental in the design and implementation of health taxes in Low- and Middle-Income Countries: localised health and economic evidence, policy championing, inter-ministerial support and global or regional momentum. Box 12.4 provides further insights into the successful implementation of SSB taxes.

Box 12.4. Innovation in fiscal policy for health: Insights from the adoption of SSB taxes

Among the most significant areas of recent innovation in global health policy has been the comparatively rapid profusion of SSB taxes, including across key emerging markets. While the literature predictably highlights the significance of specific local factors, there are also key strategic themes that emerge as enabling factors.

Fiscal crises and financial reforms as catalysts: While the prospect of a virtuous circle of enhancing health while generating additional revenues can be attractive in most contexts, the introduction of new SSB taxes has often been facilitated by governments having to confront broader fiscal pressures. This may be as part of a broader package of reforms to the taxations system (as in Mexico or South Africa), or to boost budgets in the context of a financial crisis (Hungary), while in Fiji it aimed to offset declining tariff revenues amid trade liberalisation.[116]

Whole of government approaches and diverse policy champions: Analyses of successful passage and adoption of SSB taxes highlights the importance of achieving coordinated support across ministries and departments. While the Ministry of Health is of course a key actor, its support is unlikely to be enough and in several countries the process has been led by finance ministries. In Mexico, for example, the Ministry of Finance was identified as having been an earlier, more enthusiastic and more consistent supporter of the implementation of an SSB tax than the Ministry of Health.[117]

Variable approaches to framing proposed new taxes: Similarly, it is not always the case that successful new health-relevant interventions in fiscal policy are most effectively or persuasively presented as advancing health goals. In some contexts, new tax initiatives have been presented explicitly as protecting and promoting public health, in others as more conventional tax instruments, while in other jurisdictions advocacy for new measures has drawn from across health, economic and fiscal rationales.[22]

Engaging and mobilising civil society: The significance of building effective advocacy coalitions emerges as a consistent theme within studies of contextual political factors that have facilitated SSB taxes.[22,116] A key factor here is ensuring that key health stakeholders such as civil society actors are able to engage in tax policy discussions, which was key in the case of Barbados[118]; in many jurisdictions consultations around tax policy initiatives serve to privilege private sector actors and marginalise civil society.

International support: In some contexts, the design, development and adoption of measures was clearly facilitated by access to support from diverse actors such as multilateral agencies such as WHO and its regional offices, international NGOs or from philanthropies. In Mexico, for example, the extent to which civil society were able to actively shape discourse around the proposed SSB tax was greatly enhanced by the significant financial support provided to Alianza por La Salud Alimentaria by Bloomberg Philanthropies.[119]

Countering industry opposition: The success of Bloomberg's support for health advocacy in Mexico is illustrative of the importance of actively preparing to oppose industry arguments. Industry claims that such taxes are ineffective, regressive or interfering can be predicted, and the active engagement of academics in the generation of context-specific evidence has been central to successful strategies in some jurisdictions.[22,116,120]

Because the political economy of NCD risk factors is complicated by the transnational character of its dominant firms and the diversity of actors with interests in the sales of these products, it is essential to use PCA to understand how TTCs operate at the global level and within national boundaries to influence to public health policy, especially in the growing markets of the LMICs. Recent studies of TTCs have expanded our knowledge about how these industries operate and the challenges of moving beyond attempts to address NCDs as if they could be addressed only by medical and public health measures. This chapter suggests that the political economy of health taxes needs to be understood and addressed in order to reduce the health burden of NCDs and to pay for their costs at the same time.

Key messages

- An inherent conflict of interest exists between the commercial goals of the tobacco, alcohol, unhealthy food and SSB industries and the public health and economic equity goals of national and local governments.
- The tobacco, alcohol, food and SSB industries have become increasingly concentrated into a small number of transnational corporations that account for a large proportion of the market for these products.
- With increased concentration and coordination across sectors, these industries use similar strategies and tactics to influence the policy environment for their products, especially in low- and middle-income countries.
- Corporate political activities used across these industries are very similar, as well as the arguments used against tax policy.
- Coalitions need to be built at the local, national in international levels, capable of working with or without these industries in the interests of public health.

References

1. Vigo A, Lauer J. *Estimating the Fiscal and Economic Impacts of Health Taxes on Food, Alcohol, and Tobacco.* Geneva: World Health Organization; 2017.
2. Cejudo GM, Michel CL. Addressing fragmented government action: Coordination, coherence, and integration. *Policy Sciences.* 2017; 50(4): 745–767.
3. Collin J, Casswell S. Alcohol and the sustainable development goals. *Lancet.* 2016; 387(10038): 2582–2583.
4. Pan American Health Organization. Noncommunicable Disease Risk Factors in the Americas: Considerations on the Strengthening of Regulatory Capacity. REGULA Technical Reference Document. Washington, DC: PAHO, 2015.
5. Reich MR and Balarajan Y. Political economy analysis for food and nutrition security. Health, Nutrition and Population (HNP) Discussion Paper 2011. Washington, DC; The International Bank for Reconstruction and Development/The World Bank; December 2012.
6. Freudenberg N. *Lethal But Legal Corporations, Consumption, and Protecting Public Health.* Oxford University Press; 2014.
7. Hastings G. The marketing matrix. *Journal of Social Marketing.* 2012; 2(3): 222–226, https://doi.org/10.1108/20426761211265203.
8. Jernigan D, Ross CS. The alcohol marketing landscape: Alcohol industry size, structure, strategies, and public health responses. *Journal of Studies on Alcohol and Drugs.* 2020; Supplement 19: 13–25. DOI:10.15288/jsads.2020.s19.13.
9. Cavanagh J, Clairmonte F. *Alcoholic Beverages: Dimensions of Corporate Power.* New York, St Martin's Press; 1985.
10. Euromonitor International. Alcoholic Beverages—World. 2018. Retrieved from Passport, June 14, 2019.
11. International Organisation of Vine and Wine. State of the World Vitivinicultural Sector in 2020. International Organisation of Vine and Wine April, 2021 https://www.oiv.int/public/medias/7909/oiv-state-of-the-world-vitivinicultural-sector-in-2020.pdf.
12. Collin J, Hill SE, Smith KE. Merging alcohol giants threaten global health. *BMJ.* 2015; 351: h6087.
13. Hawkins B, Holden C, Eckhardt J, Lee K. Reassessing policy paradigms: A comparison of the global tobacco and alcohol industries. *Global Public Health.* 2018. DOI: 10.1080/17441692.2016.1161815.
14. Fang J, Lee K, Sejpal N. The China national tobacco corporation: From domestic to global dragon?. *Global Public Health.* 2017; 12(3): 315–334.
15. Lee K, Eckhardt J. The globalisation strategies of five Asian tobacco companies: A comparative analysis and implications for global health governance, *Global Public Health,* 2017, 12:3, 367–379, DOI: 10.1080/17441692.2016.1273370.
16. Collin J, Hill S. Structure and Tactics of the Tobacco, Alcohol, and Sugary Beverage Industries, Background Paper, Bloomberg Task Force on Fiscal Policy for Health,

April; 2019. https://data.bloomberglp.com/dotorg/sites/2/2019/04/Structure-and-Tactics-of-the-Tobacco-Alcohol-and-Sugary-Beverage-Industries.pdf (accessed: 12 October 2020).

17. Oxfam. 'Behind the Brands': Food justice and the 10 big food and beverage companies, 2013. https://www-cdn.oxfam.org/s3fs-public/file_attachments/bp166-behind-the-brands-260213-en_2.pdf (accessed 15 May 2022).
18. Collin J, Hill SE, Smith KE. Merging alcohol giants threaten global health. *BMJ*. 2015; 351: h6087.
19. Collin J. Tobacco control, global health policy and development: Towards policy coherence in global governance. Tob Control 2012; 21: 274–80. http://dx.doi.org/10.1136/tobaccocontrol-2011-050418.
20. Jiang N, Ling P. Vested Interests in addiction research and policy. Alliance between tobacco and alcohol industries to shape public policy. Addiction (Abingdon, England). 2013; 108(5): 852–864, https://www.ncbi.nlm.nih.gov/pmc/articles/PMC3689428/.
21. Moodie R, Stuckler D, Monteiro C. et al. Profits and pandemics: Prevention of harmful effects of tobacco, alcohol and ultra-processed food and drink industries. *Lancet*. 2013; 381(9867): 670–679.
22. Elliott LM, Dalglish SL, Topp SM. Health taxes on tobacco, alcohol, food and drinks in low- and middle-income countries: A scoping review of policy content, actors, process and context. *Int J Health Policy Manag*. 2022; 11(4): 414–428. doi:10.34172/ijhpm.2020.170.
23. Schuler DA, Rehbein K, Cramer RD. Pursuing strategic advantage through political means: A multivariate approach. *The Academy of Management Journal*. 2002; 45(4): 659–672.
24. Hillman AJ, Hitts MA. Corporate political strategy formulation: A model of approach, participation and strategy decision. *Academy of Management Review*. 1999; 24(4): 825–842.
25. Savell E, Fooks G, Gilmore AB. How does the alcohol industry attempt to influence marketing regulations? A systematic review. Addiction (Abingdon, England). 2016; 111(1): 18–32. https://doi.org/10.1111/add.13048.
26. Babor TF, Robaina K, Brown K, Noel J, Cremonte J, Pantani D, Peltzer RI, Pinsky I. Is the alcohol industry doing well by "doing good"? Findings from a content analysis of the alcohol industry's actions to reduce harmful drinking. *BMJ Open*. 2018; 8: e024325. DOI:10.1136/bmjopen-2018-024325.
27. Morgan D. "Sugar Industry Expands Influence." *The Washington Post*, WP Company, 3 Nov. 2007. www.washingtonpost.com/wp-dyn/content/article/2007/11/02/AR2007110201899.html?tid=a_inl_manual&noredirect=on.
28. Monardi F, Glantz SA. Are tobacco industry campaign contributions influencing state legislative behavior? *American Journal of Public Health*. 1998; 88(6): 918–923.
29. Whyte LE. "Alcohol Distributors Ply Statehouses to Keep Profits Flowing." *Time*, May 15: https://time.com/3986536/alcohol-distributors-lobbying/.

30. Dixon V. "Interactive: How Much Are Restaurant Chains Donating to Republicans and Democrats?" *Eater*, 8 Feb. 2016. www.eater.com/2016/2/8/10904984/restaurant-PACS-political-donations.
31. Riley B. "U.S. Trade Policy Gouges American Sugar Consumers." The Heritage Foundation, *Backgrounder*, 5 June 2014. https://www.heritage.org/trade/report/us-trade-policy-gouges-american-sugar-consumers.
32. Smith KE, Savell E, Gilmore AB. What is known about tobacco industry efforts to influence tobacco tax? A systematic review of empirical studies. *Tobacco Control.* 2013; 22(2): 144–153, https://www.ncbi.nlm.nih.gov/pubmed/22887175.
33. Volz, M. (2017) How Big Tobacco stopped a Montana smoking tax. Great Falls Tribune, May 19, Associated Press. https://www.greatfallstribune.com/story/news/politics/2017/05/19/big-tobacco-stopped-montana-smoking-tax/101875332/.
34. Bakke Ø, Endal D. Alcohol policies out of context: Drinks industry supplanting government role in alcohol policies in sub-Saharan Africa. Addiction. 2010; 105(1): 22–28. DOI: 10.1111/j.1360-0443.2009.02695.x.
35. Hawkins B, Holden C. Water dripping on stone'? Industry lobbying and UK alcohol policy. *Policy Politics*. 2014; 42: 55–70.
36. "Food & Beverage: Lobbying, 2018." OpenSecrets.org, 2018, www.opensecrets.org/industries/lobbying.php?cycle=2011&ind=N01.
37. Mialon M, Swinburn B, Allender S, Sacks G. Systematic examination of publicly-available information reveals the diverse and extensive corporate political activity of the food industry in Australia. *BMC Public Health*. 2016; 16: 283.
38. Wilson D, Kerlin A. Special Report: Food, Beverage Industry Pays for Seat at Health - Policy Table. Geneva, Switzerland: Reuters; 2012.
39. Aaron D, Michael S. Sponsorship of national health organizations by two major soda companies. *American Journal of Preventive Medicine*. 2017; 52: 20–30.
40. Raebeck A, Campbell R, Balbach E. Unhealthy partnerships: The tobacco industry and African American and Latino labor organizations. *Journal of Immigrant Minor Health*. 2010; 12(2): 228–233. DOI: 10.1007/s10903-009-9269-0.
41. Balbach ED, Herzberg A, Barbeau EM. Political coalitions and working women: How the tobacco industry built a relationship with the Coalition of Labor Union Women. *Journal of Epidemiology and Community Health*. 2006; 60(Suppl 2): 27–32, https://www.ncbi.nlm.nih.gov/pmc/articles/PMC2491892/.
42. Hawkins B, McCambridge J. Industry actors, think tanks, and alcohol policy in the United Kingdom. *American Journal of Public Health*. 2014; 104(8): 1363–1369, https://www.ncbi.nlm.nih.gov/pmc/articles/PMC4103247/.
43. Harless W. "Soda Industry Outspends Richmond Tax Supporters 10-1." California Watch 14 Aug. 2012. https://www.nbcbayarea.com/news/local/soda_industry_outspends_tax_supporters_10-1_in_richmond/1924579/.
44. Liz S. "Soda Industry Steals Page from Tobacco to Combat Taxes on Sugary Drinks." *NBCNews.com*, NBCUniversal News Group, 6 Nov. 2018. https://www.nbcnews.com/health/health-news/soda-industry-steals-page-tobacco-combat-taxes-sugary-drinks-n932066.

45. Luz M. "The New Policy Battlefield: All Eyes On Coca-Cola And Social Media PR." *The Huffington Post*, 7 Dec. 2017. www.huffingtonpost.com/martin-luz/the-new-policy-battlefiel_b_470656.html.
46. Yoon S, Lam TH. The alcohol industry lobby and Hong Kong's zero wine and beer tax policy. *BMC Public Health*. 2012; 12: 717. DOI: 10.1186/1471-2458-12-717.
47. Butler S. Obstacles to the implementation of an integrated National Alcohol Policy in Ireland: Nannies, neo-liberals and joined-up government. *Journal of Social Policy*. 2009; 38(2): 343–359. DOI: 10.1017/S0047279408002870.
48. Confessore N. "Minority Groups and Bottlers Team Up in Battles Over Soda.", *The New York Times*, 13 Mar. 2013, https://www.nytimes.com/2013/03/13/nyregion/behind-soda-industrys-win-a-phalanx-of-sponsored-minority-groups.html.
49. Progressive Grocer. Tobacco Retailers Form Statewide Alliance 9 Aug. 2004. Retrieved from progressivegrocer.com: https://progressivegrocer.com/tobacco-retailers-form-statewide-alliance.
50. Campbell R, Balbach ED. Mobilising public opinion for the tobacco industry: The consumer tax alliance and excise taxes. *Tobacco Control*. 2008; 17: 351–356. https://tobaccocontrol.bmj.com/content/17/5/351.short.
51. Brownell KD, Warner KE. The perils of ignoring history: Big tobacco played dirty and millions died. How similar is Big Food?. *The Milbank Quarterly*. 2009; 87(1): 259–294. DOI:10.1111/j.1468-0009.2009.00555.x.
52. Dorfman L, Cheyne A, Friedman LC, Wadud A, and Gottlieb M. Soda and tobacco industry corporate social responsibility campaigns: How do they compare? *PLoS Medicine*. 2012; 9(6): e1001241. https://www.ncbi.nlm.nih.gov/pmc/articles/PMC3378589/.
53. Fooks GJ, Gilmore AB, Smith KE, Collin J, Holden C, Lee K. Corporate social responsibility and access to policy elites: An analysis of tobacco industry documents. *PLoS Medicine*. 2011; 8(8): e1001076. https://doi.org/10.1371/journal.pmed.1001076.
54. Jones SC, Hall S, Kypri K. Should I drink responsibly, safely or properly? Confusing messages about reducing alcohol-related harm. *PLoS ONE*. 2017; 12(9): e0184705. https://doi.org/ 10.1371/journal.pone.0184705.
55. Simon M. Clowning around with charity: How McDonald's exploits philanthropy and targets children. *Eat Drink Politics*. 2013. http://www.eatdrinkpolitics.com/2013/10/29/clowning-around-with-charity-how-mcdonalds-exploits-philanthropy-and-targets-children/.
56. Pfister, K. "Leaked: Coca-Cola's Worldwide Political Strategy to Kill Soda Taxes." *Observer*, 14 Oct. 2016, https://medium.com/cokeleak/leaked-coca-colas-worldwide-political-strategy-to-kill-soda-taxes-9717f361fb04.
57. Alsop RJ. Corporate reputation: Anything but superficial – The deep but fragile nature of corporate reputation. *Journal of Business Strategy*. 2004; 25(6): 21–29, https://doi.org/10.1108/02756660410699900.
58. Zatonski M, Hawkins B, McKee M. Framing the policy debate over spirits excise tax in Poland. *Health Promotion International*. 2016. 10.1093/heapro/daw093, https://academic.oup.com/heapro/article/33/3/515/2617566.

59. Jaichuen N, Phulkerd S, Certthkrikul N, Sacks G, Tangcharoensathien V. Corporate political activity of major food companies in Thailand: An assessment and policy recommendations. *Globalization and Health*. 2018; 14(1): 115. DOI: 10.1186/s12992-018-0432-z, https://www.ncbi.nlm.nih.gov/pmc/articles/PMC6249932/.
60. Hope A. The influence of the alcohol industry on alcohol policy in Ireland. *Nord Alkohol Narkotikatidskr*. 2006; 23: 467–481.
61. Mello MM, Pomeranz J, Moran P. The interplay of public health law and industry self-regulation: The case of sugar-sweetened beverage sales in schools. *American Journal of Public Health*. 2008; 98(4): 595–604. https://www.ncbi.nlm.nih.gov/pmc/articles/PMC2376983/ - r17.
62. Apollonio DE, Malone RE. The "We Card" Program: Tobacco Industry "Youth Smoking Prevention" as Industry Self-Preservation. *American Journal of Public Health*. July 2010; 100(7): 1188–1201. DOI: 10.2105/AJPH.2009.169573.
63. Mamudu HM, Hammond R, Glantz SA, Project cerberus: Tobacco industry strategy to create an alternative to the framework convention on tobacco control. *American Journal of Public Health*. Sept. 2008; 98(9): 1630–1642. https://doi.org/10.2105/AJPH.2007.129478.
64. Katikireddi SV, Bond L, Hilton S. Changing policy framing as a deliberate strategy for public health advocacy: A qualitative policy case study of minimum unit pricing of alcohol. *The Milbank Quarterly*. 2014; 92(2): 250–283. https://www.ncbi.nlm.nih.gov/pmc/articles/PMC4089371/ - b75.
65. Mosher JF. Joe Camel in a bottle: Diageo, the Smirnoff Brand, and the transformation of the youth alcohol market. *American Journal of Public Health*. 2012; 102(1), 56–63, https://doi.org/10.2105/AJPH.2011.300387.
66. Nixon L, Mejia P, Cheyne A. et al., "We're Part of the Solution": Evolution of the Food and Beverage Industry's Framing of Obesity Concerns Between 2000 and 2012. *American Journal of Public Health*, 105, 2228–2236, https://doi.org/10.2105/ajph.2015.302819.
67. Shields J. "Soft-Drink Industry Has Given Heavily in Council Races." *The Philadelphia Inquirer, Daily News* and *Philly.com*, 5 Jun. 2011. https://www.philly.com.
68. Moore S, Wolfe SM, Lindes D, Douglas CE. Epidemiology of failed tobacco control legislation. *JAMA*. 1994; 272(15): 1171–1175. DOI: 10.1001/jama.1994.03520150039034, https://europepmc.org/abstract/med/7933346.
69. Greenfield TK, Johnson P, Giesbrecht N. The alcohol policy development process: policymakers speak. *Contemporary Drug Problems*. 2004; 31: 627–654.
70. Nestle M. *Food Politics: How the Food Industry Influences Nutrition and Health*. Berkeley; London: University of California Press; 2002.
71. Roache SA, Platkin C, Gostin LO et al., *Big Food and Soda Versus Public Health: Industry Litigation Against Local Government Regulations to Promote Healthy Diets*, 45 Fordham Urb. L.J. 2018; 1051–1089.
72. Jernigan DH. Global alcohol producers, science, and policy: The case of the International Center for Alcohol Policies. *American Journal of Public Health*. 2012; 102(1): 80–89. DOI: 10.2105/AJPH.2011.300269.

73. Corporate Europe Observatory. A Red Light for Consumer Information: The Food Industry's €1 Billion Campaign to Block Health Warnings on Food. Corporate Europe Observatory: Brussels, 2010. https://corporateeurope.org/en/2010/06/red-light-consumer-information.
74. Waters R. "Soda and Fast Food Lobbyists Push State Preemption Laws To Prevent Local Regulation." *Forbes Magazine*, 21 Jun. 2017. https://www.forbes.com/sites/robwaters/2017/06/21/soda-and-fast-food-lobbyists-push-state-preemption-laws-to-prevent-local-regulation/?sh=4162943b745d.
75. Siegel M, Carol J, Jordan J, et al. Preemption in tobacco control: Review of an emerging public health problem. *JAMA*. 1997; 278(10): 858–863. DOI: 10.1001/jama.1997.03550100084044.
76. Mosher JF, Adler SS, Pamukcu AM, Treffers RD. Review of state laws restricting local authority to impose alcohol taxes in the United States. *Journal of Studies on Alcohol and Drugs*. 2017; 78(2): 241–248. https://doi.org/10.15288/jsad.2017.78.241.
77. Pomeranz JL, Zellers L, Bare M, Pertschuk M. State preemption of food and nutrition policies and litigation: Undermining government's role in public health. *American Journal of Preventive Medicine*. 2019; 56(1): 47–57. DOI: 10.1016/j.amepre.2018.07.027.
78. George A. *Not so Sweet Refrain: Sugar-Sweetened Beverages Taxes, Industry Opposition and Harnessing the Lessons Learned from Tobacco Control Legal Challenges*. Melbourne: McCabe Centre for Law and Cancer; 2017. https://www.cambridge.org/core/services/aop-cambridge-core/content/view/55A55799892CF1CFFFECA7F7D4B12996/S1744133118000178a.pdf/not_so_sweet_refrain_sugarsweetened_beverage_taxes_industry_opposition_and_harnessing_the_lessons_learned_from_tobacco_control_legal_challenges.pdf.
79. Nixon ML, Mahmoud L, Glantz SA. Tobacco industry litigation to deter local public health ordinances: The industry usually loses in court. *Tobacco Control*. 2004; 13: 65–73, https://tobaccocontrol.bmj.com/content/13/1/65.
80. Bødker M, Pisinger C, Toft U, Jørgensen T. The rise and fall of the world's first fat tax. *Health Policy*. 2015; 119(6): 737–742. DOI: 10.1016/j.healthpol.2015.03.003.
81. Mialon M, Mialon J. Analysis of corporate political activity strategies of the food industry: Evidence from France. *Public Health Nutrition*. 2018; 21(18): 3407–3421. DOI: 10.1017/S1368980018001763.
82. Shamasunder B, Bero L. Financial ties and conflicts of interest between pharmaceutical and tobacco companies. *JAMA*. 2002; 288(6): 738–744. DOI: 10.1001/jama.288.6.738, https://jamanetwork.com/journals/jama/fullarticle/195192.
83. Bero LA. Tobacco industry manipulation of research. Public Health Reports (Washington, D.C.: 1974). 2005; 120(2): 200–208. https://www.ncbi.nlm.nih.gov/pmc/articles/PMC1497700/.
84. Ulucanlar S, Fooks GJ, Gilmore AB. The policy dystopia model: An interpretive analysis of tobacco industry political activity. *PLoS Medicine*. 2016; 13(9): e1002125.
85. Tselengidis A, Östergren P-O. Lobbying against sugar taxation in the European Union: Analysing the lobbying arguments and tactics of stakeholders in the food and drink industries. *Scandinavian Journal of Public Health*. 2019 July; 47(5): 565–575.

86. Gilmore AB, Fooks G, Drope J, Bialous SA, Jackson RR. Exposing and addressing tobacco industry conduct in low-income and middle-income countries. *The Lancet.* 2015; 385(9972): 1029–1043.
87. Taillie LS, Reyes M, Colchero MA, Popkin B, Corvalán C. An evaluation of Chile's Law of Food Labeling and Advertising on sugarsweetened beverage purchases from 2015 to 2017: A before-and-after study. *PLoS Med.* 2020; 17(2): e1003015. https://doi.org/10.1371/journal.pmed.1003015.
88. Robaina K, Babor T, Pinsky I, and Johns P. The alcohol industry's commercial and political activities in Latin America and the Caribbean: Implications for public health. NCD Alliance, Global Alcohol Policy Alliance, Healthy Latin America Coalition, and Healthy Caribbean Coalition, 2020.
89. AmBev. Q2 2012 CIA BEBIDAS DAS AMERICAS AMBEV Earnings Conference Call - Final. (C. Transcriptions, Compiler), 2012. Retrieved April 6, 2015, from global.factiva.com.
90. McCambridge J, Daube M, McKee M. Brussels declaration: A vehicle for the advancement of tobacco and alcohol industry interests at the science/policy interface? *Tobacco Control.* 2019; 28: 7–12.
91. Gneiting U, Schmitz HP. Comparing global alcohol and tobacco control efforts: Network formation and evolution in international health governance. *Health Policy and Planning.* 2016; 31 (Suppl 1): i98–i109. https://doi.org/10.1093/heapol/czv125.
92. Bump JB, Reich MR. Political economy analysis for tobacco control in low- and middle-income countries. *Health Policy and Planning.* March 2013; 28(2): 123–133, https://doi.org/10.1093/heapol/czs049.
93. Crosbie E, Bialous S, and Glantz SA. Memoranda of understanding: A tobacco industry strategy to undermine illicit tobacco trade policies. *Tobacco Control.* 2019; 28(e2): e110-e118.
94. Collin J, LeGresley E, MacKenzie R, Lawrence S and Lee K. (2004) Complicity in Contraband: British American Tobacco and Cigarette Smuggling in Asia. *Tobacco Control,* 13(Supp 2): ii96–ii111.
95. World Health Organization. Protocol to eliminate illicit trade in tobacco products. ISBN 978 92 4 150524 6 (NLM classification: HD 9130.6), World Health Organization 2013.
96. Armendares PE, Shigematsu LMR. Política fiscal y control del tabaco: Una oportunidad única para beneficiar a la salud pública y al erario [Fiscal policy and tobacco control: A unique opportunity to benefit public health and the public treasury]. *Salud Publica Mex.* 2006; 48(Suppl. 1): S167–S172.
97. World Health Organization. Strategy meeting on the use of fiscal policies for public health, Geneva, Switzerland, 4–5 December 2017. Geneva: World Health Organization (WHO/HGF/EAE/HealthTaxes/2017/MeetingReport) Licence: CC BY-NC-SA 3.0 IGO, 2018.
98. World Health Organization. Safeguarding against possible conflicts of interest in nutrition programmes: draft approach for the prevention and management of conflicts

of interest in the policy development and implementation of nutrition programmes at country level: report by the Director-General. World Health Organization Geneva: WHO; 2017. https://apps.who.int/iris/handle/10665/274165.

99. World Health Organization. *Time to Deliver: Report of the WHO Independent High-Level Commission on Noncommunicable Diseases*. Geneva: World Health Organization; 2018. Licence: CC BY-NCSA 3.0 IGO.

100. Ralston R, Hill S, Gomes F, Collin J. Towards preventing and managing conflict of interest in nutrition policy? An analysis of submissions to a consultation on a draft WHO tool. *International Journal of Health Policy and Management*. 2020. DOI: 10.34172/ijhpm.2020.52.

101. WHO. Guidelines for implementation of Article 5.3 of the WHO Framework Convention on Tobacco Control on the protection of public health policies with respect to tobacco control from commercial and other vested interests of the tobacco industry. November, 2008. https://apps.who.int/iris/bitstream/handle/10665/80510/9789241505185_eng.pdf?sequence=1 (accessed 12 October 2020).

102. Task Force on Fiscal Policy for Health. Health Taxes to Save Lives: Employing Effective Excise Taxes on Tobacco, Alcohol, and Sugary Beverages. Chairs: Michael R. Bloomberg and Lawrence H. Summers. New York: Bloomberg Philanthropies, 2019. Available at: https://www.bloomberg.org/program/public-health/task-force-fiscal-policy-health/.

103. Babor TF, Robaina K. Public health, academic medicine, and the alcohol industry's corporate social responsibility activities. *Am J Public Health*. 2013; 103(2): 206–214.

104. Babor, TF. Conflict-of-Interest Policies in Addiction Science: The Spirit and Letter of the Law. *Journal of Studies on Alcohol and Drugs*. 2019; 80(2), 145–148. https://doi.org/10.15288/jsad.2019.80.145.

105. Mialon M, Swinburn B, Sacks G. A proposed approach to systematically identify and monitor the corporate political activity of the food industry with respect to public health using publicly available information. *Obesity Reviews*. 2015; 16(7): 519–530.

106. Kickbusch I. Addressing the interface of the political and commercial determinants of health. *Health Promotion International*. 2012; 27(4): 427–428.

107. Peña S, Cuadrado C, Escobar MT, et al. Proposal of the Front for a Healthy Tax Reform 2006. *Tobacco Free Chile*. https://www.chilelibredetabaco.cl/que-puedes-hacer/

108. Castellblanch R. Challenging pharmaceutical industry political power in Maine and Vermont. *Journal of Health Politics*. 2003; 28: 109–132.

109. Pracht E, Moore W. Interest groups and state Medicaid drug programs. *Journal of Health Politics*. 2003; 28: 9–39.

110. Wiist W. The corporate play book, health, and democracy: The snack food and beverage industry's tactics in context. In: Stuckler D, Siegel, K, editors. Sick Societies: Responding to the global challenge of chronic disease. Oxford: Oxford University Press, 2011.

111. World Health Organization. WHO global coordination mechanism on the prevention and control of noncommunicable diseases: final report: WHO GCM/NCD working

group on the alignment of international cooperation with national NCD plans (Working group 3.2, 2016–2017). World Health Organization.2018. https://apps.who.int/iris/handle/10665/312273.

112. Guiding Principles on Businesses and Human Rights: Implementing the United Nations Protect, Respect and Remedy Framework. UNHCR, 2011. HR/PUB/11/04k.
113. Kickbusch I, Allen L, Franz C. The commercial determinants of health. *The Lancet Global Health*. 2016; 4(12): e895–e896.
114. Schmitz HP. The global health network on alcohol control: Successes and limits of evidence-based advocacy. *Health Policy and Planning*. 2016; 31(Suppl. 1): i87–i97.
115. Page SE. The difference: How the power of Diversity creates better groups, firms, schools, and societies. Princeton, NJ: Princeton University Press. 2007.
116. Baker P, Jones A, Thow AM. Accelerating the worldwide adoption of sugar-sweetened beverage taxes: Strengthening commitment and capacity: Comment on "The untapped power of soda taxes: Incentivizing consumers, generating revenue, and altering corporate behavior". *International Journal of Health Policy and Management*. 2018; 7(5): 474.
117. Carriedo Lutzenkirchen AA. A policy analysis of the 2014 Mexican soda tax. PhD thesis, London School of Hygiene & Tropical Medicine; 2018. DOI: https://doi.org/10.17037/PUBS.04648204.
118. Healthy Caribbean Coalition. The Implementation of Taxation on Sugar-Sweetened Beverages by the Government of Barbados: A Civil Society Perspective, July; 2016. http://www.healthycaribbean.org/wp-content/uploads/2016/07/HCC-SSB-Brief-2016.pdf (accessed 12 October 2020).
119. Bonilla-Chacín M, Iglasias R, Agustino S, Claudio T, Claudio M. Learning from the Mexican Experience with Taxes on Sugar-Sweetened Beverages and Energy-Dense Foods of Low Nutritional Value: Poverty and Social Impact Analysis. Health, Nutrition and Population Discussion Paper. Washington, DC: World Bank, 2016.
120. Carriedo A, Lock K, Hawkins B. Policy process and non-state actors' influence on the 2014 Mexican Soda Tax. *Health Policy and Planning*. 2020; 35(8): 941–952.

https://doi.org/10.1142/9781800612396_0016

Special Focus 4

The Role of Civil Society in Tobacco Tax Reform in the Philippines

Filomeno Sta Ana[*], **Angeli Vigo**[†], **and Jeremias Paul**[†]

SF 4.1. Seismic shift: The 2012 tobacco tax reform in a nutshell

On 20 December 2012, the President of the Philippines signed the Sin Tax Law (Republic Act 10351), which mandated, amongst others, fundamental reforms on excise taxes on tobacco starting January 2013. After numerous attempts to reform spanning 15 years, Congress finally passed a law that addressed fundamental weaknesses in tobacco excise tax structures. It was an arduous process with the same law passing the Senate with a narrow margin of one vote.

Prior to the passage of the law, cigarettes sold in the Philippines were considerably cheaper than those sold in neighbouring countries.[a] The system was frustratingly complex and protected legacy brands, which existed in the country in 1997. The 2012 reform corrected the structural weaknesses that kept cigarettes affordable and which diminished revenues in real terms.

* Action for Economic Reforms (AER), Philippines.

† World Health Organization, Switzerland.

[a] World Health Organization. *Tobacco and Poverty in the Philippines*. Geneva, Switzerland: WHO Press; 2008.

Fig. SF4.1. Comparison of tobacco tax rates per pack.

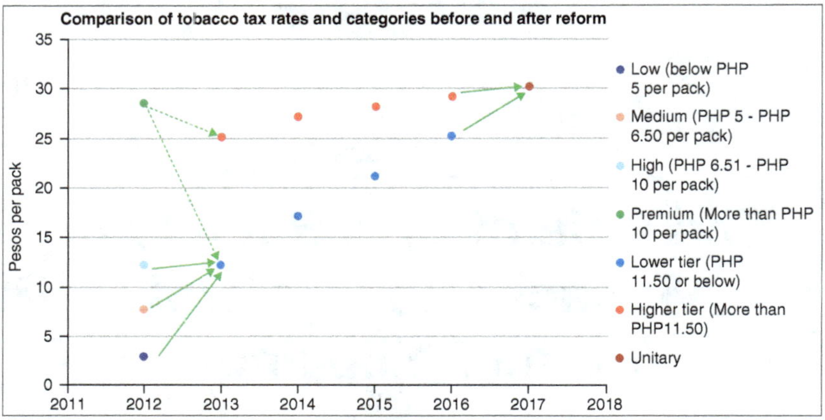

Multi-tier taxes, which produced non-optimal revenue and encouraged downshifting of consumption to lower priced brands, were gradually phased out over a period of 5 years. Instead, a unitary tax (regardless of cigarette net retail price) was imposed. This new structure simplified tax enforcement while delivering significant health and revenue impacts (Figure SF4.1).

The price-classification freeze that used cigarette prices in 1997 as a basis for tax classification was also removed, and tax rates became automatically indexed to inflation. This helped ensure that cigarettes prices would be maintained in real terms. Finally, the tobacco tax increases also supported the expansion of universal health coverage by having approximately 85% of the incremental revenues from the tobacco tax earmarked for health programs, including the Philippine Health Insurance Corporation (PhilHealth), the implementing agency of the National Health Insurance Program, which was established to provide health insurance coverage for all Filipinos.

The challenges faced by Filipino tax reform advocates were not unique. First, the proposition of raising any type of taxes has always been politically unpopular. In fact, the President at that time explicitly promised that the government would not impose new taxes. Second, the affected industries had massive war chests and were determined to oppose taxes that would discourage consumption of the taxed products.

The Philippine experience illustrates how these challenges can be addressed by a broad coalition among stakeholders with a unified strategy.

This case study will focus on the pivotal role of one of the key actors in the tobacco tax reform saga: civil society organisations (CSOs).

SF 4.2. Citizen groups in the Philippines

Within the last three decades, Philippine CSOs' influence in the public affairs has grown significantly. Their strength may be due in part to their sheer number: the Asian Development Bank reports that the 'Philippines has the largest number of NGOs per capita in Asia'.[b] Many of these organisations include sustainable development as part of their mission and so there is a semblance of a unified purpose and strategy.[c] Philippine CSOs also have strong expertise and experience which makes them more effective advocates.

However, the issue of reforming tobacco taxes cuts across multiple fields of discipline: public health, economics, governance. Therefore, it requires a coordinated response from CSOs in these different fields. These groups have different backgrounds and perspectives. How were they able to mount a coordinated, effective push for tobacco tax reform?

SF 4.3. Lessons from the Philippine experience

SF 4.3.1. Health sells

The key to the successful campaign was positioning tobacco taxation reform as a health measure. In previous attempts, proposed tobacco tax increases were always designed and promoted as revenue-raising measures, which proved to be a narrow approach.

The year 2012 saw a significant shift in strategy. This time, advocates focused on the health impact of the tax increases: improved health through reduced consumption and a stronger healthcare system through increased revenue from the taxes.

Emphasising the health impact of tobacco excise tax reform created the broadest reform coalition possible. The campaign attracted a diverse group of supporters and more than a 100 organisations joined the 'sin tax coalition'.

---

[b] Asian Development Bank. *Civil Society Briefs*. Manila, Philippines; 2013.

[c] *Ibid*.

This movement consisted of doctors, nurses and other health professionals, tobacco-control activists, women, youth, urban and rural poor, persons with disabilities, academics, economists and former senior government officials.

> "This is the most important health care, medical bill that will probably be discussed in Congress."
>
> Dr Enrique Ona, Secretary of the Department of Health (2010–2014)
>
> Source: Macaraig, A. Ona backs inhibition call for Recto, Marcos. Rappler. 28 November 2012. (https://www.rappler.com/nation/ona-backs-inhibition-call-for-recto-marcos; accessed 23 November 2020)

Table SF4.1. Overview of CSOs in Philippine sin tax coalition.

Medical professionals	These groups are composed of physicians, nurses, as well as professors of medical schools.	• Skilled in health advocacy campaigns • Strong links with Department of Health • Connections with personal physicians of legislators
Fiscal and development policy experts	The coalition includes a group of economists and lawyers specialising in economic and governance issues.	• Expertise in analysis of economic measures • Strong relationships with Department of Finance and Bureau of Internal Revenue • Strong presence in media
Tobacco control groups	These groups push for tobacco tax reform as part of their commitment to support the implementation of the WHO FCTC, including Article 6.	• Skilled in health advocacy campaigns • Can draw on regional and global networks for support and coordinated action
Other sectors	Women, urban poor, public sector employees, persons with disabilities and elderly and youth and students are also represented in the coalition.	• Provides the 'human face' of tobacco taxation reform

Making health as the primary objective of the tobacco tax increase boosted popular support for the measure. As a World Bank report correctly observed, 'Who could argue with a health measure that promised to save lives?'[d]

SF 4.3.2. Tobacco taxation as the main target

Faced with a daunting task and limited resources, advocates had to make several strategic decisions.

First, a decision was made to dedicate more resources in pushing for tobacco tax reform. Advocates believed that tobacco use was the more pressing health problem, given that there is no safe level of tobacco consumption.

Second, advocates recognised that there was a need to concentrate efforts on defeating the more formidable adversary; in the Philippines, tobacco-friendly groups wielded more influence compared to the alcohol industry. In fact, the Philippine tobacco industry was described at one point, as the 'strongest tobacco lobby in Asia.'[e]

Third, the advocates used the WHO Framework Convention on Tobacco Control (WHO FCTC), which the Philippines ratified, as an argument. Citing the WHO FCTC provided a stronger legal basis for imposing higher taxes on tobacco. There is no similar binding legal instrument, which puts pressure on countries to raise taxes on alcohol or sugary drinks.

As explained in Chapter 13 of this book, the diversity and well-established links among the various tobacco control groups globally allowed Philippine civil society groups, already exceptionally well-organised and influential in the public sphere, to exchange knowledge and experience and thus gain deeper insights. This resulted in more effective local strategies.

---

[d] Kaiser K, Bredenkamp C, Iglesias R. *Sin Tax Reform in the Philippines: Transforming Public Finance, Health, and Governance for More Inclusive Development. Directions in Development.* Washington, DC: World Bank. License: Creative Commons Attribution CC BY 3.0 IGO; 2016.

[e] Alechnowicz K, Chapman S. The Philippine tobacco industry: 'The strongest tobacco lobby in Asia'. *Tobacco Control.* 2004; 13(Suppl 2): ii71–ii78.

SF 4.3.3. Unity in diversity

Independent experts who belong to CSOs are not bound by the same constraints as government officials. Thus, they can provide technical expertise as well as perform sensitive tasks which cannot be done by reform advocates within government.

CSOs made bold public statements in support of the measure and publicly rebuked out-of-line politicians. A few weeks before the passing of the tax reforms, taking the cue from the broad coalition, more than 30 medical associations (part of what the coalition fondly called the 'white army'), signed a strongly worded manifesto calling for the inhibition of pro-tobacco legislators.[f]

CSOs also gathered support for the measure through personal conversations with potential allies. The medical professional associations sought out the personal physicians of legislators, 'taking advantage of the personal authority of physicians and leveraging the medical weight of a patient visit for national policy reform'.[g]

To complement the efforts made by health groups, fiscal policy experts engaged their contacts within the Department of Finance and other government agencies. The CSOs' economic impact analyses informed the proposed legislation and supported the implementation of a single tax rate.

SF 4.4. Tobacco tax reform: Improving health, equity while increasing revenues

The gains from the tobacco tax reforms are solid: the reduction of smoking prevalence, the increase in revenues and the increase in the health budget.[h]

[f] Macaraig, A. Ona backs inhibition call for Recto, Marcos. Rappler. 28 November 2012. https://www.rappler.com/nation/ona-backs-inhibition-call-for-recto-marcos (accessed 23 November 2020).

[g] Bhalla K, Bump J, Frost L, Glassman A, McQueston K, Pratt BA, Pierre-Louis AM, Harman N, Meiro-Lorenzo M. Building the foundation for healthy societies: influencing multisectoral action for health phase I (Vol. 2). Case Studies on Multisectoral Action. 2014; 111.

[h] It goes without saying that the impact of the 2018 and 2019 legislation on health and revenues is still early to tell.

Fig. SF4.2. Average tax price and tobacco excise tax revenue as a percent of GDP.

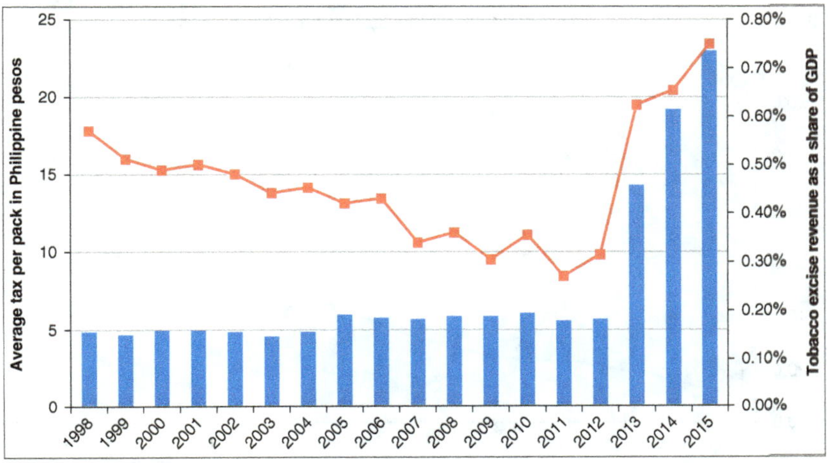

Figure SF4.2 shows the steep increase in tobacco excise tax revenues (in constant prices) starting in 2013, when the 'Sin Tax Law' was implemented. Before the passage of the 2012 law, tobacco excise tax revenues as a percentage of GDP was declining in real terms.

Figure SF4.3 shows a similarly sharp increase in the Philippine government's health budget. Note that as a result of the tobacco tax reform, a big share of the incremental revenues from the excise taxes on cigarettes and alcohol products has been earmarked for universal health care programs. Cigarettes, more than alcoholic beverages, have accounted for a much larger portion of incremental revenues allocated for health.

Figure SF4.4 presents the significant reduction of the smoking prevalence rate, which is correlated with the sharp increase in tobacco taxation. One can confidently attribute the decline in smoking prevalence principally to the tobacco tax since no other major tobacco-control intervention happened during this period. Although the law requiring graphic health warnings (Republic Act 10643) was enacted by Congress in 2014, it was not immediately implemented. It took at least 2 years for the executive agencies to finalise the implementing rules and regulations and operationalise the law.

Fig. SF4.3. Department of health budget – 2007–2016.

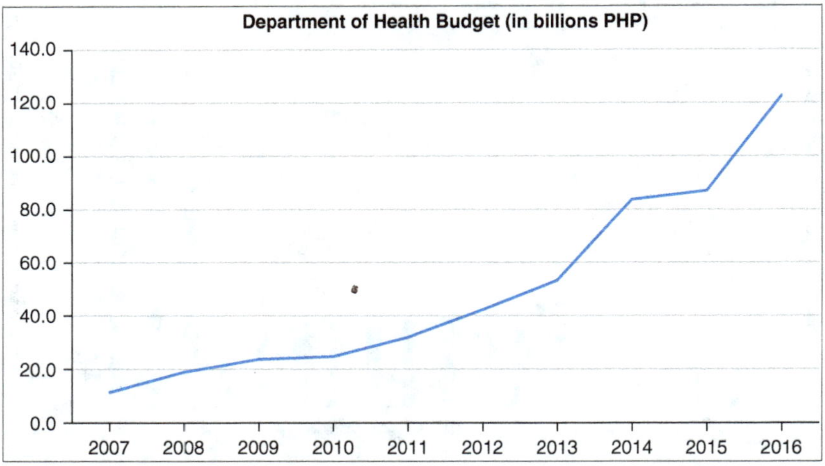

Source: Department of Finance.

Fig. SF4.4. Adult smoking prevalence.

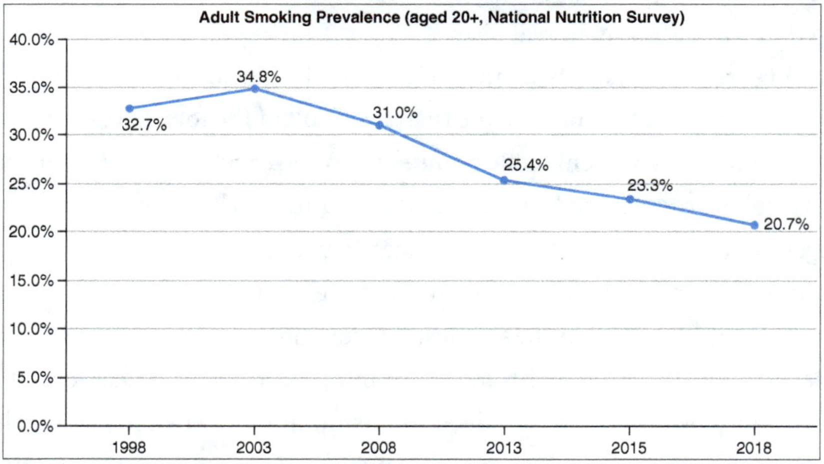

Source: National Nutrition Survey for different years, as published by the Food and Nutrition Research Institute of the Department of Science and Technology.

SF 4.5. Capitalising on momentum: CSOs push for related laws

The tobacco tax reform resulted in effects beyond the achievement of its stated goals. It energised the CSO coalition, which continued to campaign for other health-related measures.[i]

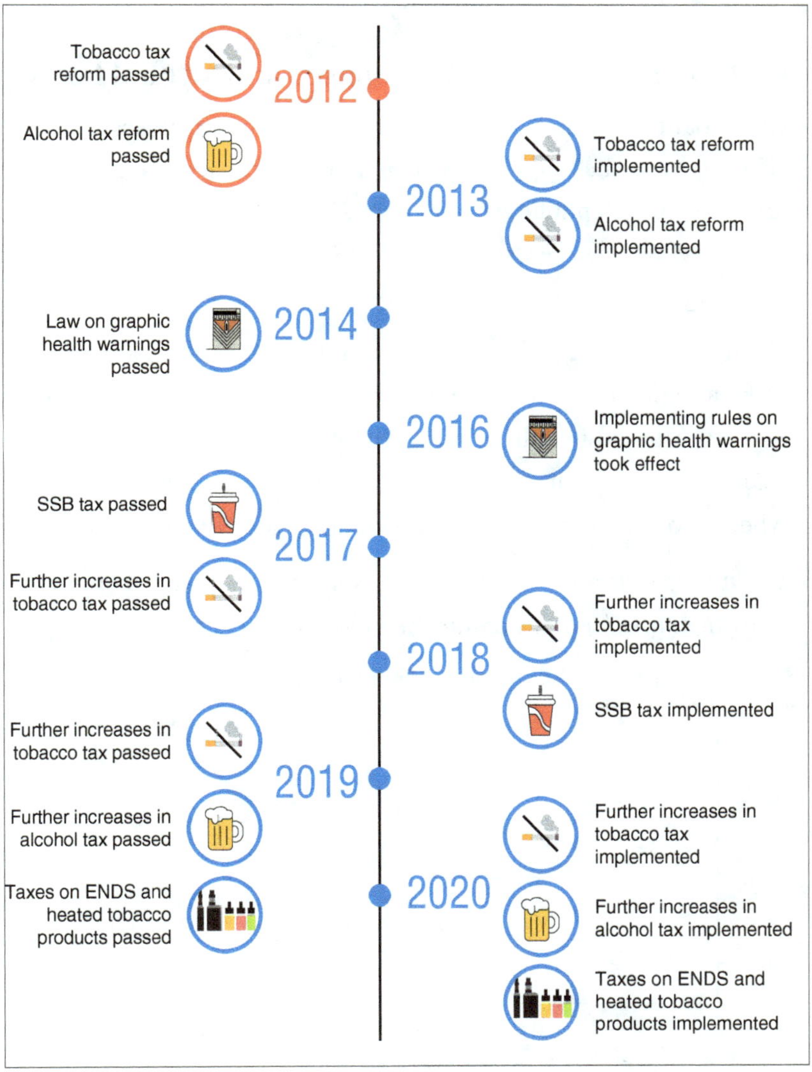

[i] Diosana J-A. Raising tobacco taxes: The Philippine experience. *Asian Pacific Journal of Cancer Prevention*. 2020; 21: 27–31.

Law on graphic health warnings (Republic Act 10643). The CSO coalition supported the proposed measure requiring manufacturers to display graphic warnings on 50% of the front and back of cigarette packs.

The law on graphic health warnings was passed (Republic Act 10643) in 2014, and the signing of its Implementing Rules and Regulations (IRR) happened in 2016.

SF 4.5.1. Further increases in tobacco and alcohol taxes

The CSO coalition continued calling for additional increases in tobacco and alcohol taxes. The Philippine Congress raised tobacco taxes twice after the 2012 reforms (Republic Act 10963 in 2017 and Republic Act 11346 in 2019). The latest amendments which took effect in 2020 (Republic Act 11346) mandated significant tax increases (Figure SF4.5).

> "High prices and graphic health warning on cigarettes are going to be an effective tandem to help reduce tobacco consumption. A picture-based health warning, the public's counterpart of the cigarette industry's marketing arm, is going to truly empower people when it comes to their right to information and right to health."
>
> *Behind the Colors of Tobacco Advertising* by Action for Economic Reform, https://aer.ph/behind-the-colors-of-tobacco-advertising/

Fig. SF4.5. Comparison of tobacco tax rates.

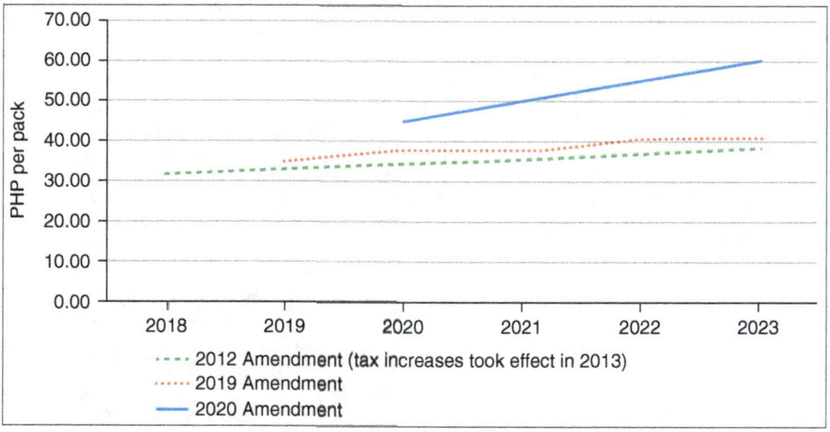

Fig. SF4.6. Comparison of tax rates for cheapest beer.

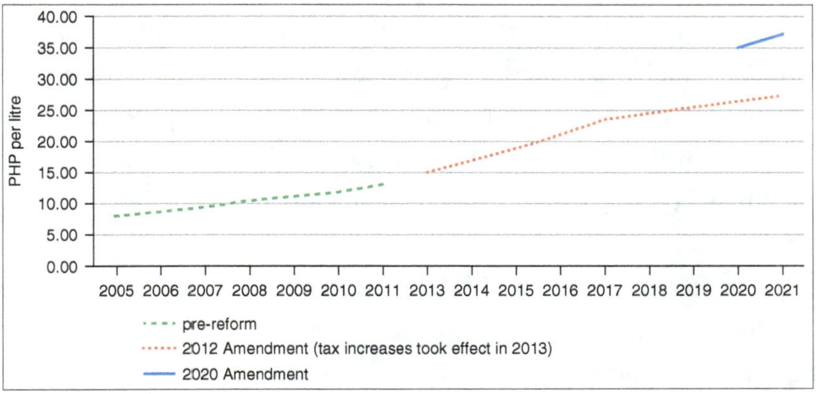

Although alcohol excise taxes, together with tobacco taxes, increased in 2013 by virtue of Republic Act 10351, CSOs remained steadfast in their campaign to push for further alcohol tax increases. Consequently, alcohol taxes increased in 2020, in line with Republic Act 11467. As illustration, Figure SF4.6 describes the change in the tax rates for the cheapest beer, a widely consumed alcoholic beverage in the Philippines.

SF 4.5.2. Expansion of sin taxes

CSOs likewise pushed for broadening the coverage of sin taxes to include sugar-sweetened beverages (SSBs), heated tobacco products (HTPs) and electronic nicotine delivery systems (ENDS). Congress eventually imposed taxes on these products: SSB taxes, signed as law in 2017, took effect in 2018 (Republic Act 10963); the year after, taxation was imposed on HTPs and ENDS (Republic Act 11346), which was followed by executive decrees regulating these products.[j]

[j] Executive Order 106 required that all e-liquids, solutions or refills forming components of electronic nicotine and non-nicotine delivery systems (ENDS/ENNDS), heated tobacco products (HTPs) should be registered with the Food and Drug Administration (FDA). It also required a designated area for users of ENDS/ENNDS.

Epilogue

The 2012 tobacco tax reform was a historic achievement. It corrected the fundamental weaknesses of the old law and paved the way for bigger economic and social gains, such as creating broader fiscal space that enabled sustained growth and contributing to the establishment of universal health care. While these impacts are beyond the scope of this case study, these have been documented in other reports.[k]

Years after the reform, the Philippines continues to build on the success of the 2012 reforms. In 2021, the Tobacconomics' 'Cigarette Tax Scorecard' ranked the Philippines seventh among 170 countries in total performance, taking into account absolute price, cigarette affordability, share of prices in retail price and tax structure.

---

[k] Sidel J, and Faustino J. *Thinking and working politically in development: Coalitions for change* in the Philippines. The Asia Foundation; 2020.

https://doi.org/10.1142/9781800612396_0017

Chapter 13

The Future of Health Taxes: Helping It Happen

Angeli Vigo*, Jeremy A Lauer†, Franco Sassi‡, and Agnes Soucat§

13.1. How this book can be used, and by whom

This book has been designed to meet the needs of a diverse audience, serving two main purposes. The first is to help those who wish to establish a case for health taxes, providing economic arguments and empirical evidence in support of their adoption. The second purpose is to set out key considerations in the design and implementation of health taxes, conveying sufficient technical knowledge to inform key choices faced by decision-makers in policy development.

An important message of this book is that not any tax, and not even any consumption tax, can be a health tax, that is, a tax designed to improve health. If health ministries have one exclusive prerogative in the field of health taxes, this is the entitlement to claim a health rationale for a fiscal policy. Health ministries should apply that claim sparingly and should set the bar high in granting their seal of approval for taxation measures. Not only a poorly or

* World Health Organization, Switzerland.

† University of Strathclyde, UK (formerly World Health Organization, Switzerland).

‡ Imperial College London, UK.

§ Agence Française de Développement, France (formerly World Health Organization, Switzerland).

unsuitably designed tax will bring no health benefits, but also it will be counterproductive for the cause of public health and for health taxes more widely. In this final chapter, we reiterate and summarise what a health tax is, and what it is not, bringing together arguments that have been developed throughout the book. We summarise the guiding principles of the design of health taxes and the political economy considerations that can determine the success, or failure, of health taxes. Finally, we look at the future of health taxes and how they can become a mainstream policy tool in countries worldwide.

13.2. Understanding what health taxes are; when taxes are not health taxes

Consumption is a key driving force in the growth model of most modern economies. Social welfare returns on increasing consumption, however, have been diminishing, with greater negative externalities being generated, especially to the detriment of the natural environment, and also greater negative long-term impacts on health, largely unaccounted for in people's consumption choices. Even essential consumption, such as food consumption, a key enabler of human development and well-being, has developed in ways that make it a leading cause of environmental degradation and depletion of natural resources, as well as a leading cause of disease burden worldwide.

A very large share of consumption by households and individuals, in many countries the majority of it, has impacts on health. This includes both consumption that has direct and immediate health impacts, such as the consumption of tobacco and alcohol products, as well as the consumption of goods and services ranging from food to energy, from housing to transport, that has less immediate or less direct, but no less important, health impacts. Consumers are aware of, and understand, only a small part of the health impacts generated by the above forms of consumption, and well-documented cognitive biases prevent them from coherently balancing present benefits and future consequences, resulting in consumption choices that are typically inconsistent with long-term individual and social welfare.

In the current context, the idea that consumption taxes should cause the least distortion to consumer choices, sounds, at best, like a missed opportunity. In fact, the practice of consumption taxation is rife with deviations from the 'least distortion' principle and consumption tax rates are often differentiated across products in alignment with policy goals, including health in some instances, but mostly in response to externalities and income inequalities. However, governments throughout the world have shown an increasing interest in using consumption taxes to address a wider range of the spill-over impacts of consumption. This trend strengthens the case for health taxes, that is for aligning the differentiation of consumption tax rates with health goals.

Health taxes are fundamentally fiscal policies aimed at addressing the negative health spill-overs of people's consumption choices, including spill-overs affecting other people (externalities), those affecting the same consumers or their households in the future (internalities), as well as future generations more widely (e.g. in terms of health system sustainability).

A key goal of health taxes is to incentivise consumers to make healthier choices through the differentiation of consumption tax rates. In most instances so far, health taxes have been designed as excise taxes, adding to general consumption taxes like value-added taxes. Nonetheless, even general consumption taxes can qualify as health taxes if their rates and bases are suitably differentiated to serve health goals. In other words, what makes a consumption tax a health tax is its health rationale.

A health rationale cannot be claimed when taxes are not designed to achieve a meaningful reduction of the detrimental health spill-over effects of specific forms of consumption.

13.3. Designing effective taxes, mitigating unintended impacts

Effective health taxes are designed to create both demand-side and supply-side incentives by changing market prices and profit margins for taxed products. In principle, price increases will incentivise consumers to reduce their consumption of taxed products, while shrinking profit margins will incentivise manufacturers to change their products, where possible, in ways that would prevent the application of the tax or mitigate its impact. In practice, we have seen in this book that both consumers' and manufacturers' responses may offset some, or all, of the benefits of health taxes. Consumers may substitute taxed products with others that have similar or worse health impacts; manufacturers may adopt strategies to limit the transfer of taxes onto prices faced by consumers, while minimising impacts on their profits. Designing effective health taxes requires awareness of such potential responses and the ability to prevent them by adopting smart tax-design solutions.

Health taxes are meant to provide incentives for behaviour change, so they must be sufficiently large to motivate change and impact affordability. While official (WHO) recommendations exist, at least for tobacco products, on the size of total taxes as a proportion of retail prices, the appropriate size of each health tax needs to be determined with reference to the specific context in which the tax is to be implemented and to the health goals the government is pursuing.

When faced with price hikes caused by taxation, consumers typically will first seek substitutes within the same product category and then consider wider substitutions. Ideally, prices should be aligned with potential health impacts, especially within product categories. Higher prices should correspond to the least healthy products. The reality is different, and much more complex; for example, in some product markets price is seen by consumers as a signal of quality. Taxes cannot ensure that prices are aligned with health impacts, but they can influence prices and reduce price differentials, where they exist, between cheap unhealthy options and more expensive and healthier options, increasing the relative affordability of the latter. For this purpose, specific excises are often recommended over ad valorem taxes, and taxation according to the quantity of an unhealthy component in a product (e.g. ethanol for alcohol beverages) is preferred over taxation by the quantity of product.

With the exception of tobacco products, the principle of using taxation to incentivise reductions in the unhealthy components in products by manufacturers has been increasingly applied in the design of health taxes. Most health taxes can incentivise manufacturers to change their products, but some do so more than others. Tiered taxes based on sugar content, for instance, have been effective in incentivising soft drink reformulation when appropriately designed. But the responses health taxes can elicit from manufacturers are also driven by structural factors and market competition, all of which need to be foreseen and accounted for in tax design.

13.4. Understanding and managing the political economy of health taxes

Health taxes are fundamentally different from other public health policies. Taxes can increase prices for consumers and decrease profits for suppliers. Health taxes involve different benefits as well as different costs for various stakeholders, and this triggers complex, and often divisive, political economy dynamics. Many consumers loathe having to pay more for products they value, and whose risks they do not fully perceive. Manufacturers often find the stigmatisation of their products, marked as unhealthy by the levying of health taxes, as even less acceptable than the economic losses caused by taxation. Goals and views often diverge within governments too. The proponents of health taxes face formidable challenges, for which they need to be well prepared, however strong their case may be. This book illustrates such political economy challenges and provides tools and examples that proponents of health taxes may use to navigate the complexity of adopting, designing and implementing health taxes.

13.5. Taxes can be used to promote health

The evidence shows that health taxes are effective fiscal measures for reducing the harmful consumption of products such as tobacco, alcohol and SSBs and are an important tool for reducing the burden of non-communicable diseases and other consumption-related adverse outcomes.

The pathway for change is described in detail in *Chapter 3: Protecting and promoting health through taxation: Evidence and gaps.* Health taxes change relative prices of taxed versus untaxed products which, in turn, affect consumption behaviours. The reduced consumption of these products translates into improvements in health: evidence shows that higher cigarette prices and taxes are associated with lower levels of cancer and respiratory disease and lower overall mortality and higher prices/taxes for alcoholic beverages are associated with reduced health risks (e.g. liver cirrhosis) and reduced risks of other harms (e.g. accidents, violence). There is also emerging evidence that links sugary beverages and other unhealthy food prices/taxes to negative health outcomes, and there are some studies that have demonstrated associations with reduced body mass index.

It is important to note that the change in consumer behaviour varies depending on demographic and socioeconomic status (SES). For instance, in the case of tobacco, SSBs and other selected foods, the evidence suggests that lower-income populations are relatively more price sensitive compared to their higher-income counterparts. Finally, the chapter also explains how substitution and tax avoidance behaviours may affect the net impact of the taxes.

Chapter 3 emphasises that behavioural changes are triggered when the prices of taxed goods increase relative to untaxed goods. Thus, it is important to determine whether the taxes are absorbed by the manufacturer, or whether these are passed on to the consumers. The commercial responses of the taxed industries are explored in *Chapter 4: Supply-side responses to health taxes.* Empirical studies show that taxes on tobacco, alcohol and SSBs are usually passed on to consumers, sometimes exceeding the amount of the tax. The extent of tax pass-through can vary widely, depending on factors such as type of product, package size, brand characteristics, store type, market structure and others. The same chapter also describes how taxes can encourage manufacturers to reformulate their products in response to the tax.

While the focus of much of this book is on taxes on tobacco, alcohol and SSBs, *Chapter 7: Expanding health taxation to other unhealthy behaviours and harmful activities* explores taxation of other activities that may have a negative health impact. The chapter describes the challenges and advantages of using taxes as a way to address the negative health effects caused by air pollution, land use, gambling and farming practices.

13.6. Health taxes can have economic benefits

Economic impacts are not the principal objective of health taxes, but they are nevertheless socially important outcomes that policymakers need to consider. Indeed, many arguments advanced against health taxes do not attempt to rebut their positive health impacts but rather to convince policymakers that the negative economic impacts of health taxes outweigh their health benefits.

Policymakers often grapple with the question: if taxes on these products are designed with a health goal in mind, can these measures be relied upon to generate stable revenue for countries? The revenue-raising potential of health taxes is explored in *Chapter 2: The place for health taxes in the wider fiscal system*. The chapter explains that taxes on tobacco and alcohol have a long history and raise significant amounts of revenues across countries. On average, health tax revenues account for 0.8% of GDP. Empirical evidence shows that increasing health tax rates is expected to increase tax revenues since in many countries, the tax rates are very likely not set at their revenue maximising point. In addition to increasing health tax rates, there might be substantial revenue potential from extending health taxes to other products that generate negative externalities linked to health. Scope exists to enhance the role of health taxes, but health tax reform needs to be embedded within the design and functioning of the broader tax system.

Apart from revenue impacts, policymakers also need to consider how health taxes may affect the labour market. Opponents of health taxes claim that these measures will result in negative labour impacts and economic downturn, particularly in lower-income contexts. *Chapter 5: The labour market impact of health taxes* explains how these claims are based on studies that use inappropriate methodology, thus showing only the partial, gross impacts. While affected industries might incur job losses from reduced consumption, and the economy will incur transient restructuring costs, consumer spending on other goods and services and spending of increased government tax revenue can drive a sectoral shift that results in either minimal, neutral job losses or even gains. Furthermore, the implementation of health taxes can help reverse the indirect costs to an economy from productivity losses attributable to morbidity and mortality from consumption of tobacco, alcohol and SSBs/energy dense foods.

13.7. Health taxes can support the achievement of broader development goals

The reduction in consumption of harmful products triggered by increases in health taxes has effects in multiple development dimensions beyond the health and economic impacts described in the previous chapters. *Chapter 6: Impacts of health taxes on the attainment of the SDGs* looks at the broader societal impacts of these measures. Most of the literature on health taxes and sustainable development has focused on the effect these taxes have on income inequalities and the discussion about their progressive or regressive nature. The chapter shows that the effects extend beyond income inequalities; in general, health taxes positively affect the three systems that sustain human life, namely, the global society, the earth's physical system and the world's economy.

13.8. To reap the benefits of health taxes, tax design and implementation require careful consideration

Apart from considering health taxes within the broader fiscal framework, the technical aspects of tax design must also be thoughtfully studied.

As explained in *Chapter 8: The design of effective health taxes,* in designing a health tax policymakers must consider: the type of tax to be applied; what products are to be taxed (i.e. the tax base); the tax structure (i.e. how the products are taxed); and the tax rate to be applied. The chapter discusses the current state of evidence regarding the implications of tax structure.

To further maximise the benefits of health taxes, the design and implementation of these measures should also be analysed within the context of countries' overall tax and governance systems.

One of the important issues policymakers face is how to utilise the revenue from health taxes, and countries have adopted various ways of earmarking health taxes. From a political economy perspective, soft earmarking has helped to advance the adoption of new health taxes in some settings. *Chapter 9: Public governance and financing, and earmarking health taxes* explains these points, as well as other considerations related to public financial management in further detail.

The systematic monitoring of health taxes is also a key component in the effective implementation of health taxes. It is important to monitor health taxes to ensure that they are achieving the goal of decreasing the affordability of the taxed products. In many LMICs, alcohol and SSBs are becoming dramatically more affordable due to rapidly growing incomes and progress on reducing the affordability of tobacco is insufficient. Monitoring can help identify weaknesses in the tax scheme and will inform decisions for further action. *Chapter 10: Monitoring and measuring health taxes* not only explains the importance of monitoring health taxes but also proposes an approach for monitoring taxes on alcohol and SSBs adapting the WHO methodology for collecting data on tobacco taxation.

13.9. Challenges to the implementation of health taxes

Health taxes, like any government policies, require a careful examination of the political economy landscape of the country. The industry sectors involved in the production, distribution and promotion of tobacco, alcohol, unhealthy foods and SSBs have historically opposed health taxes because they can decrease the demand for their products and reduce profits. However, industry is by no means the only source of challenges to health taxes.

Challenges may even come from outside the country. Trade law arguments are sometimes used to dissuade countries from implementing health taxes. Opponents of health taxes have claimed that increasing taxes would contravene countries' obligations under international trade law, since these result in discriminatory effects for imported products. However, as explained in *Chapter 11: Health taxes and trade law*, even where a health tax has the effect of favouring domestic products, it may still be lawful under trade agreements, so long as that effect is justifiable in terms of protecting human health.

However, there are also many other stakeholders involved constructively in the development and implementation of health taxes, including government agencies, non-governmental organisations, civil society groups, public health professionals, and the scientific community. Thus, while health-tax advocates face powerful foes, they can find allies in other sectors.

To achieve this goal, there is a need to build coalitions at the local, national and international levels capable of working collaboratively in the interests of public health. *Chapter 12: A political economy analysis of health taxes* provides a useful resource for policymakers by providing a description of the relevant actors, strategies employed to oppose taxes and recommendations for engaging with these different groups.

13.10. The future of health taxes

Our current understanding of health taxes has extended beyond the concept of a collection of excise taxes on a limited number of consumption goods. The emerging conception of health taxes encompasses the potential for the development of an innovative agenda based on centring health in fiscal policy, in line with the principle that health taxes are fiscal policies aimed at addressing the negative health spill-overs of consumption choices, including spill-overs affecting other people, those affecting consumers or their households in the future, as well as those affecting future generations. Our confidence in the innovative potential of the health-taxes agenda stems from three facts. First, for purely fiscal reasons differentiated consumption taxes are likely to become an increasingly important part of public policy. Second, the linkage of health taxes with the broader goals of public policy, that is, not those required merely for the purposes of financing the state but also for the sake of preserving both human health and the planetary environment, is inevitable. Third, the increasing need to demonstrate the political legitimacy of the public sector, including the ability to link, both conceptually and in practice, the revenue and expenditure sides of the fiscal system, both complements and reinforces the trend towards centring health in fiscal policy.

13.10.1. Health taxes in three key domains (tobacco, alcohol, SSBs)

Despite their demonstrated positive impact on health, public finance and broader development objectives, health taxes are underutilised globally. In particular, taxes on tobacco, alcohol and SSBs show substantial potential for further extension and development. At global scale, health goals cannot be said to be always at 'the centre' of existing taxation of tobacco, alcohol and SSBs, although there may be exceptions for some products in some jurisdictions (e.g. tobacco taxes in Australia). That said, it is likely that, even in a hypothetical future of optimal health taxation of tobacco, alcohol and SSBs, tax design and rates will differ across jurisdictions in order to take account of product- and market-specific characteristics, as well as differing health goals according to product and burden of disease.

13.10.2. New avenues for health taxes

Although the main focus of this book has been taxes on tobacco, alcohol and SSBs, we have also touched on other potential areas for the application of health taxes, in particular on the (health) taxation of fossil fuels as a primary source of urban air pollution (Chapter 7). Though there is no substitute for socially optimal carbon pricing, differentiated taxes on the major sources of microscopic particulate matter and of other noxious pollutants, particularly in urban areas, is a promising avenue for the development of health taxes. Health taxes on fossil fuels not only have obvious synergies with limiting the adverse effects of climate change, but they also make salient to individuals the concrete benefit of improved health, in addition to the more remote (both conceptually and in time) benefits people legitimately care about when thinking exclusively of planetary health.

Through the lens of planetary health, it is obvious that a number of areas of traditional environmental concern also have major health implications. An important area in which synergistic fiscal incentives can be created to promote both human and planetary health is food. Food and diet are key determinants of health and major sources of greenhouse gas emissions and depletion of natural resources such as land and water. Fiscal policies have shown great promise when applied to SSBs. Using SSB taxes as a proof of concept, a case can be built for the wider use of consumption tax rate differentiation on food and non-alcoholic beverages, which would complement and reinforce other policies aimed at incentivising consumers towards food and dietary choices that are conducive to health and environmental sustainability.

13.10.3. Towards a more holistic approach to health taxes

A more holistic approach to health taxes seems possible, though this goes beyond the traditional definition of health taxes as corrective taxes as set out previously. The development of such a programme, however, would depend on advances in economic theory about which we can only speculate.

The following seems probable in outline: there will be extensions to optimal tax theory as we now know it. Though there are technical difficulties to be surmounted, the avenues of development might involve:

i. relaxing the usual assumption of complete and perfect markets underlying the indirect (i.e. income-mediated) utility models on which existing optimal tax theory rests,
ii. inferring the internal 'market' dynamics of individuals' optimising behaviour regarding investment in and/or consumption of health capital versus other forms of investment and consumption, and
iii. internalising in a shadow-pricing system the major sources of internalities (e.g. hyperbolic discounting, uncertainty, incomplete and asymmetric information, myopia and other recognised sources of irrational decision-making).

Extending these thoughts somewhat, health capital can be thought of as an idealised asset that jointly determines longevity and wage income. As noted in the introductory chapter, there is no ready metric of prospective and intrinsic health status (i.e. of 'health capital') rather only retrospective measures of health-capital realisations (e.g. outcomes such as longevity and wages). The further study of health capital, therefore, seems a promising avenue for reframing, and to a certain extent, rethinking health taxes: since internal 'market failures' exist (whence the term 'internalities'), it is doubtful whether individuals can even in principle optimise their investment and consumption choices regarding an idealised asset that cannot be directly observed. What sort of 'tax policy' would render health capital salient for individuals?

Another avenue for reconceptualisation would be to go beyond the traditional welfarist emphasis on benefits realised by individuals (as it were, in isolation). When 'centring health in fiscal policy', there thus seems scope for giving increased attention to the production and consumption of emergent and/or collective goods, especially those with the potential for network effects (such as communities of various kinds). Many such goods can be understood as public goods in the neoclassical tradition (e.g. when their production is not guaranteed without collective action), but others might be better described as common goods (e.g. when overuse is guaranteed in the absence of collective action). Both public and common goods present coordination problems, and in the absence of emergent collective action, they require the appointment of an agent to act on behalf of those who will benefit from enhanced coordination in the use of the resource. In the present context of fiscal measures for health, the agent is the state.

Nevertheless, with the progressive loss of credibility and opportunity for both the social theory of the state (i.e. one emphasising collective mechanisms of protection against life-course risks faced by all members of society) and the more minimalistic neoliberal theory of the state (i.e. emphasising the liberty of the individual in the context of a collective that serves primarily to protect individual property rights), a more compelling conception of the social contract has yet to emerge. One promising formulation proposes the state as the provider and protector of Common Goods for Health.[1] In the sense used in that publication, 'common goods' encompasses both goods and services economists have traditionally called public goods (i.e. with supply failures), as well as common goods per se (i.e. with demand failures). The notion of 'common goods for health' is defined as 'population-based functions or interventions that require public financing', including:

- Policy and coordination
- Regulation and legislation
- Taxes and subsidies
- Information collection, analysis and communication and
- Population services

Recent failures of collective action in global health can be attributed in part to the attrition, over decades, of state-sponsored mechanisms for the financing and provision of common goods for health, which has operated either under the banner of austerity or in the name of a radical reconceptualisation of the social theory of the state along neoliberal lines.

Notwithstanding these failures (or because of them), according to the IMF's Fiscal Monitor, since early 2020 and as of September 2021 additional amounts equivalent to US$ 17 trillion in public expenditure (accounting for more than 20% of annual gross world output) had been disbursed in direct and indirect economic support ('stimulus') as a result of the pandemic. Given that health taxes are not only 'common goods for health' in their own right by the above definition but can in addition be used to finance other common goods for health on the list given above, there would seem to be substantial scope to broaden both the theoretical and practical basis of our understanding of health taxes.

13.10.4. Need for coordination with other fiscal measures

Some of the controversy surrounding health taxes has been fostered by the tendency for health taxes (or for that matter environmental taxes) to be seen in isolation, rather than as merely one component of a complex fiscal system. Any tax in isolation should not be judged as regressive or progressive without consideration of the entire range of fiscal measures in place, including expenditure measures.

Admittedly, certain elements of the fiscal system have the advantage (or misfortune) of being more 'visible', either to consumers or to producers. The visibility of fiscal measures functions effectively as a form of (conceptual) concentration, of either the benefits or costs of such measures. Excise taxes are highly visible; as noted earlier in this chapter, they could not be called health taxes without this feature. Yet many of the least transparent (i.e. least visible) fiscal measures also deserve attention in the context of centring health in fiscal policies. For example, tax expenditures (i.e. deferrals, deductions, credits, exemptions and concessionary tax rates) make up more than half of the effective subsidies of fossil fuels (i.e. excluding unpriced externality costs, which might also be considered a subsidy).[2]

Although tax expenditures, which are foregone government revenues, act similarly in economic terms to actual government expenditures, they do not appear in the balance sheet, and they are not subject to any regular budgetary or appropriations discipline; they are usually, therefore, implemented in the complete absence of any of the basic principles of public financial management.

13.11. Health taxes in the immediate post-pandemic era

At the time of writing, the near-to-medium-term future threatens to be increasingly multi-polar and unstable. The words of the Chief Economist of the IMF, quoted in the introductory chapter to this book, seem, with a few nuances, as relevant now as when they were written.

Whatever disruptions have so far been experienced along the lines of those foreshadowed by the IMF in 2020 are, moreover, merely a foretaste of the scale of upheavals to the social fabric and to social cohesion, of the chaotic incoordination and too-little-too-late responses that have characterised national attempts to address supranational issues, and of the social and political polarisation that will be witnessed when the effects of the climate emergency become generalised and severe.

Health taxes by themselves are insufficient to address such problems, or even to achieve the totality of the Sustainable Development Goals, but they can play an important role as an enabler and facilitator of related policy goals, such as the SDG commitments to Universal Health Coverage. Earlier in this chapter, we recalled that work presented in Chapter 2 showed, globally and on average, that 0.8% of GDP was being collected in the form of health taxes. In 2020, world output stood at approximately US$ 85 trillion, implying that health taxes were generating revenues in the order of US$ 680 billion per year. For comparison, achieving Universal Health Coverage in 67 low- and middle-income countries has been estimated to require resources in the order of 1.2% of gross world product, according to WHO estimates.[3] Without much effort, therefore, health taxes can (and, in our view, must) play an important role in financing key components of the SDGs.

References

1. Financing common goods for health. Geneva: World Health Organization, 2021.
2. International Monetary Fund. Fossil fuel subsidies [https://www.imf.org/en/Topics/climate change/energy subsidies]. International Monetary Fund, 2021.
3. Stenberg K, Hanssen O, Edejer T, Bertram M, Brindley C, Meshreky A. et al. Financing transformative health systems towards achievement of the health sustainable development goals: a model for projected resource needs in 67 low-income and middle-income countries. *Lancet Global Health.* 2017; 5: 875–887.

https://doi.org/10.1142/9781800612396_bmatter

About the Editors

Jeremy A Lauer joined Strathclyde University in February 2020 as a professor of management science following a career (1995–2020) as an economist with the World Health Organization (WHO). Jeremy has a bachelor's degree (AB, 1986) in mathematics and philosophy from St John's College in Annapolis, Maryland, master's degrees (MA, MSc, 1991) in economics and in agricultural and applied economics from the University of Wisconsin, Madison, and a doctorate (PhD, 2009) in health policy and management from Erasmus University Rotterdam. Jeremy has contributed to an influential body of work on the cost effectiveness of interventions against cardiovascular risk factors and disease, respiratory conditions, cancers, maternal and child health, HIV/AIDS, malaria, tuberculosis and chronic diseases, as well as on health systems research and topics in epidemiology, modelling and statistics. Jeremy, working with his WHO colleagues, finalised a major update on the cost effectiveness of 500 interventions covering 20 areas of disease and risk factors for WHO-CHOICE in 2020. Jeremy has served as principal investigator and co-investigator on research projects in breast-cancer and chronic-disease control while at the WHO and has been a member of Steering Committees or Technical Advisory Groups at the University of Stellenbosch (SACEMA), the University of Basel (Swiss TPH) and the University of Bergen (CIH). In 2016, Jeremy advised the UN Secretary-General's High-Level Commission on Health Employment and Economic Growth on fiscal space for health workforce expansion in lower- and lower-middle income countries. In 2018, Jeremy was invited to advise the G20 health ministers' working group on synergies between the health system and the economy. In 2018, he led the economic analysis for the flagship 2019 WHO publication *A Healthier Humanity*. In 2016, while at WHO, Jeremy initiated and subsequently led a global WHO project on health taxes, health financing and fiscal reform for health. This book is a product of that work.

Franco Sassi graduated with a degree in economics and a doctorate in health economics from the University of London in 2000. He is currently chair in International Health Policy and Economics and director of the Centre for Health Economics & Policy Innovation at Imperial College Business School, after leaving the position of senior health economist and head of the Public Health Programme at the OECD. Previously, he was senior lecturer in Health Policy at the London School of Economics and Political Science (LSE), and held adjunct and visiting positions at a number of universities in the United States, including the University of California at Berkeley, Harvard University, the University of California at San Francisco and Duke University – as well as at the Université de Montréal in Canada and at the Università Cattolica del Sacro Cuore in Rome. Professor Sassi's research focusses on economic analysis of health services, the economics of chronic disease prevention and measuring inequalities in access to healthcare. He has been principal investigator and project coordinator of the EU project Science & Technology in Childhood Obesity Policy (STOP). He is the lead author of *Obesity and the Economics of Prevention: Fit Not Fat* (OECD and Edward Elgar, 2010), editor and author of *Tackling Harmful Use: Economics and Public Health Policy* (OECD, 2015) and *Promoting Health, Preventing Disease: The Economic Case* (OUP, 2015); and author of a large number of publications on the economics of chronic disease prevention. He was awarded a 2000–2001 Commonwealth Fund Harkness Fellowship in Health Care Policy.

Agnès Soucat is the director of the Division of Health and Social Protection of the French Development Agency (Agence française de développement). She was previously the director of the Department of Health Systems, Governance and Financing at the WHO. Prior to that, Dr Soucat held the position of director for Human Development for the African Development

Bank, where she was responsible for the health, education and social protection activities of the Bank for 53 African countries; she also held the position of global lead economist for the Health, Nutrition and Population Global Practice Group of the World Bank. She has over 30 years of experience in poverty reduction and health, covering more than 70 countries in Africa, Asia and Europe. Dr Soucat was a pioneer in several fields of innovations in healthcare financing, including community-based financing and performance-based financing, and she has authored seminal publications on these topics. She is also a co-author of the *World Bank's World Development Report 2004: Making Services Work for Poor People*, and of the Lancet Commission report *Global Health 2035: A World Converging Within a Generation*. Dr Soucat was a Commissioner on the recent Lancet and Rockefeller Commission on Planetary Health. She also did extensive work on the labour market dynamics of the health workforce in Africa. This book on health taxes is the direct result of her leadership on innovative financing while at WHO. Dr Soucat holds an MD and a master's degree in nutrition from the University of Nancy in France as well as a master's of public health and a PhD in health economics from Johns Hopkins University.

Angeli Vigo is responsible for parliamentary engagement and co-manages the inter-agency collaboration on health taxes at the WHO. After training in law at the University of the Philippines, Angeli was admitted to the Philippine Bar in 2012. She worked at the Supreme Court of the Philippines and taught at De La Salle University and Lyceum University in Manila, before moving to WHO headquarters in Geneva in 2015. She worked in tobacco product regulation for two years, during which she managed the development of the technical report series of the 'WHO Study Group on Tobacco Product Regulation' (WHO TobReg). These reports provide the WHO Director-General with scientifically sound, evidence-based recommendations for Member States about tobacco product regulation. In 2017, Angeli authored the background paper on the economic implications of health taxes for the WHO strategy meeting held that year – which was the first time that tobacco, alcohol and sugar-sweetened products were considered under the same policy umbrella. Since then, she co-manages the joint activities of a multi-agency collaboration on health taxes composed of a dozen international organisations, including the World Bank, the OECD and the Asian Development Bank and is responsible for parliamentary outreach to several countries in Africa and Asia.

www.ingramcontent.com/pod-product-compliance
Lightning Source LLC
LaVergne TN
LVHW010325220926
848484LV00004BB/843